Essentials for Ophthalmic Lens Work

Clifford W. Brooks, O.D.

Essentials for Ophthalmic Lens Work

Clifford W. Brooks, O.D.

The Professional Press, Inc.
Chicago, Illinois

© 1983 by The Professional Press, Inc.

ISBN 0-87873-049-4

Library of Congress Catalog Card Number 82-061248

Published by The Professional Press, Inc.
11 E. Adams St., Suite 1209, Chicago, IL 60603

Printed in the U.S.A.

Dedication

To Him who by wisdom founded the earth;
And by understanding established the heavens.

Proverbs 3:19

Acknowledgements

The author wishes to thank Gordon G. Heath, Dean of the Indiana University School of Optometry, for his encouragement of faculty development and work in arranging for the sabbatical leave that proved so necessary for beginning a project like this.

Special thanks go also to Jacque Kubley, for original photography and his many illustrations; Robert Ruff, for resource help in certain practical aspects; Lois Selk, for assistance in locating library resource materials; and Cindy Stantz, Lori Bell, Gloria Jean, Connie Strange, Vickie Stryker, and Debbie Spicer, for help in manuscript preparation.

Appreciation for ideas, materials, and information pertaining to this text, current classroom information, and future publications go also to Harry Cook, Bill and Al White, James Dirheimer, and many of the other employees of Quality Optical in Cincinnati; Bernie Joubert and Fred N. Winters, Jr., of American Optical Corporation; Eldon Weinhaus and Salvator Ruta of Midland Optical Co., St. Louis; Rob Johnson and Tracy Dunn of Tulsa Lens Specialists; Ernest Fulford, Harry Goaz, Joseph Tusinski, Leo Elsky, and Arlon Wimpey of Coburn Optical Industries; Joel and Sylvan Ray of Associated Optical; Michael Gumnick of Omega Optical; Rodney Tahran and Jacques Stoerr of Multi-Optics Corporation; Jack Dworetzky of Shieldalloy Corporation; Walter L. Silvernail, Technical Services, West Chicago; David Beach of National Optronics Incorporated; George Rybeck and Joel Friedman of AIT Industries; and Patricia Junkin of the Optical Laboratories Association.

Sincere appreciation goes to Josef Reiner, director of the Höheren Fachscule für Augenoptik in Cologne, Germany, where I spent two enjoyable years teaching. His gracious arrangements for my visit seven years later opened up many valuable sources of information.

Thanks as well go to Wilhelm Kempkes, also of the Cologne school, for providing information and serving as a model for some of the photographs.

An extension of appreciation goes to C. Dieter Beuthien of Wernicke and Co., GmbH, Düsseldorf, Germany, for allowing the use of WECO equipment during and after the writing of the text.

Appreciation for hospitality shown, ideas given, and materials and information exchanged is also extended to Helmut Bittner, Hans G. Schubert, and Rolf W. Both of Carl Zeiss, Aalen, West Germany; Gerhardt Kasparek of Marwitz and Hauser, Stuttgart, West Germany; Michael Liese, Werner Köppen, Toni Lindermier, and Herr Schwertfirm of Rodenstock, Munich, West Germany; Eugen Stratemeyer of Eugen Stratemeyer GmbH. and Co., Bochum, West Germany; Heinz Simon, Cologne, West Germany; Marc Alexandre and Louis Grosperrin of Essilor, Paris; John Wylde and Roy Parsons of J. and S. Wylde Ltd., Croydon and Leatherhead, England; M. Jalie and Henri Obstfeld of City and East London College; and Mabel Nisted and John Ross, The City University, London, England.

But perhaps most of all, real thanks go to my wife, Vickie, whose constant encouragement continues to prove invaluable, and my children Debbie and Andrew, who are a delight to me.

Preface

It was originally my intent to create a text that would encompass all aspects of the lens fabrication process. After beginning the work it soon became apparent that, because of the demand for completeness and scope of the material, confinement to one volume was impractical. Thus, the material appearing here represents the first book in a series. The remainder of the series is to cover those other aspects of lens fabrication not considered here. It is also to include at least one volume devoted exclusively to the practical aspects of ophthalmic lens optics. A practical understanding of this area is an absolute necessity for all individuals who intend to function competently in the community of ophthalmic professionals.

I hope that this present text will take readers through a step-by-step understanding of lens finishing, serving not only those who are to be daily exercising their skills in this area, but also those who would gain an understanding of and respect for what takes place in another vital part of the optical profession.

Table of Contents

Chapter 1

An Overview of the Fabrication Process

An optical laboratory actually consists of two separate facilities. One is involved with creating the needed lens power by grinding and polishing the surface of the lens; this facility is referred to as a *surfacing laboratory*. The second facility takes the surfaced lens and finishes it by centering it optically and grinding the edges so that the lens fits the shape of the chosen frame. This facility is known as the *finishing laboratory* (see Figure 1–1). It is the finishing aspect of lens fabrication with which this text primarily concerns itself.

The finishing laboratory has the versatility of being able either to be closely associated with a surfacing laboratory, or to be at another location independent from it.

OPTIONS IN OBTAINING LENSES

Whenever possible, single vision lenses are edged from lenses kept in stock at the *finishing laboratory*. If the stock lens proves too small for the frame, or if a great deal of prism is prescribed, then a lens must be produced in the surfacing laboratory.

Normally, all multifocal lenses are individually processed by a surfacing laboratory. (It is best to send along all frame dimensions. This ensures that the lens will neither be ground thicker than necessary nor end up being too small for the chosen frame.) Some finishing laboratories order prefinished spherical bifocals[1] for spherical lens prescriptions. This is usually done only when *both* left and right eyes are spherical. Attempting to match one nonspherical lens from a surfacing laboratory with a prefinished bifocal from another source can create unnecessary problems and mismatches—the exact position of the optical center in relationship to the near segment must be known, accurately duplicated, and appropriate for the wearer.

USING THE SMALLEST STOCK LENS

It is generally advisable to use the smallest possible stock lens for each prescription. For cases of *minus lenses* this is only a matter of economics, since larger lenses are generally more expensive than smaller ones. Figure 1–2 shows that in its final form the finished lens will have exactly the same center and edge thickness regardless of whether the lens chosen was large or small (because both center thicknesses are the same).

The situation with *plus lenses* is no longer just a matter of cost. Because of lens optics, as the lens becomes larger, the center must also increase in thickness (see Figure 1–3). Unnecessary use of large lenses just to be certain that the lens will cut out results in thick centers, thick edges, and glasses that magnify the wearer's eyes unnecessarily. It is much better to use one of several lens blank size determiners available in combination with the frame, as is done in dispensing[2] or the formula

$$MBS = ED + 2 \text{ (dec.)}$$

where:

MBS is the Minimum Blank Size
ED is the Effective Diameter
and 2 (dec.) is twice the decentration per lens.[3]

---

[1]Instead of being custom made, prefinished spherical bifocals may be mass produced with both inside and outside surfaces already ground and polished.

[2]See Clifford W. Brooks and Irvin M. Borish, *System for Ophthalmic Dispensing*, Chicago: The Professional Press, 1979.

[3]If the reader is new to optical terminology and experiences difficulty, Chapter 3 should help to explain fully the concept of centration and its associated terminology.

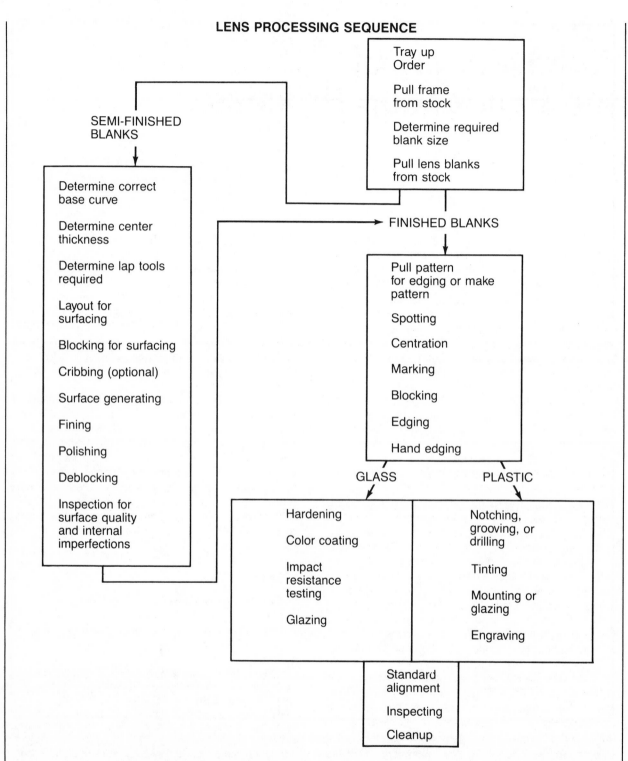

Figure 1–1. *The processes list on the righthand side in the main column sequence may be performed in the finishing laboratory. The processes in the lefthand "loop" are a function of the surfacing laboratory.*

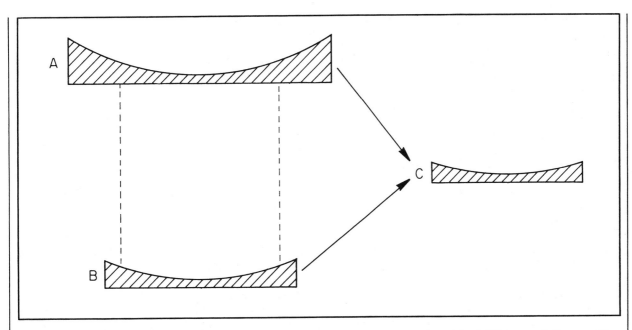

Figure 1–2. *Whether a large uncut minus lens blank (A) or a small uncut lens blank (B) is used, the resulting edged lens is exactly the same (C). Dotted lines show the diameter being cut to produce lens* C.

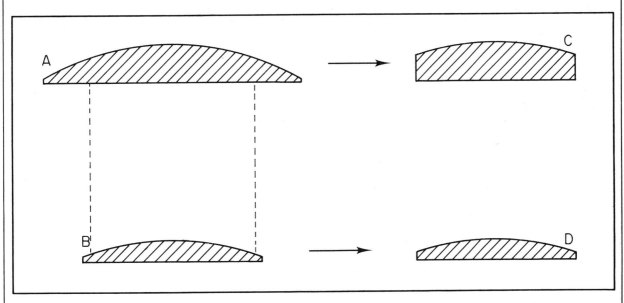

Figure 1–3. *When a plus lens blank much larger than necessary is used (A), the result is a lens too thick in both center and edge (C). The smallest possible blank (B) should be chosen, as a much better functional and cosmetic result is obtained (D). Dotted lines indicate the diameter being cut from the blank to produce the finished lens.*

This formula makes no allowance for edge chipping. (As will be discussed in later chapters, it is wise to allow an extra 2- to 4-mm safety factor to avoid possible lens waste due to an unanticipated chip during edging.)

An assumption made in determining the minimum blank size in this manner is that there is no prism called for in the prescription and that the lenses are stock single vision lenses.

AN OVERVIEW OF THE EDGING PROCESS

Edging is often used to denote the entire lens finishing process. In actuality, edging is preceded by many steps, described in more detail in later chapters.

Location of Lens Axis and Major Reference Point

A lens measuring device is used to determine lens cylinder axis and major reference point; it is referred to as a *Lensometer, focimeter,* or *lens analyzer,* depending upon the manufacturer. This instrument allows a precise location of the lens axis, as well as the *optical center* (that point on the lens where no prismatic effect is found). When prism is desired, the *major reference point*[4] (that point on the lens where the correct amount of prescribed prism is manifested) must be located. Thereafter, both horizontal orientation of the 180-degree meridian and the major reference point may be indicated by three inked dots placed on the surface of the lens. The process is commonly referred to as *spotting of lenses* because of these three inked "spots" placed on the lens

---

[4]British Standards use the term *centration point* instead of *major reference point.*

surface. See Chapter 2 for a complete discussion of spotting.

Centration of the Lens

Since the pupil of the eye is seldom found to be directly in line with the middle of the frame's lens opening, the major reference point of the lens must be moved. This process, known as decentration, is done with the aid of a centration device. Using the three reference dots previously placed on the lens, a technician can now reposition it to allow for correct horizontal and vertical positioning in the frame. Once the lens has been positioned, it may be marked for correct orientation. These two stages, spotting followed by centration (marking), comprise *lens layout.* Chapter 3 describes centration of single vision lenses, followed by a discussion of multifocal lens centration in Chapter 4.

Blocking of the Lens

To ensure accurate edging, the lens must be mechanically secured to prevent slippage. This may be done with several methods, which are compared in Chapter 5. Some methods allow blocking directly from the centration device, while others use a set of reference lines placed on the lens by the device itself.

Edging the Lens

The blocked lens is now placed in the edger and a pattern used to guide shaping (see Chapter 7). After making the necessary setting for size, the lens is edged.

As each of these steps have several variations and may be performed somewhat differently depending upon the type of lens being used, they will be considered individually in detail.

PROFICIENCY TEST QUESTIONS

1. T or F   Lenses are surfaced in a finishing laboratory.

2. T or F   Bifocal lenses are not available in finished, stock form.

3. T or F   If finished stock bifocals are used, they
are best used when *both* left and right
distance powers are spherical.

4. Apart from price considerations, when is it critical
that the smallest possible lens blank be used?
   a. When the prescription is minus in power
   b. When the prescription in plus in power
   c. Apart from economic considerations, it isn't
critical in either case.
   d. It is critical for both plus and minus prescriptions.

5. Using the generalized formula for minimum blank
size, what is the minimum blank size required for
a frame having an effective diameter of 53 and a
decentration of 3 mm per lens when *no allowance*
is made for chipping?
   a. 54 mm
   b. 59 mm
   c. 62 mm
   d. 68 mm
   e. 71 mm

6. Arrange the steps in the edging process in their
correct order.
   1. blocking
   2. centration
   3. edging
   4. location of axis and MRP
   a. 2,3,1,4
   b. 2,4,1,3
   c. 1,2,3,4
   d. 4,2,1,3
   e. 4,3,2,1

Chapter 2
Spotting of Lenses

SPOTTING AND POWER VERIFICATION OF SINGLE VISION LENSES

Two processes are carried out simultaneously in this first operation in the lens finishing procedure. The first process is lens verification; the second, lens spotting. Regardless of whether the lens in question has been surfaced in-house or was received from another supplier in finished form, verification of lens power and optical quality is essential.

Checking for Optical Quality

To check the optical quality of an uncut lens, its front surface quality, back surface quality, and internal lens characteristics are checked. Surface quality is inspected using an unfrosted incandescent bulb and holding the lens as if it were a mirror (see Figures 2–1 and 2–2). The lens is tilted so that all areas of the lens surface are inspected. The image of the light bulb filament must be sharp and clear on all areas of the lens surface. The lens is then turned over and the second surface is inspected in a like manner.

Internal lens properties may be checked for foreign material by looking at the lens with a dark background and a light such as a 40-watt, incandescent clear (unfrosted) bulb positioned 12 inches (305 mm) from the lens, striking it at an angle from behind (see Figures 2–3 and 2–4). Any foreign substance in or on the lens will scatter the light, causing the area of the foreign substance to be visible.

Assuming that it is free of surface deficiencies or

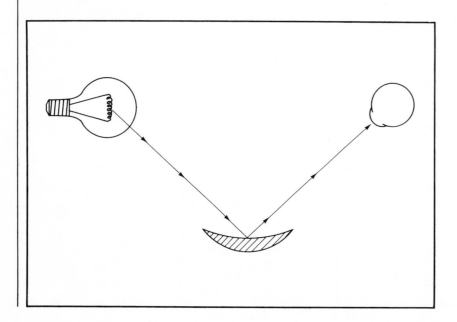

Figure 2–1. *When the lens is held such that its surface acts as a mirror, surface irregularities cause the reflected unfrosted light bulb's filament image to appear irregularly distorted.*

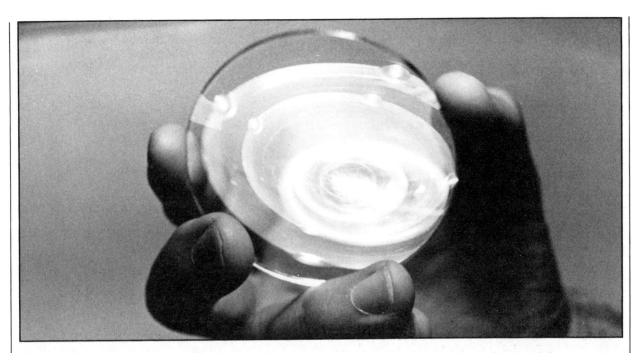

Figure 2–2. *Look at the bulb filament and tilt the lens slightly to inspect the entire surface rapidly.*

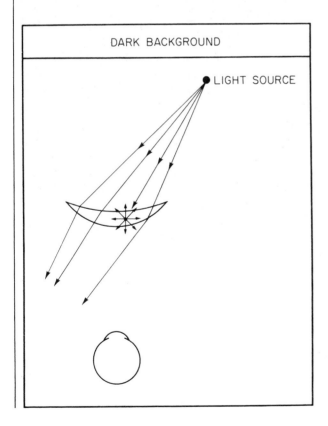

DARK BACKGROUND

● LIGHT SOURCE

Figure 2–3. *A defect within the lens causes a scattering of light. By positioning the light source off to the side and viewing the lens against a matte black background, the main body of a clean, unblemished lens will almost disappear. Any defect becomes easily visible. This method of inspection is used by inspectors wearing white gloves for factory quality control.*

internal foreign matter, the lens may now be checked for power variations. This may be done while observing a straight line such as the edge of a fluorescent tube through the lens. If the straight edge is vertical, the lens is moved left and right along one of its major meridians* (see Figure 2–5). If the lens has any refractive power, the line observed through the lens will appear to curve as the lens is moved (see Figure 2–6). It should curve evenly, however, because an unevenness in the curve indicates a power variation within the lens. Possible causes of the variation are a wavy surface or nonuniformity of refractive index within the lens material.

*The major meridians of a lens are along the cylinder axis and 90 degrees away from the axis.

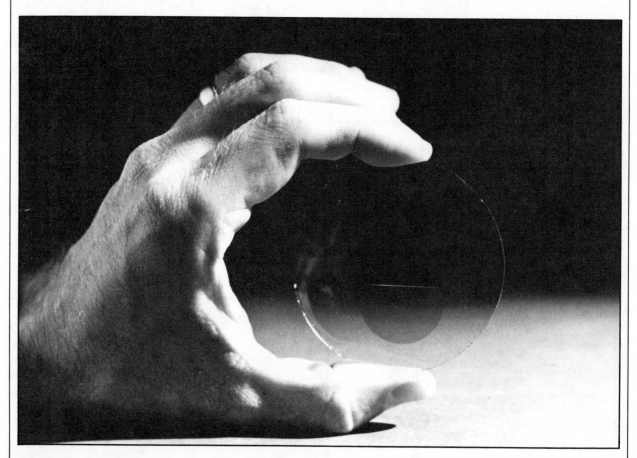

Figure 2–4. *Inspecting a lens in oblique illumination against a matte black background.*

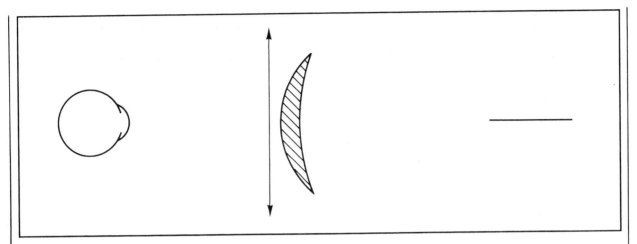

Figure 2–5. *In this top view, the operator checks for waviness by moving the lens left and right and observing a vertical straight edge. The distance between the straight edge and lens will vary, depending upon lens power.*

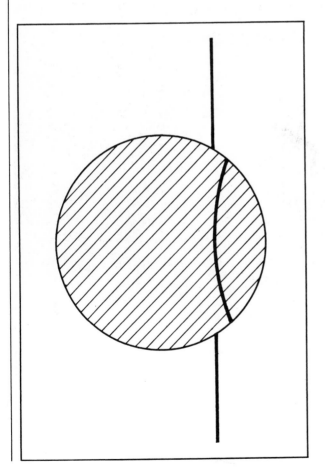

Figure 2–6. *Lenses free from waviness (caused by either poor surface manufacture or an irregularity in the refractive index of the material) will display a uniformly curved image of the straight edge as the lens is moved to either side. This is caused by the refractive characteristics of the lens. Defects discovered in this manner may also be evident through the Lensometer. The lens is moved while the focused target is viewed through the instrument. Defective areas in the lens will cause a degradation in target clarity.*

USE OF THE LENSOMETER

The power of a lens may be measured using an instrument that is variously referred to as a lensmeter, Lensometer, focimeter, vertometer, and vertexometer. For clarity, this book will use *Lensometer*[1] when referring to any of these instrument types.

Before attempting to read the power of a lens using a Lensometer, the operator must first focus the eyepiece. An eyepiece not focused for the eye of the individual using it will cause an inaccurate reading.

Focus by turning the eyepiece outward, then slowly rotate it inwards until the cross hairs and rings appear to *first* focus. The eyepiece location should be noted, as it will vary from individual to individual (see Figure 2–7).

_____

[1]This is the tradename for American Optical's lens measuring instrument.

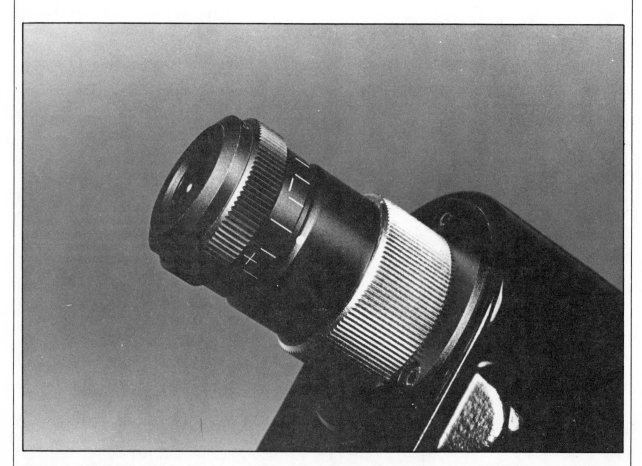

Figure 2–7. *The Lensometer eyepiece is set for "zero." Turning the eyepiece outward adds plus power to the system; inward adds minus power. For practitioners who themselves have only a small spherical eyeglass correction and wish to use the instrument without their glasses, the instrument allows this versatility. The eyepiece should, in any case, be adjusted for the most plus power through which the mires can be seen sharply.*

10

Neutralizing in Minus Cylinder Form

To "neutralize," or measure, the power of a lens such that the prescription may be written directly in minus cylinder form,* the lens is placed in the instrument and the power wheel turned to high plus (see Figure 2–8). One looks through the eyepiece and turns the power wheel slowly in the minus direction until the target within the instrument begins to focus.

The target consists of two sets of lines that run at right angles to each other, forming a cross. One set is either narrowly spaced or a single line (Figure 2–9); this set is known as the *sphere line(s)*. The set at right angles is a triple set (see Figure 2–10). These lines are referred to as the *cylinder lines*.

As the power wheel is being turned in the minus direction, either

1. both set of lines will focus simultaneously, indicating that the lens is spherical (as in Figure 2–11), or
2. one set of lines will begin to focus before the other, indicating that a cylinder component is present.

If the prescription is spherical, then when the lines first focus, the refractive power is read directly from the power wheel.

To find the power when a cylinder component is present involves using the axis wheel, shown in Figure 2–8. As one set of lines begins to clear, rotate the axis wheel while viewing the target. As a major meridian is approached on the axis wheel, one set of lines begins to clear. In order to obtain the correct values, first focus the sphere line(s). (If the cylinder lines are clearing instead of the sphere line(s), rotate the axis wheel 90 degrees.)

Once the sphere line is clear, the sphere and axis components of the prescription have been determined and can be recorded directly from the power and axis wheels.

Now slowly turn the power wheel once more in the minus direction until the cylinder lines clear. (Do *not* rotate the axis wheel.) Note the power wheel reading. The cylinder value is the difference between the first reading (sphere line) and the second reading (cylinder lines) and is recorded as a minus value.

The procedure may be more thoroughly described by the following example. The lens is placed in the

*The minus cylinder form of lens prescription writing expresses the cylinder component of the lens as a negative number, whereas the plus cylinder form expresses it positively.

Lensometer and the power wheel rotated to +15.00D. While slowly rotating the power wheel back in the minus direction, it is noted that the cylinder lines are beginning to clear. Because these are the wrong lines to start with, the axis wheel is rotated from 180 degrees to 90 degrees, so that now the sphere line begins to clear. As the power wheel is slowly turned toward minus (away from plus) and the axis wheel slightly adjusted, maximum clarity is obtained. The power wheel reads +2.50D and the axis wheel reads 87 degrees. The prescription can be ⅔ written as

sph	cyl	axis
+2.50		87

Now the power wheel is turned once again in a minus direction. The cylinder lines come into focus when the power wheel reaches +1.00D. Because the cylinder value is the *difference* between the two major meridians, the correct value is 1.50D and is recorded as a minus number. The prescription now reads

sph	cyl	axis
+2.50	−1.50	87

Neutralizing in Plus Cylinder Form

In the event that a prescription is to be written in plus cylinder form, the lens can be neutralized in the Lensometer such that the power may be written directly from Lensometer values without having to convert or *transpose* the prescription from minus to plus cylinder form. Direct plus cylinder neutralization is carried out as follows.

1. Turn the power wheel into the high *minus* numbers.
2. Slowly advance the power wheel in the plus direction.
3. Rotate the axis wheel to cause the sphere line(s) to come into focus first.
4. When in focus, record the sphere and axis values.
5. Move the power wheel a second time, still in the plus direction, until the cylinder lines come into clear focus.
6. The difference between first and second power readings is the cylinder and is recorded as a plus value.

Note that the procedure is identical to minus cylinder neutralization, with the exception of the direction of power wheel movement.

11

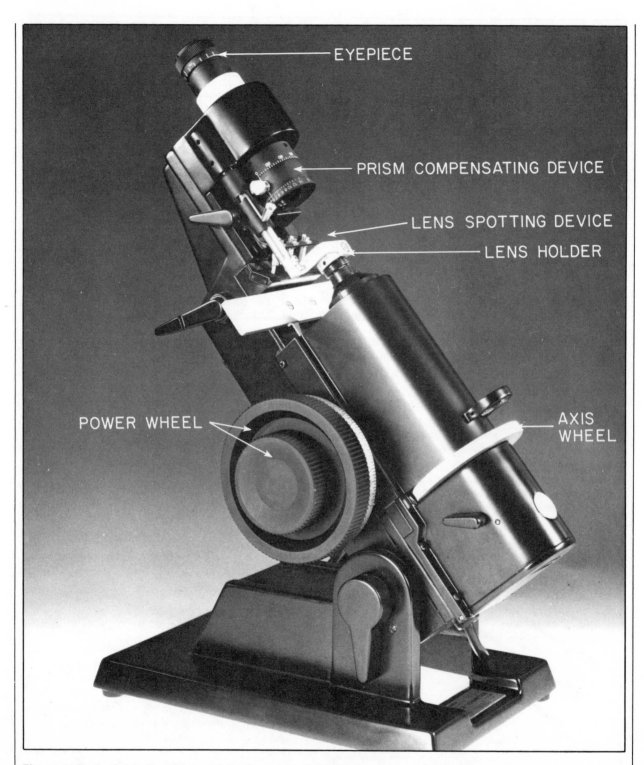

Figure 2–8. *Available through a variety of sources, the basic lens measuring instrument is a necessary part of every optically related profession. (Photo courtesy of Marco)*

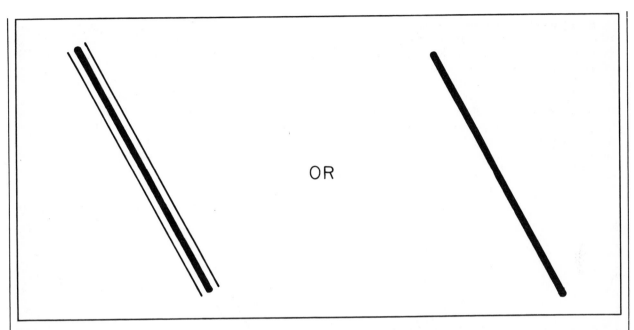

Figure 2–9. *The exact configuration of the sphere line(s) varies from instrument to instrument. (Some instruments do not use lines at all, but rather a circle of dots that elongate into a circle of short lines when cylinder power is present in the lens.)*

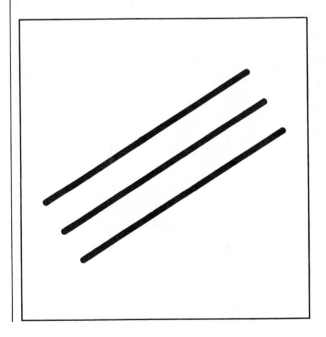

Figure 2–10. *Cylinder lines appear at right angles to the sphere lines and are usually visible simultaneously, except in the case of extremely high cylinder values. (Instruments using a circle of dots will show elongation of the dots 90 degrees from the direction of elongation as evidenced when the target was viewed with the instrument set for the correct sphere power.)*

Power Verification and Spotting of Spheres

When the lens is of known power, it is not necessary to carry out the entire neutralization process. Instead the power is simply checked. This is done by setting the Lensometer for the expected sphere value. If the lens is a sphere, the target should be immediately clear, indicating a lens of the correct power. If the target is unclear, the lens may have been mismarked and the proper power may be found by adjusting the Lensometer power wheel.

Occasionally the Lensometer target will not appear clean and crisp after being focused correctly. The best focus may nevertheless indicate a correct power reading. If this is the case, the lens is not well polished and should not be used.

When the lens has been determined to be of acceptable quality, center it optically in the Lensometer by moving the lens until the center of the target crosses the center of the crosshairs in the Lensometer eyepiece or on the Lensometer screen (see Figure 2–11). The marking device is then swung into position and the front surface of the lens spotted

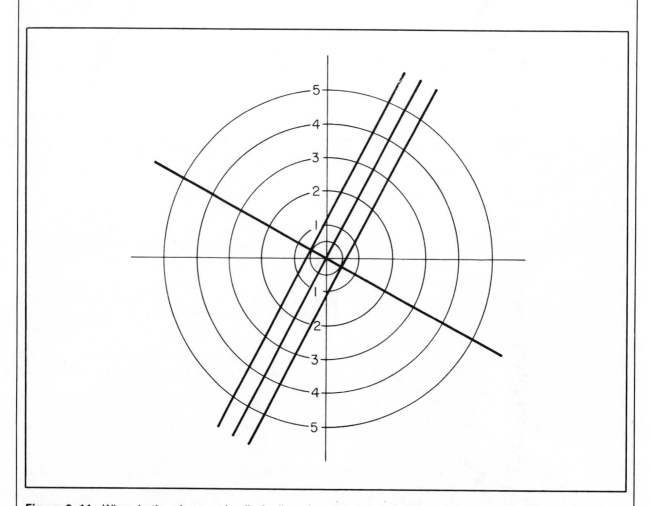

Figure 2–11. *When both sphere and cylinder lines focus at the same time, the lens has a uniform power in all meridians and is spoken of as being* spherical. *(Instruments using a circle of dots will show no elongation in any direction. The focused target appears to be the same as when there is no lens in the instrument and the power wheel registers zero.)*

If the sphere and cylinder lines do not intersect at the center of the mires, the lens optical center is not before the Lensometer aperture and prism is being manifested.

(see Figure 2–12).

Power Verification and Spotting of Spherocylinders

When verifying spherocylinder lenses, the Lensometer power wheel is turned to the expected sphere power as was the case with simple sphere lenses. In addition, however, the cylinder axis wheel is also turned until the axis indicated by the prescription is correctly positioned. Now the single vision lens is placed in the instrument and rotated (as in Figure 2–13) until the sphere lines of the Lensometer target are sharp and unbroken. (The lens may also be moved horizontally and vertically in an effort to begin centering the target lines over the central crosshairs of the eyepiece or screen). Then turn the Lensometer power wheel in the appropriate direction for checking the cylinder power, (i.e., in the minus direction when fabricating with minus cylinder notation).

Assuming the lens to be of correct refractive power, carefully move the lens left, right, upward, and downward until the target is accurately centered. (In the case of high cylinder powers it may be necessary to rock the power wheel between sphere and cylinder readings to achieve a correct centration, as only one set of target lines may be visible at a time.) Care also must be taken not to rotate the lens and thereby cause the axis to be incorrectly positioned. As in Figure 2–14, when the target is accurately centered, the lens may be spotted.

As soon as the lens is spotted, it should be removed from the Lensometer and marked for the right or left eye. Lenses are marked on the inner surface with a china marker or similar marking device suitable for writing on glass or plastic. (The marker must not be of the type that is absorbed into

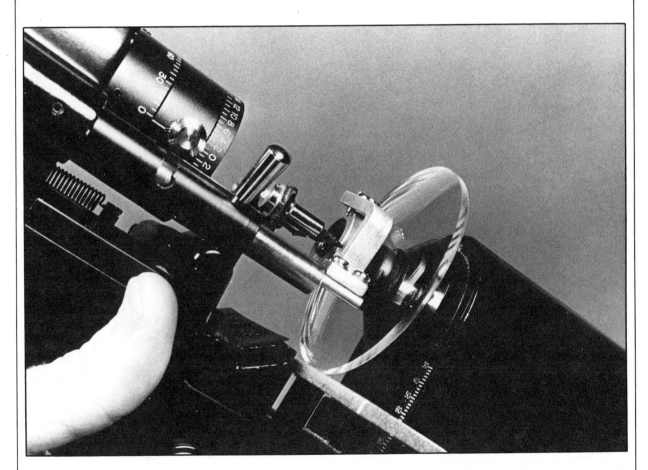

Figure 2–12. *The inking mechanism places three horizontally aligned dots on the lens. All subsequent steps are based on these dots.*

plastic lens material.) The letter *R* or *L* in uppercase letters is written in the upper half of the lens, above the three spots. Figure 2–15 shows that the letters are written normally (not in mirror image as is commonly done in surfacing procedures). The lens is then returned to its tray with the back (concave) side down. Placing the lens front side down risks scratching the front lens surface as the lens slides in the tray. By convention the right lens is always placed in the right side of the tray, the left lens in the left side (as in Figure 2–16). In the production process, each practitioner expects the right lens to be on the right side. If it is not, lenses can be marked or edged for the wrong eye, since any reversal in placement is unanticipated and can be easily overlooked.

Spotting with Autolensometers

Autolensometers perform in much the same manner as the manual variety, their chief advantages being speed of operation when measuring lenses of unknown power and a reduced training time for new operators.

Use of an autolensometer for spotting lenses requires no presetting of the instrument. When the lens is placed in the instrument, a sphere, cylinder, and axis appear on a digital display. The spherocylinder lens must be rotated until the correct axis appears. A horizontal and/or vertical arrow will appear (see Figure 2–17) to indicate in which direction the lens must be moved to achieve the correct optical centration. When this has been achieved, the

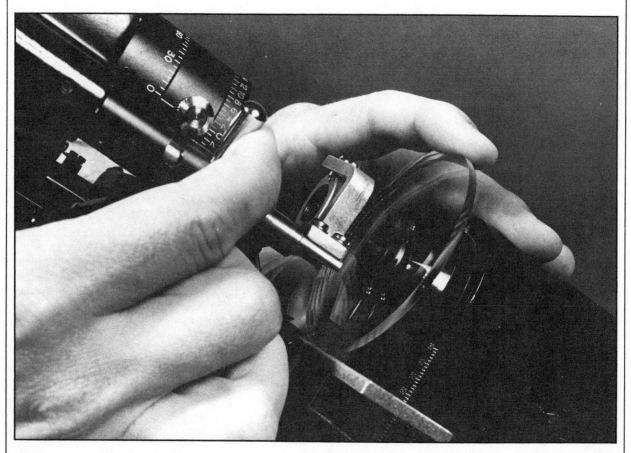

Figure 2–13. *When a practitioner moves or rotates a lens, the lens holding mechanism is retracted to facilitate movement and avoid possible scratching.*

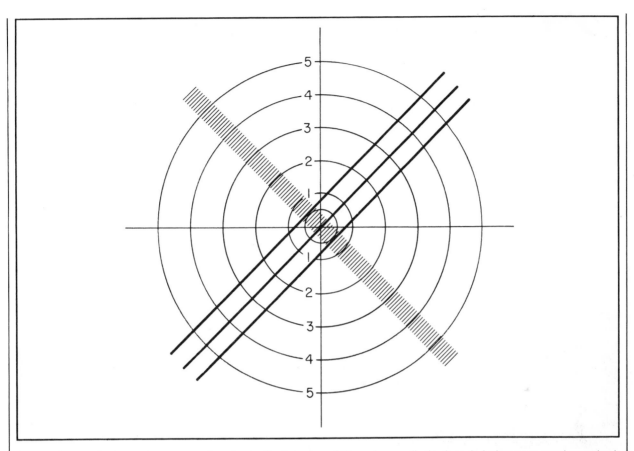

Figure 2–14. *Take care to ensure that the optical center of the spherocylinder lens is being accurately marked. It is always advisable to oscillate the power wheel back and forth between sphere and cylinder meridians to assure that no prismatic effect will be present after edging.*

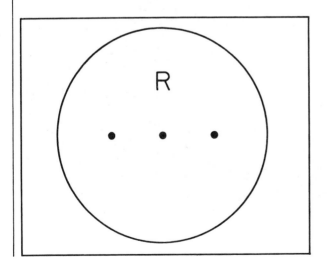

Figure 2–15. *The lens designation (R or L) is always marked on the upper half of the lens so that the lens will not be blocked upside-down. Though not as critical for nonprismatic single vision lenses, an inverted prism lens or multifocal would be worse than useless when inverted!*

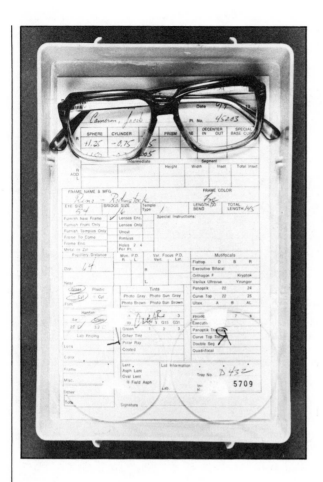

Figure 2–16. *By convention the right lens is placed on the righthand side of the tray and is always face up to avoid scratching the front surface. In spite of the convention, the lenses should still be checked before each step in the fabrication process to verify that the correct lens is being used.*

lens may be spotted in the same manner as with manual models.

OC VS. MRP

Up to this point the procedure described has been limited to single vision lenses with no prism power indicated in the prescription. The *optical center* (OC) has been diligently marked in such a manner that, when the process has been completed, it will be positioned directly before the pupil of the eye.

Whenever the eye looks through a lens at a point other than the optical center, a lateral and/or vertical displacement of the image occurs. This displacement is the *prismatic effect* of the lens. In some instances a prescription indicates that a prismatic

effect of a given value is required. The proper prismatic effect must be incorporated into the finished pair of glasses so that it will be directly in front of the pupil. That point on the lens where both the prescribed refractive *and* prismatic power are located is known as the *major reference point* (MRP).[2] For prescriptions that include prism, the OC and MRP are separate points and do not coincide. When no prism is indicated, the OC and MRP are one and the same point.

The distance in centimeters between the OC and the MRP for a desired prismatic effect depends

---

[2]British equivalent of the major reference point is the *centration point* (CP).

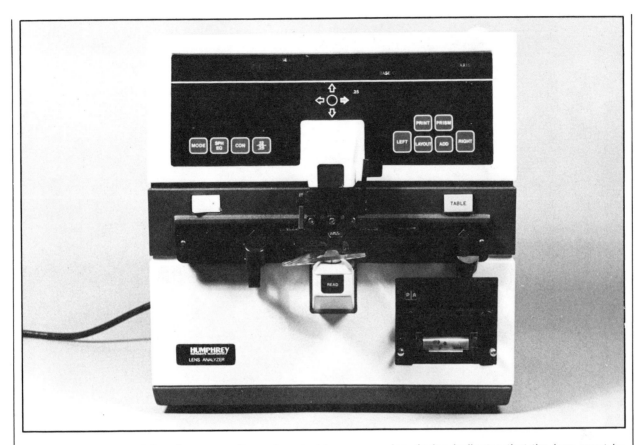

Figure 2–17. *The righthand arrow on the automated lens measuring device indicates that the lens must be moved to the right to arrive at the optical center.*

upon the power of the lens. It can be calculated using Prentice's rule for decentration, which states that

$$\Delta = cF,$$

where

Δ = prism diopters at the point of reference,

c = distance in centimeters,

and

F = power of the lens.

For spherical lenses the calculation is straightforward.[3] For example, how far away from each other will OC and MRP be for a -3.00 lens when a 1.5Δ prismatic effect is desired?

Since F = -3.00D
and Δ = 1.5Δ,
therefore Δ = cF or c = $\dfrac{\Delta}{F}$
and c = $\dfrac{1.5}{3}$ = 0.5 cm
or 5 mm from OC to MRP.

---

[3] For decentration of plano cylinder lenses along major meridians, the power used is the power of the cylinder in the meridian of decentration. If a cylinder is oriented at an oblique axis and decentration is horizontal or vertical, the prism will be induced with its base-oriented obliquely. For more information on the optical effects of decentration, see the companion book by the same author, Clifford W. Brooks and Irvin M. Borish, *System for Ophthalmic Dispensing,* Chicago: The Professional Press, 1979.

19

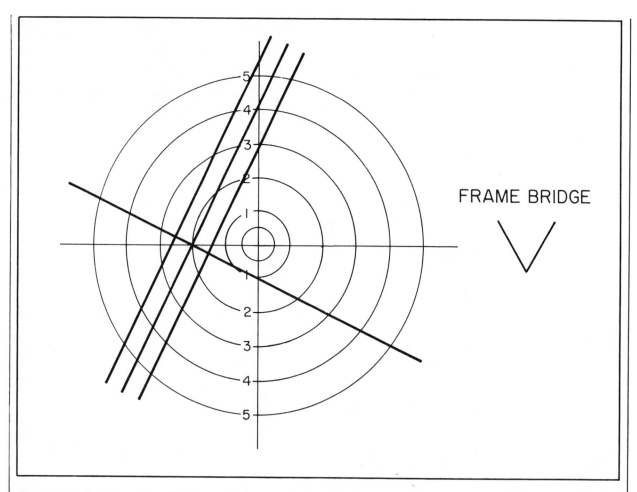

FRAME BRIDGE

Figure 2–18. *Prismatic effect can be created by decentering the lens in the Lensometer until the sphere/cylinder line intersection is positioned for the indicated amount. (Achievement of desired prism by decentration is limited by lens size and refractive power.)*

SPOTTING OF SINGLE VISION LENSES WITH PRISM

The procedure of spotting single vision lenses with prism is identical to that of nonprism lenses, with the exception of target centration. Instead of centering the intersection of target sphere and cylinder lines at the center of the crosshairs, the target lines must be positioned to correspond to the desired prismatic effect. If, for example, the right lens calls for 2.0Δ base-out prism, then the target intersection must be on the circular mire marked 2.0Δ where it crosses the horizontal 180-degree line as shown in Figure 2–18. Once this position is achieved in conjunction with a correct axis position, the lens may be spotted.

Figure 2–19 indicates that the center Lensometer ink spot will no longer be at the center of the uncut lens, but will indicate the location of the major reference point.

In a case in which both horizontal and vertical prisms are called for simultaneously in the same lens, the target must be moved both laterally and vertically until it reaches the desired position. That position is one where the target center is directly above (or below) the required horizontal prism reading. It is also exactly left or right of the required vertical prism reading. For example, Figure 2–20 shows that for a right eye that requires 4.0Δ base out and 2.0Δ base up, the target must be four units to the left of center *and* two units above center.

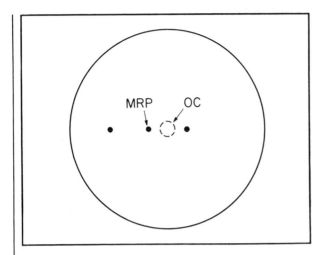

Figure 2–19. *The major reference point (MRP) of a lens will ultimately be positioned directly before the wearer's pupil center. If prism is indicated in the prescription, the optical center (OC) is displaced purposely. Therefore, the point that will be important in centration and is consequently spotted is the major reference point—not the optical center.*

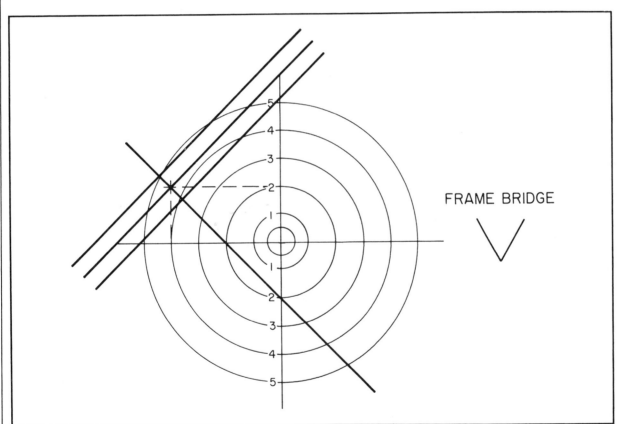

FRAME BRIDGE

Figure 2–20. *In positioning a prismatic lens, the only important reference is the origin of sphere and cylinder lines. Where other parts of those individual lines may cross the circular mires is of no consequence.*

In the example shown, the sphere/cylinder line origin must be directly above or below the place where the 4.0Δ circle crosses the horizontal line farthest from the "nose." The sphere/cylinder line origin must simultaneously also be exactly at the same level as the upper crossing point for the 2.0Δ circle. (Essentially this duplicates the vector sum of horizontal and vertical prism components.)

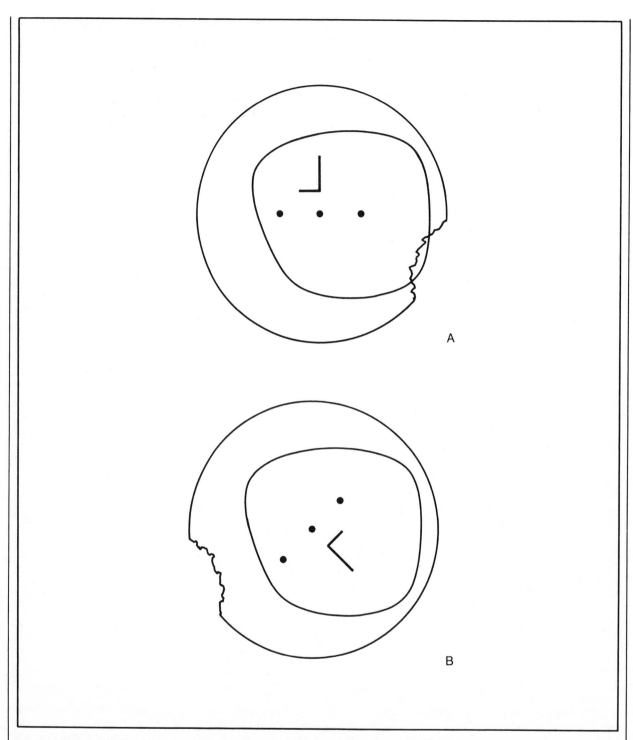

Figure 2–21. (A) *The lens will be ruined if edged as marked. By turning this spherical lens, the same optical endpoint is achieved without sacrificing quality. (B) The lens should be remarked so that in marking and blocking the chipped portion will be positioned as shown.*

MAKING THE MOST OF A BLEMISHED LENS

Occasionally lenses become chipped or scratched in handling, shipping, or surfacing. By taking full advantage of lens optical properties it may be possible to use the lens without compromising the quality of the finished product. The crucial factor here is the location of the imperfect or damaged portion in relation to the final lens shape and lens power.

The most versatile lens type is the spherical lens. Because it is of uniform power in all meridians, it can be rotated around its optical center to any angle without changing its optical characteristics. Therefore, if a large chip were to be broken from its edge, as shown in Figure 2–21 (A), the lens need only be turned so that during the edging process this chipped portion will be edged away (B). If the person spotting lenses is familiar with the frame shape, the correct position can be indicated right away. By the same reasoning, if it is obvious that the defect is too large for the frame called for, it can be put back right away before more time is lost.

The spherocylinder lens is somewhat less adaptable, but nevertheless has two possible orientations. The decision on how best to orient a slightly damaged spherocylinder is made after spotting the lens, but before it is marked with L or R.

For example, take a prescription for the right eye of power +2.00 −1.00 x 10. The lens is verified and spotted as shown in Figure 2–22(A). If the operator realizes the frame shape required, it will become evident (B) that this orientation is unacceptable. Turning the lens upside-down in a 180-degree rotation does not effect the optics, since a 10-degree axis is the same as a 190-degree axis. (For this reason only axis notation up to 180 degrees is utilized.) Turning the lens also repositions it so that the scratch will be completely ground away (C). The lens may now be designated in the "new" upper half with the appropriate *R*.

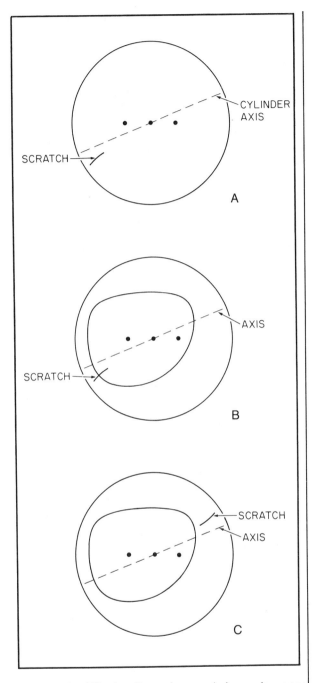

Figure 2–22. *A scratch on a lens may not make the lens unusable. Whether it can be used depends upon scratch location, frame size, and, in the case of cylinder lenses, axis orientation. In A, the lens is marked for edging (no prism). If used as oriented, the scratch will appear on the edged lens. However, because a spherocylinder without prism can be rotated 180 degrees without any change in optical effect, this lens is still useful. (Any rotation of the lens must be done* after *spotting and* before *the lens is marked.)*

If the lens proved to be unacceptable in both B *and* C, *it may still be useful later for a frame with a smaller eyesize or a prescription having a different axis orientation.*

23

Standard lens blanks that must be positioned for prescribed prism can also be rotated, but only before the MRP is marked.[4] Spherical lenses can be rotated until the optimum position is located, then moved horizontally and/or vertically to achieve a prismatic effect. Spherocylinders can be turned 180 degrees if desirable, but again, only *before* moving the target off center to achieve a prismatic effect.

SPOTTING AND PRESCRIPTION VERIFICATION OF MULTIFOCAL LENSES

Multifocal lenses are checked for surface defects and internal deficiencies in the same manner as are single vision lenses. They should also be spotted, thus marking the major reference point and the 180-degree line. This line indicates the horizontal plane of the lenses and is not the axis of the cylinder, but rather the line from which the axis of the cylinder is measured.

For multifocals with spherical distance portions, the bifocal should be oriented as it will be when mounted in the frame. In the instance of flat top bifocals, the segment top should be oriented horizontally. Keep in mind, however, that in the case of spherical lenses, the 180-degree line may be tilted during the next step of centration to accommodate near segment positioning. The central dot marking the OC is the only fixed point at this stage.

For multifocals with spherocylinder distance portions, the axis of the cylinder has been custom ground for that particular lens. Therefore, if the near segment is positioned to approximate the orientation it should have in the frame, the lens need only be slightly rotated to achieve its specified cylinder axis. After the lens has been spotted, the 180-degree line should be parallel to the upper edge of a flat top segment. If it is not, the cylinder axis was surfaced improperly, as the example in Figure 2–23. In such an instance it will be impossible to mount the lens in the frame with both its segment top straight and the cylinder axis correct. Only in the case of an extremely low-powered cylinder might an error like this fall within acceptable quality standards.

In order to mark the MRP and 180-degree line for multifocals with round segments and a spherically powered distance portion, simply rotate the lenses to

---

[4]Lenses that have been specifically surfaced to obtain a prismatic effect could not have been achieved by decentration of a standard lens blank have only one possible orientation. They can neither be rotated as a sphere would be, nor turned 180 degrees.

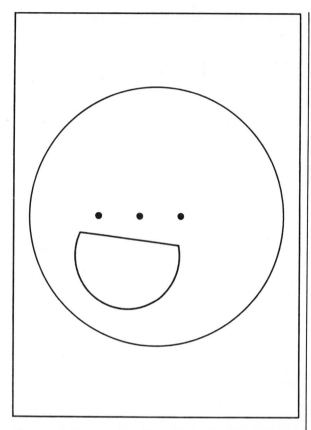

Figure 2–23. *Non-parallelism of dots and segment top indicate problems for all but spherical lenses. Either the cylinder axis will be incorrect or the segment top crooked. Both instances are unacceptable.*

the estimated segment position. Because segments are rotated inward toward the nose as the right lens faces the Lensometer operator, it is rotated so that the segment is slightly right of center. The left lens segment will be likewise rotated somewhat left of center.

For spherocylindrical round segment multifocals the lens is turned to the correct cylinder axis and the MRP and horizontal line spotted. Whether the cylinder axis is acceptable in reference to the near segment positions can only be judged during the centration process that follows.

Invisible segment or "blended bifocal" lenses have

round segment areas whose borders have been blended to make them unnoticeable. These are spotted in exactly the same manner as are round segment lenses, but are not to be confused with the so-called progressive addition lenses that will be considered shortly.

Verify all segments for accuracy of the near addition power after the lens is spotted. Once this is completed, remove the lens from the instrument and mark it with an *L* or *R* in the conventional manner.

When the Major Reference Point Enters the Segment Portion

When a bifocal or trifocal is ordered with its top higher than the geometric center of the edged lens, matters become more complicated. Recall that the normal location of the MRP is halfway between the top and bottom of the edged lens. This means that unless specific provisions are made, the major reference point will be right in the segment area! Because the segment top is higher than this midpoint, when using the Lensometer, the MRP becomes "lost" in the segment.

To get around this problem, lens power measurements may be made above the segment, as is done with progressive addition lenses. Unfortunately, spotting of the lenses cannot be done accurately because of the lateral and vertical prismatic effect of the segment upon the distance lens optics. For all but round segments, though, centration can be carried out normally without ever spotting the lenses. For round segments, the following process can be used.[5]

1. Verify distance power just above the segment and, while taking care to keep the cylinder axis correct, move the lens laterally until there is no horizontal prism (or if prism is prescribed, until the correct amount appears).
2. Spot the lens at this elevated point. The vertical position of the multifocal lens depends only upon how high the segment top will be. This is determined later in the centration process. As long as the three dots on the lens are kept horizontal, the cylinder axis will be right.

---

[5]There are several factors that can prevent this process from being entirely accurate, such as the horizontal prism that may be induced by the presence of a strong oblique cylinder. Yet because the near add can, with higher powers, affect the apparent cylinder axis as well as induce horizontal and vertical prism of its own, the method shown remains a viable compromise.

SPOTTING OF PROGRESSIVE ADDITION LENSES

Progressive addition lenses have certain hidden etch marks used in lens orientation. Lenses coming from the surfacing laboratory may be premarked, in which case they need only be verified before edging. They need not be marked again.

To check distance lens power, position the lens in the Lensometer so as to look through the area above the MRP. (See Figure 2–24.) Near lens power is checked through a point well into the near zone, so that no intermediate progressive power is measured. To check for prism, conventional methods are used at the MRP. Note, however, that the Lensometer target may not be altogether clear because of the effects of a beginning progressive zone.

Verify the near addition using the specified area well into the near progressive zone. Failure to drop far enough into the near zone causes erroneous readings because of the constantly changing power in the progressive zone.

In terms of lens spotting, the progressive addition lens is treated exactly like any other. The OC or MRP is located and the lens turned until the axis is correct. After spotting, check the lens to be certain that the spotted MRP corresponds to the already present markings painted on the lens. The three Lensometer dots shown in Figure 2–25, signifying the 180-degree line, must also parallel the painted markings. The location of these painted marks is based on the hidden etch marks present on the lens.

When Lenses Are Not Premarked

In the event that a progressive addition lens leaves the surfacing lab without visible markings, the finishing lab should reconstruct the manufacturer's recommended system of identifying marks. This is done as follows:

1. Locate the hidden etch marks by holding the lens under an incandescent bulb. (The background should be matte black to help etch marks stand out. Two small etched circles are usually found at about 1.5 cm from either side of the lens center.)
2. Dot the centers of the etched circles with a marking pen.
3. Place the lens on a verification card provided by the manufacturer and turn the lens so that the dots fall at the indicated "engraved circle" points of the card. Alternately, a flexible template suitable for tracing may be placed on the lens.
4. Trace the appropriate lines on the lens from the master markings found on the verification card (Figure 2–26) or template (Figure 2–27).

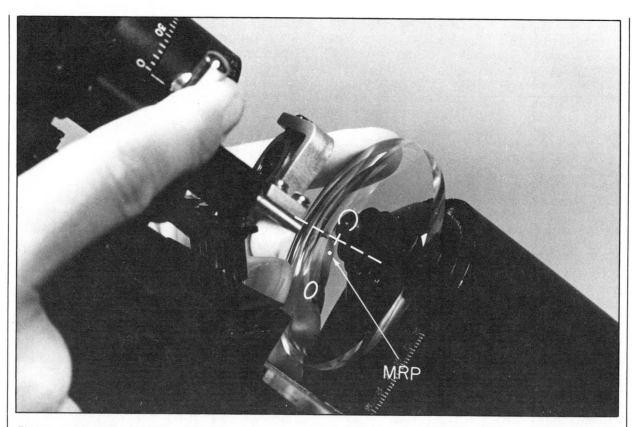

Figure 2–24. *If the power of a progressive add lens is not checked above the major reference point, erroneous readings may result. This is due to the fact that the major reference point marks the beginning of a change in power where the progressive zone or corridor leads down into the near portion.*

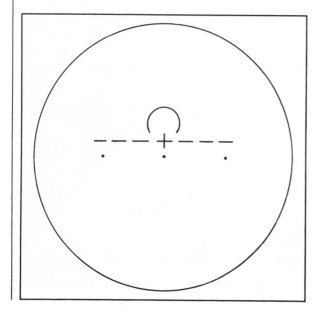

Figure 2–25. *For this progressive addition lens, the three dots are parallel to the premarked horizontal. With nonspherical progressive addition lenses, failure of the three dots to parallel the marked horizontal indicates possible misplacement of both the progressive corridor and near zone, reducing wearer usability of the lens.*

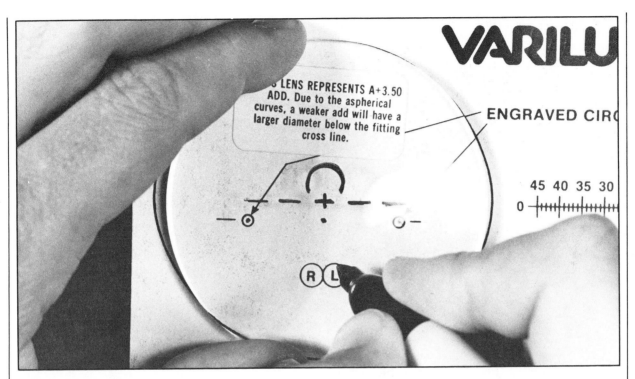

Figure 2–26. *When the engraved circles on the lens are located and dotted, the guide marks can be reconstructed for use in layout (when the fitting cross system is used) and in power verification.*

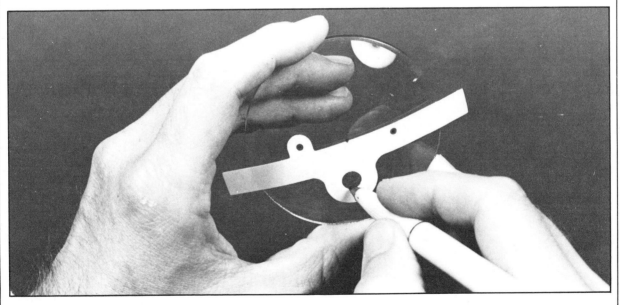

Figure 2–27. *A template placed on the lens in accordance with previously located etch marks allows remarking of progressive addition lenses.*

PROFICIENCY TEST QUESTIONS

1. *Internal* lens deficiencies are inspected for by
   a. looking at the filament of an unfrosted light bulb as it reflects from the surface of the lens.
   b. observing a straight line through the lens as the lens is moved back and forth.
   c. looking through the lens at a black background under indirect illumination.
   d. all of the above methods are correct.
   e. methods b and c above are correct.

2. A prescription is $-2.00 -1.25 \times 30$. What *two* power wheel readings appear when first sphere, then cylinder lines are brought into focus?
   a. -2.00
   b. -0.75
   c. -3.25
   d. -1.25
   e. $+0.75$

3. T or F When using the Lensometer to neutralize a lens of unknown power and obtain results directly in plus cylinder form, the power wheel is turned into the high minus numbers and slowly moved in the plus direction until the cylinder lines are first brought into sharp focus.

4. The Lensometer power wheel is turned into the high plus power and returned until the sphere lines are clear. (Power wheel reads $+2.00D$, axis wheel reads 12.) The power wheel is turned further into the minus until the cylinder lines clear. (Power wheel reads -1.00.) What is the prescription?
   a. $+2.00 -1.00 \times 12$
   b. $-1.00 +2.00 \times 12$
   c. $+2.00 -1.00 \times 102$
   d. $+2.00 -3.00 \times 12$
   e. $-1.00 +2.00 \times 12$

5. The Lensometer power wheel is turned into the high plus power and returned until the *cylinder* lines are clear. (Power wheel reads $+4.00D$, axis wheel reads 180.) The power wheel is turned further into the minus until the *sphere* line clears. (Power wheel reads $+3.00D$.) What is the prescription?
   a. $+4.00 -1.00 \times 90$
   b. $+4.00 -3.00 \times 180$
   c. $+4.00 -1.00 \times 180$
   d. $+3.00 -1.00 \times 90$
   e. $+3.00 -1.00 \times 90$

6. When spotting a single vision lens for edging, in reference to *edged lens orientation,* the Lensometer ink dots will be on
   a. the sphere meridian.
   b. the cylinder meridian.
   c. the 180-degree meridian.
   d. the cylinder axis.

7. T or F When spotting a lens using plus cylinder notation instead of minus cylinder notation, the lens is turned 90 degrees from where it would otherwise be.

8. By convention, lenses in the finishing lab are marked for right *(R)* or left *(L)* on the
   a. outside surface, in mirror image, on the upper half.
   b. inside surface, on the lower half.
   c. inside surface, on the upper half.
   d. outside surface, on the lower half.
   e. outside surface, on the upper half.

9. T or F Because lenses are placed convex side up in the lab tray, the wearer's right lens will be in the lower left half of the tray and the left lens in the lower right half of the tray.

10. For high cylinders in which either the Lensometer sphere or the cylinder lines are visible one group at a time, but not simultaneously, the major reference point
    a. is found by centering on the sphere line.
    b. is found by centering on the center cylinder line.
    c. is found by alternately centering on first the sphere line, then the center cylinder line.
    d. is found by using a lens center locator.
    e. cannot be found by any of the above methods.

11. Which point should *always* appear exactly in front of the wearer's pupil?
    a. OC
    b. DBC
    c. geometric center
    d. MRP
    e. IOP

12. For which of the following prescriptions is there a difference in the physical location of the optical

28

center and the major reference point?
a. -4.00D sphere
b. $-4.00 -2.00 \times 180$
c. -4.00D sphere with 0.5Δ base-in prism
d. $-4.00 -2.00 \times 180$ with 0.5Δ base-up prism
e. The optical center and major reference point are synonomous terms and hence, are always at the same point on a lens.

13. A flat top bifocal is spotted for the MRP, and it is immediately evident that the three dots are *not* parallel to the segment line. In which Rx is this of no consequence?
a. It is *always* of consequence.
b. $-1.00 -1.00 \times 180$
c. pl -1.00×70
d. -2.25D sph

14. T or F If the MRP "disappears" into the segment, the lens is spotted by changing the Lensometer power wheel so that the target lines clear through the segment. The MRP, which "vanished," can now be found and spotted.

15. T or F Spotting a pre-marked progressive addition lens is only done for verification purposes, as the later centration process can be accomplished using only the marks already on the lens.

16. T or F There are "invisible" engravings on progressive addition lenses that allow the desired MRP and near portions of the lens to be exactly located.

17. How far away from the MRP must the OC be moved to create the proper prismatic effect by decentration for the following lens?
$+1.50 -1.50 \times 90$ 0.5Δ base out
a. 3.33 mm
b. 30 mm
c. 0 mm
d. The distance can't be figured from the measurements provided.

18. How far away from the MRP must the OC be moved to create the proper prismatic effect by decentration for the following lens?
$+1.50 +1.50 \times 90$ 0.5Δ base out (notice the form of the Rx)
a. 1.67 mm
b. 3.33 mm
c. 0 mm
d. The distance can't be figured from the measurements provided.

19. The Rx is
R: -6.00D sph 1.0Δ base out. The lens is in the Lensometer (convex side facing the operator) with the Lensometer target exactly centered. In which direction must the lens be moved before it may be correctly spotted?
a. It is correct as is and need not be moved.
b. Left
c. Right
d. Up
e. Down

Matching
(More than one answer may be appropriate.)

20. $+4.00$D sph_____ a. After this lens has been spotted, it will be *un*affected by any lens rotation around the center spot.

21. $-4.25 -1.00 \times 35$ _____ b. After spotting, this lens will be *un*affected if the lens is rotated *exactly 180 degrees around the center spot.*

22. $-1.00 -2.00 \times$ 182Δ base in _____ c. After spotting, this lens will be *affected* by any *lens* rotation.

Chapter 3
Centration of Single Vision Lenses

PURPOSE OF CENTERING

During the edging process the lens rotates around a central point while being ground to a specific shape to fit the frame. This central point of rotation corresponds to a hole in the pattern. This hole should always be in the middle of the pattern used on the edger to generate the shape. This middle point, the *geometric* or *boxing center* of the lens, is defined as being the center of the smallest rectangle which encloses the lens shape using horizontal and vertical lines. As Figure 3–1 shows, if the pattern is correctly made for the boxing system of measuring frames, lenses, and patterns, the point around which the spectacle lens rotates during edging becomes the geometric or boxing center of the edged lens.[1]

In order for the major reference point of the lens to end up before the wearer's pupil, the lens must be moved, or *decentered* away from this central point. Take great care here, as the slightest error during this centration process will mean inaccuracy in the finished product.

THE MECHANICS OF LENS CENTRATION

The first part of the centration process involves figuring out exactly where the major reference point of the lens will be in relationship to the boxing center of the edged lens. If these two points are not coincident, the lens is said to be *decentered*. The distance and direction of this decentration[2] must be calculated to ensure that the lens optics will be positioned properly before the eye.

How to Calculate Horizontal Decentration Using the Boxing System
There are two measurements required in the calculation of decentration. One depends on the wearer, the

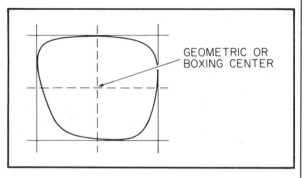

GEOMETRIC OR BOXING CENTER

Figure 3–1. *During the edging process the lens rotates around a given point. For the boxing system this becomes the geometric or boxing center of the edged lens.*

second on the frame being worn. The first measurement is how far apart the person's pupil centers are from each other. This is known as the *interpupillary distance* (PD). The second measurement is the distance between the geometrical (boxing) centers of the frame's two lens openings. This is known as the

---

[1] When British Standards are used, the pattern (former) rotates around the *datum center*. For a diagrammatic explanation of boxing, British, and GOMAC Systems, see Appendix 1.

[2] *Decentration* is a term applied to any lens movement required to achieve a certain optical effect. For example, a lens optical center is decentered with reference to the eye to achieve a desired prismatic effect. In surfacing the lens, it is decentered to situate it properly for grinding of the optical center at a given location. In short, any time a lens blank is moved prior to some surfacing or edging procedure, the term *decentration* may be applied.

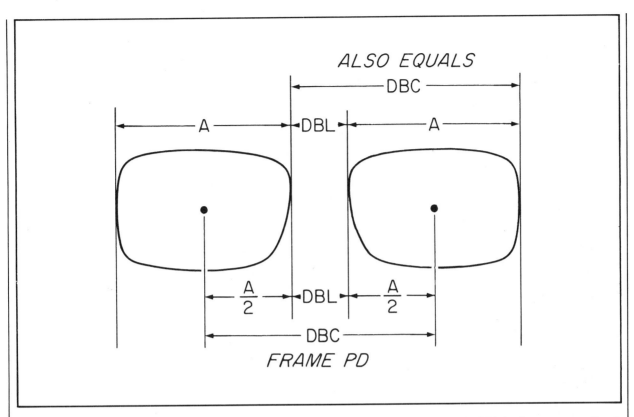

Figure 3–2. *It can be seen from the figure that the distance between centers (DBC) is the same as the A dimension (eyesize) plus the DBL (bridge size). Since the DBC cannot be measured directly, it may be measured as shown in the upper righthand corner of the figure.*

distance between centers (DBC).[3] (The distance between centers is also commonly referred to as the *frame PD*.)

Determination of the Distance Between Centers

For frames that conform to the boxing system of measurement, the DBC is equal to the eyesize (abbreviated *A*) plus the *distance between lenses* (DBL). This is true because the geometrical center is located halfway across each lens opening.

Since the *A* dimensions of right and left lenses are equal,

---

[3]The distance between centers is the term used by the American National Standards Institute. Alternate terms with the same meaning are *geometrical center distance* (GCD), *frame center distance, boxing center distance,* and *frame PD.*

$$DBC = \frac{\text{right lens } A \text{ dimension}}{2} + DBL +$$

$$\frac{\text{left lens } A \text{ dimension}}{2}$$

then

$$DBC = A + DBL.$$

This is shown in Figure 3–2.

If the frame itself is available the DBC can be measured. Start at the most nasal point on the right lens opening and measure on a straight horizontal to the plane of the most temporal point on the left lens opening, as in Figure 3–3. As one of these two

31

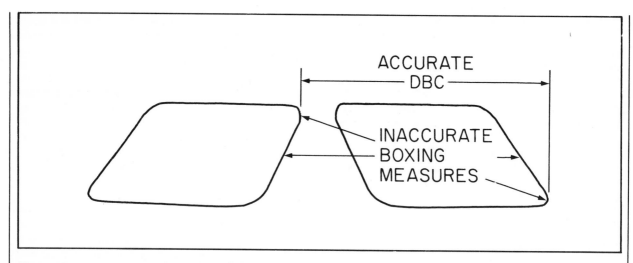

Figure 3–3. *It can be seen by actually holding a ruler to the illustrated dimensions that a great deal of difference in size may result from the two methods of measurement. (This diagram applies to the commonly used boxing system only.)*

points may be higher or lower than the other, simply measuring in the middle of the frame is not likely to be accurate.[4]

Decentration per Lens

Most commonly the wearer's PD will be less than the frame PD. This will require that the lenses be decentered inward (nasally) toward the center of the frame. The amount of decentration per lens can be determined by subtracting the wearer's PD from the DBC (frame PD) and dividing by two.

$$\frac{DBC - \text{wearer PD}}{2} = \text{decentration per lens.}[5]$$

---

[4]The student using British Standards will, in fact, measure exactly across the center of the frame to obtain the datum center distance (DCD). By substituting datum center distance for distance between centers (DBC), "datum length" for *A,* and "datum DBL" for "boxing DBL" throughout, the student will find decentration measures will work well in the ophthalmic laboratory using British Standards. A thorough study of Appendix 1 on standards should be made to avoid confusion.

[5]*Decentration* (or *decentration per lens*) refers to the amount one lens is moved. *Total decentration* refers to the sum of both left and right decentrations. Therefore total decentration = GCD − wearer PD.

Example:

Suppose the order form indicates that the wearer's PD is 64 mm. The frame size indicated is 53 □ 17. In other words, the eye size is 53 mm and the DBL 17 mm. The □ symbol indicates that the dimensions are listed according to the boxing system. If the frame is known to conform to boxing measure standards, what is the decentration per lens required?

Solution:

In order to initially determine the difference between the DBC and wearer's PD, we must know the DBC. By definition,

$$DBC = A + DBL.$$
$$\text{Since } A = 53 \text{ mm,}$$
$$\text{and DBL} = 17 \text{ mm,}$$
$$\text{then DBC} = 53 + 17$$
$$= 70 \text{ mm}$$

Now because it is known that

$$\text{decentration per lens} = \frac{DBC - PD}{2}$$

In this instance we see that

$$\frac{70 - 64}{2} = \frac{6}{2} = 3 \text{ mm per lens.}$$

In the unusual case where the wearer's PD is greater than the DBC, a negative decentration will result from the calculations. This indicates that decentration outward is required and the MRP of the lens will be decentered temporally.

Determining Decentration from Monocular PD's.
Occasionally a prescription specifies the wearer's PD in reference to each eye individually. This measure is referred to as the *monocular PD;* it uses for its reference point the center of the nose. Instead of a more conventionally measured *binocular PD* of, for example, 64, we may have a right monocular PD of 31 and a left monocular PD of 33. This difference between left and right PD's is not unusual considering the asymmetry of facial features of many normal individuals.

For a monocular PD, decentration is determined by first dividing the distance between centers (DBC) of the frame by 2, then subtracting the monocular PD; thus

$$\text{decentration} = \frac{\text{DBC}}{2} - \text{monocular PD.}$$

Decentration for Reading Glasses.
In most cases it will not be evident to laboratory personnel whether the prescription being fabricated is for distance vision or for near vision. A single number given for PD could be either the distance PD or the "near PD." This near PD designates a smaller separation of the MRP's of the finished lenses to allow for convergence, which is an inward turning of the person's eyes that occurs when he or she does close work. Occasionally, however, an order for single vision lenses is received that lists both distance and near PD's. This would be written as 65/62, for example. Unless otherwise noted, it must be assumed that the distance PD (65) is desired, even if the prescription is for low plus lenses. When the order form also contains the instructions, "for reading glasses," the smaller measure is chosen (62), as this is the separation of the lines of sight of the eyes at the plane of the prescription lenses.

When in doubt as to which measure to use, direct contact with the originator of the prescription is in order.

Horizontal Centration of Lenses by Hand
It is possible to carry out the centration of lenses with only a minimal amount of equipment. If care is taken, it may be done quite accurately, but requires a steady hand. The only equipment needed is a sheet of millimeter-ruled graph paper and a lens marking pen. It is helpful if the graph paper is marked with a central cross. The intersection of the two lines can then serve as the location of the boxing center.[6] (In actual fact, when centration is done by hand a *lens protractor* is used, as illustrated in Figure 3–4. This protractor can be used in both surfacing and finishing. However, for instructional purposes the concept can be further simplified by the use of graph paper.) The operation is performed as follows:

Step 1.
The previously spotted right lens is placed face down (front surface down). The front surface is placed down to avoid error by parallax[7] that can be introduced when the lens is placed convex side up with the center dot thereby considerably further from the surface of the graph paper. (Because this parallax error can be avoided through the use of centration devices, the experienced lab technician should be able to center the lens beginning with either the concave or the convex side of the lens up.)

Step 2.
The three spots on the lens are aligned with the main horizontal line. The central dot is placed at the intersection of the cross (see Figure 3–5).

Step 3.
The lens is decentered left or right in accordance with the number of millimeters calculated and the required direction of decentration.

In the example previously given, the required decentration was 3 mm per eye nasally—that is, 3 mm in. If this right lens is to be decentered in accordance with the example given, it must be moved to the left three millimeters such that the three dots remain on the horizontal line and the central MRP dot is 3 mm to the left of the intersection (see Figure 3–6).

---

[6]For students using British Standards, the datum center is the reference point.

[7]*Parallax* is the phenomenon that occurs when someone attempts to visually align an object with a scale when the object is not directly in contact with the scale. If the viewer's eye is not on a line directly perpendicular to the correct reading on the scale above or below the object, an error results. (The most common example of a parallax error occurs when the front seat passenger attempts to read the speedometer of a car.)

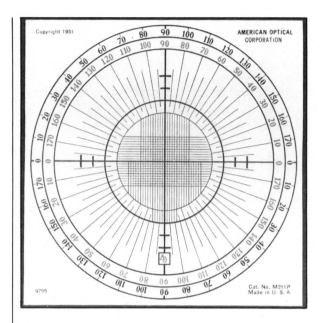

Figure 3–4. *A lens protractor maintains the simplic-ity of graph paper, but adds degree markings. These are used mainly in the lens surfacing process. The inner degree scale is used when the lens is placed convex side up (as when glasses are being worn). The outer scale is appropriate when the convex side is facing down.*

Step 4.
Dot the lens with the marking pen near its edge at four points—two at either end of the 180-degree line and at the top and bottom along the 90-degree line, as Figure 3–6 shows.

Step 5.
Now using the two 180-degree dots as a guide, draw a long horizontal line through the central part of the lens while holding a flexible ruler on the back side of the lens (see Figure 3–7). This line is the *cutting line.*

Step 6.
Draw a shorter, vertically intersecting line across this first horizontal line, using the 90-degree dots as a guide. Figure 3–8 shows the vertical line, which need be only 10 mm long. The difference in length be-tween the two lines gives an immediate visual cue as to the orientation of the lens. The intersection of the two lines shows exactly where the lens will be blocked and normally indicates the future boxing center of the edged lens.

Vertical Centration of Lenses
When there is no preference expressed on the order form as to a vertical location of the major reference points, it is assumed that they are to be left in their standard position. In most cases this will be in the same plane as the boxing center of the edged lens. Therefore, unless otherwise specified, the three dots on the previously spotted lens will remain on the 180-degree line throughout the centration operation.

When a lens order specifies a preference for the vertical height of the major reference point, then in addition to the lateral decentration previously de-scribed, there must be a vertical decentration of the MRP.

How Vertical Placement May Be Specified
One method for specifying vertical MRP location is in millimeters above or below the horizontal midline of the frame's lens opening. This is represented on the graph paper by the horizontally drawn reference line. If the order form specifies "2 above," then the MRP is moved (decentered) 2 mm up, in addition to its lateral decentration (as shown in Figure 3–9). It is imperative that the three lens dots remain parallel to the horizontal reference line.

The second method gives the vertical height of the MRP in terms of the distance from the lower line of the box enclosing the shape of the lens to be manu-factured. This vertical height must then be respecified in terms of its distance above or below the horizontal midline so that the lens may be marked. This hori-zontal midline is the *datum line.* In order to make the conversion, the vertical dimension of the frame must be known. When it is, conversion may be done by

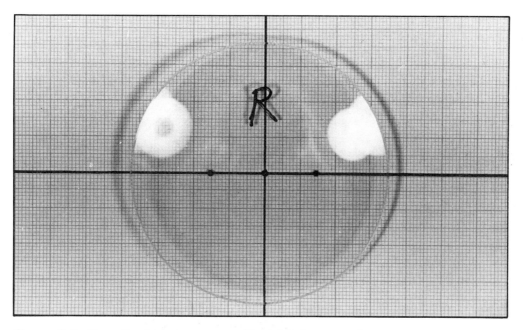

Figure 3–5. *Here the lens is seen positioned before any decentration occurs. Graph paper is used, since this "grid" is the basis for even the most complex centration device.*

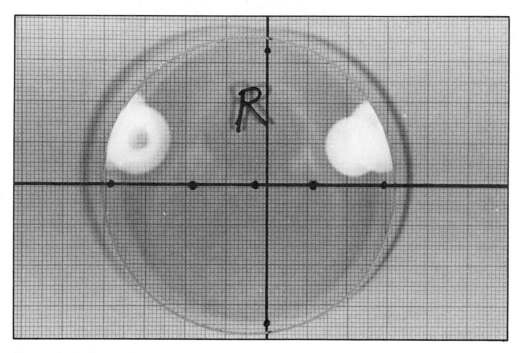

Figure 3–6. *For a right lens with its concave side up, the direction of decentration is inward (left) toward the nose. The boxing center of the lens must be marked. (This is the point around which the lens will rotate during edging.) In preparation for hand marking a lens (the old-fashioned way), the lens is dotted near the edges on the x,y coordinates of the grid.*

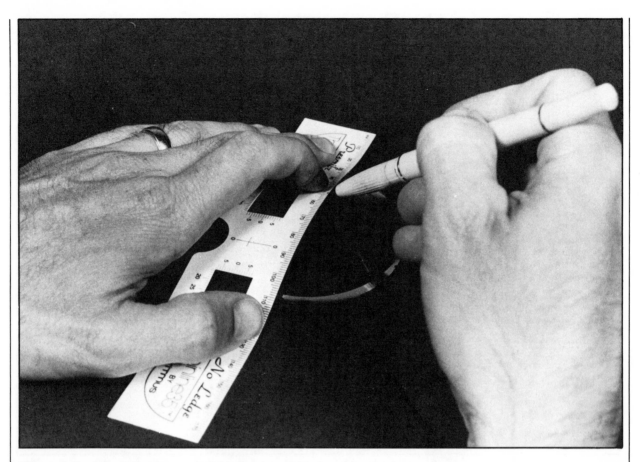

Figure 3–7. *A flexible ruler or straightedge is used to hand mark a lens.*

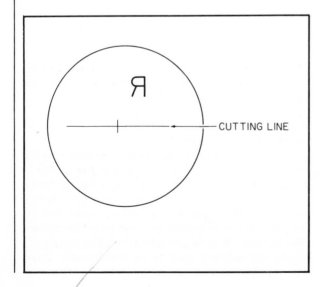

CUTTING LINE

Figure 3–8. *It will be noted that because of decentration, the cross is no longer at the geometric center of the lens. Is the lens concave side up or convex side up?*

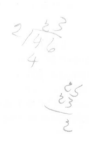

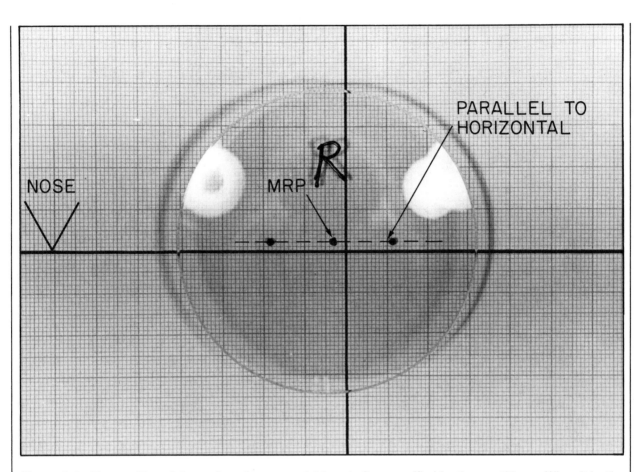

Figure 3–9. *The position of the major reference point is not often specified by the practitioner. When it is, the procedure is carried out through a simple raising or lowering of the central Lensometer dot, exercising care to maintain parallelism between the three dots and the X axis of the grid.*

subtracting half the vertical dimension of the frame (abbreviated as *B*) from the specified MRP height.

$$\text{vertical decentration} = \text{MRP height} - \frac{B}{2}.$$

Take the illustration of an order specifying an MRP height of 25 mm and using a frame having a vertical dimension (*B*) of 46 mm. The height above (or below) the horizontal midline of the lens may be visualized from Figure 3–10. In this example, vertical decentration is calculated as

$$25 \text{ mm} - \frac{46}{2} = 2 \text{ mm}.$$

It can be seen that since the MRP height is greater than half the *B* dimension, the vertical decentration is positive and the lens is moved up by 2 mm.

Exceptions to the Rule in the Vertical Centration Process

Some patterns used in the edging process may not conform to standards specifying that the center of rotation of the pattern be at the boxing center. When deviations from this standard occur it is in the vertical positioning of the pattern's rotational center. For example, a frame manufacturer may be of the opinion that because of its design a certain frame usually will cause the wearer's eyes to be considerably above the vertical midpoint of the lens. In an attempt to

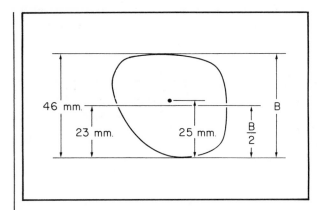

Figure 3–10. *If the position of the major reference point is given in terms of height from the lowermost portion of the shape, the needed drop or raise can be calculated using one half of the B dimension.*

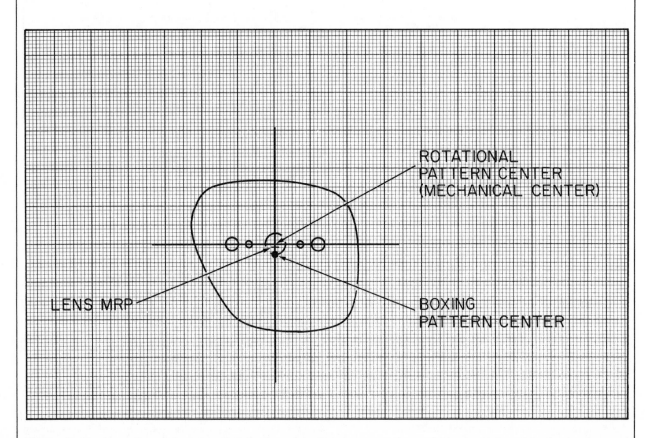

Figure 3–11. *Here it may be seen that in the centration process, the main horizontal and vertical reference lines always correspond to the rotational center of the pattern.*

38

compensate for this, the rotational center is moved above the boxing center of the pattern. When both left and right lenses are made using this pattern, both lens optical centers will be above center an equal amount. However, when a certain MRP height is specified, additional compensation must be made in order to arrive at that height.

When patterns have their rotational center above the boxing center, the difference between these two locations must be taken into consideration when attempting to place the MRP at a specific height. If this rotational center *is* above the boxing center, the distance between these two centers must be subtracted from the normally calculated MRP raise or drop. (Were the rotational center to be *below* the boxing center, the difference would be *added* to the otherwise calculated height.)

For example, suppose the vertical decentration required is 2 mm above the boxing center. A pattern with its center of rotation 3 mm above its boxing center will automatically cause the MRP to be 3 mm above the boxing center of the edged lens. Therefore, in order for the correct result to be obtained, 3 mm are subtracted from the normally calculated vertical decentration.

$$+ 2 \text{ mm} - 3 \text{ mm} = -1 \text{ mm}.$$

In other words, when this particular pattern is used, the MRP must be positioned 1 mm below the horizontal 180-degree reference line to make the lens center properly, as Figure 3–11 shows.

The Lens Protractor

As stated previously, when lenses are laid out for marking by hand, the most commonly used aid is a lens protractor rather than a sheet of graph paper. Some lens protractors have three raised pegs that hold the surface of the lens without allowing it to come directly in contact with the face of the protractor. These pegs both hold the lens steady, keeping it from rocking, and also prevent the ink spots on the lens from smearing or rubbing off.

The degree scales on a lens protractor are mainly used for marking the lens axis for surfacing. They theoretically could be used in finishing, were the axis of the cylinder used as a reference instead of the 180-degree line. The lens protractor scale which increases in value in a counterclockwise direction is intended for use when the front surface of the lens faces the operator. The clockwise numbered axis scale is for use when the front surface of the lens is placed face down on the protractor. The presence of a third scale of degrees, normally 90 degrees away

from the other two, is used for reference purposes if the lens protractor must be turned sideways to decenter lenses horizontally.

Marking a Single Vision Lens with a Lens Marking Device

A lens marking device has several advantages over hand marking of lenses, although the process itself is basically the same. These advantages are:

1. The optical system of the instrument eliminates parallax problems.
2. Internal illumination makes viewing of marks on the lens and segments of the lens easier.
3. The system contains a lens marking stamp that always strikes at the same place, giving a consistant, straight set of marks.
4. A second vertical line within the instrument that may be moved left or right permits prealignment for horizontal decentrations.

Following are the steps involved to mark a single vision lens on a centering device:

1. Turn on the internal illumination system.
2. Calculate the amount of decentration required.
3. Adjust the movable vertical line for the correct amount and direction of decentration.
4. Put the lens in the device and center the MRP on the movable reference line at the height indicated on the Rx, making certain that the three dots on the lens are horizontally aligned.
5. Mark the lens.

(From time to time, view a marked lens through the instrument *before* it is removed to determine if the lens is being accurately marked along the 180-degree meridian.)

For lenses over plus 6.00D, it may aid in accuracy to also lightly mark the front surface of the lens as well. This helps to minimize parallax error when blocking.

To demonstrate the mechanics of the marking system it is helpful to use illustrations.

For example, a frame has an eyesize (A) of 54 mm and a DBL of 20 mm. The PD of the wearer measures 66 mm. The lenses are already spotted and must be marked.

Assuming that the instrument is on and in good working order, decentration is calculated.

$$\text{decentration per lens} = \frac{A + DBL - PD}{2}$$

$$= \frac{54 + 20 - 66}{2}$$

$$= \frac{8}{2} = 4 \text{ mm}.$$

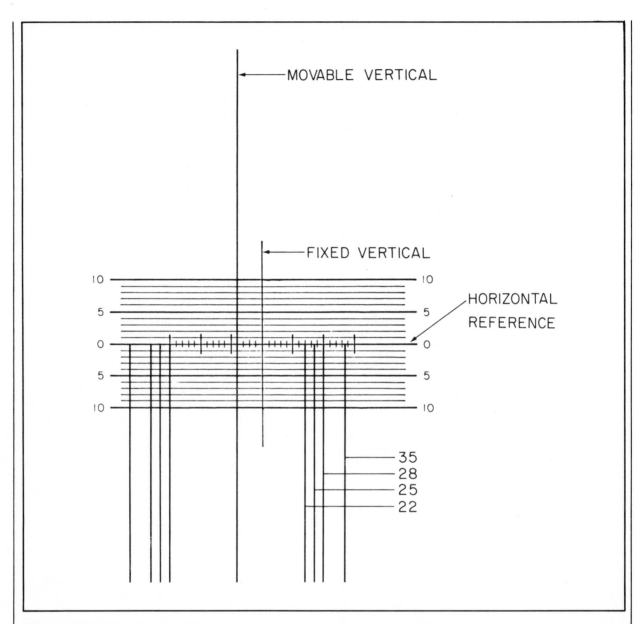

Figure 3–12. *In the case of single vision lenses, the movable line indicates the positioning of the major reference point and the fixed vertical line the position of the geometric center of the lens after edging.*

To preadjust the device for the right lens, first learn in which direction the major reference point will be moved. Because decentration is positive—with the wearer's PD smaller than the frame PD—the lenses will decenter nasally. In this instance the lens will be placed convex side down, meaning that since it is a right lens it will be moved to the left. As Figure 3–12 shows, the movable vertical line therefore is positioned 4 mm to the left of the central reference line.

Now place the lens face down in the instrument and align it such that the central dot is at the intersection of the fixed horizontal and movable ver-

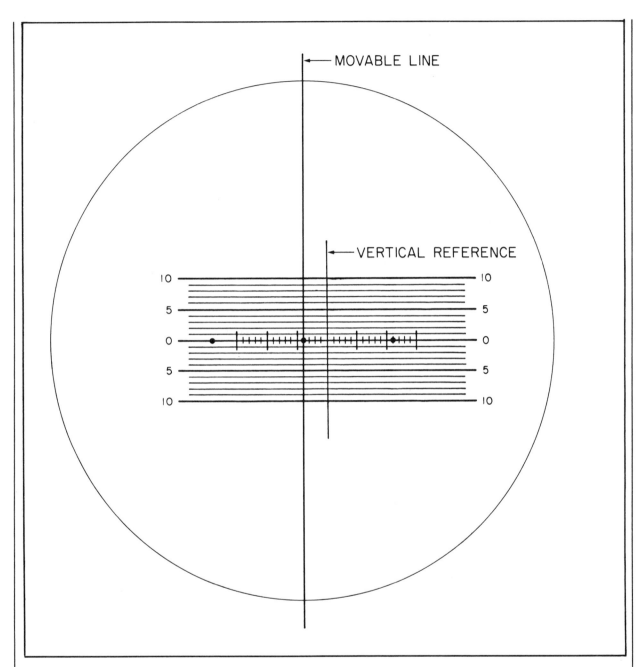

MOVABLE LINE

VERTICAL REFERENCE

Figure 3–13. *The movable line is preset to the correct decentration. This helps to prevent the dot on the lens from getting "lost" on the grid since it is more difficult to see than the line. With the movable line pointing out the desired MRP location, the lens is positioned as shown.*

tical lines. Figure 3–13 indicates that the other two dots must fall directly on the horizontal reference line.

Stamp the lens to denote the 180-degree line and the point that will become the boxing center (see Figure 3–14).

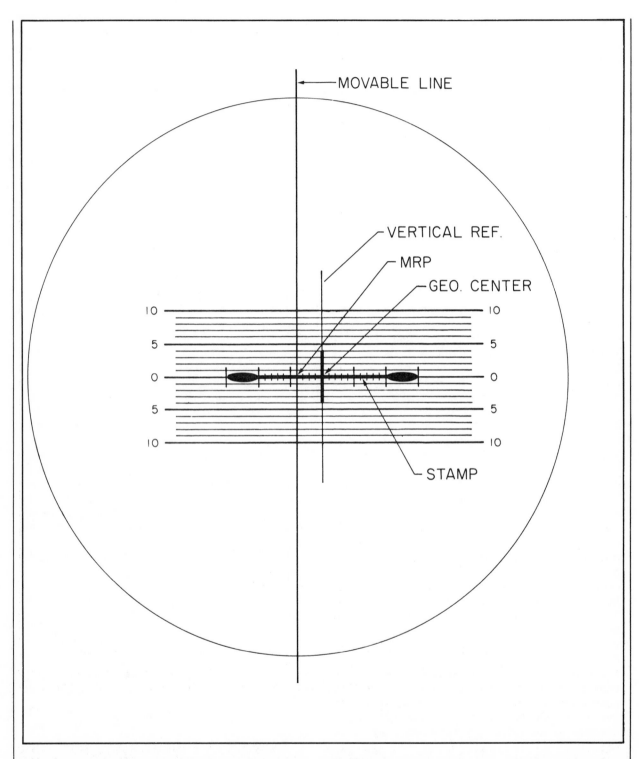

Figure 3–14. *On the centration device, the stamp always places its mark at the origin. The MRP dot is obliterated by the stamp that now marks the future geometrical or boxing center of the edged lens.*

Some older lens markers have a decentration scale on the horizontal line which, for excessively large eyesizes, does not extend far enough to allow a marking of the lens in one step. If this is the case, move the lens to the end of the scale, mark it, then decenter for the remainder of the amount using the just-marked spot as a reference point. Then mark the lens a second time. The vertical portion of the first mark may be wiped away or crossed out using a marking pen.

IS THE LENS BLANK LARGE ENOUGH?

In order to save on both material cost and time, attention should be given at each stage as to whether or not the final product will be suitable for dispensing. With many marking devices it is possible to use the instrument in determining if the lens blank chosen is indeed large enough to make the prescription for the frame ordered. It goes without saying that for a child's frame a smaller lens blank can be used. A larger one will be necessary for a full grown adult, even if the two prescriptions are the same.

A significant difference in the size of the lens blank needed will depend not only on the eyesize, but also on the shape of the edged lens and the wearer's PD. Even though these factors should be taken into consideration initially when the lens is chosen from stock, errors can occur.

To help avoid edging a lens that is not quite large enough, some centering devices use a system that visually compares the blank to the required size. There are two main systems.

The first system is a series of circles of known diameter that appear on the screen of the instrument (see Figure 3–15). These show possible *effective diameters*. The *effective diameter* (ED) required for a given frame shape and size is the minimum size blank that would be required with the geometrical center of the uncut blank at the boxing center of the frame's lens opening (that is, with no decentration). The ED is found by measuring the distance from the boxing center of the lens opening to that portion of the lens groove that is farthest away from it. This distance is then doubled.

The ED circles on the target screen of the centration device are used as follows: When properly positioned for marking, the decentered lens blank must completely enclose the circle having the same diameter as the ED of the frame, as Figure 3–16 illustrates.

A second system used in centration devices to ensure that a lens is large enough is that of super-

imposing the shadow of the pattern to be used upon the screen of the centering device. The operator simultaneously sees the scale used in decentration, the outline of the lens, and the shadow of the pattern. This system works best when the pattern is exactly the same size as the finished lens will be. If the pattern size duplicates the required size of the finished lens, then the shadow of the pattern must be completely enclosed by the decentered lens blank. If it is not, any part of the pattern found outside of the lens blank (see Figure 3–17) will end up as an "air space" between lens edge and frame.

This pattern shadow system can be used with patterns somewhat larger or smaller than the finished lens, but compensation must be made. To compensate, the size of the pattern must be known. This can be measured directly or can be calculated by adding the absolute value of the "set number" printed on the pattern to 36.5 mm.

To illustrate, suppose that the eyesize of the frame is 4 mm larger than the pattern itself. If the pattern were placed on top of the finished lens and centered, the lens would be 2 mm larger than the pattern in every direction. This means that a visual estimate can be made using the pattern shadow system even if the pattern is smaller than the eyesize to be edged. The edge of the lens blank must clear the pattern shadow by half the difference between pattern size and eyesize. If this amount of clearance is not present, the lens will not cut out.

If a lens of eyesize 58 were to be edged, first the lens blank would be placed on the centering device and positioned correctly. The pattern, measured according to the boxing system, would be measured and found to be 52 mm in size. It could be viewed through the instrument (see Figure 3–18). Would the lens cut out of the blank provided?

To find the minimum distance from the edge of the pattern to the edge of the lens, take

$$\frac{\text{eyesize} - \text{pattern size}}{2}$$

or

$$\frac{58 - 52}{2} = 3 \text{ mm}.$$

Applying this to Figure 3–18, there is less than 3 mm between pattern edge and lens edge, meaning that the lens will not cut out.

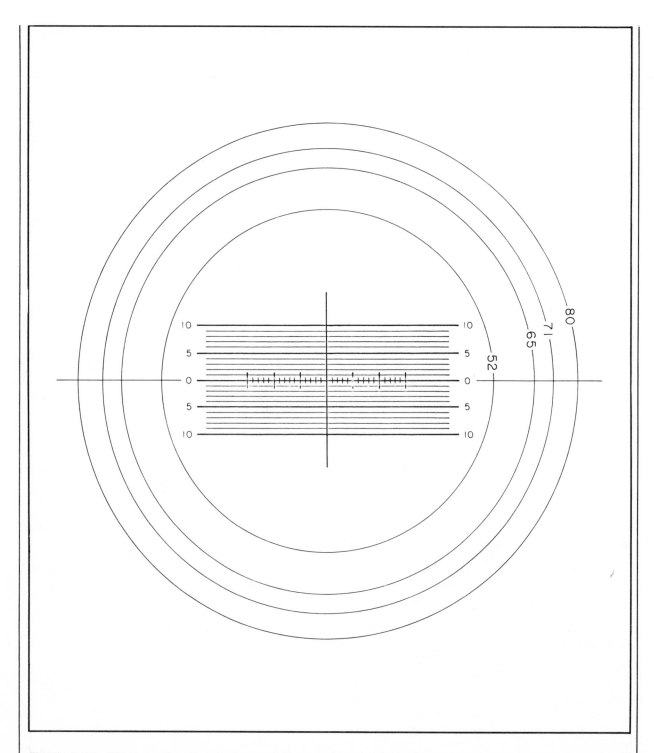

Figure 3–15. *When a centration device contains a series of concentric circles, the correctly centered uncut lens must completely enclose the circle equal to the effective diameter (ED) of frame. (It cannot be assumed that because the circle equal to the frame eyesize is enclosed, the uncut lens will be large enough.)*

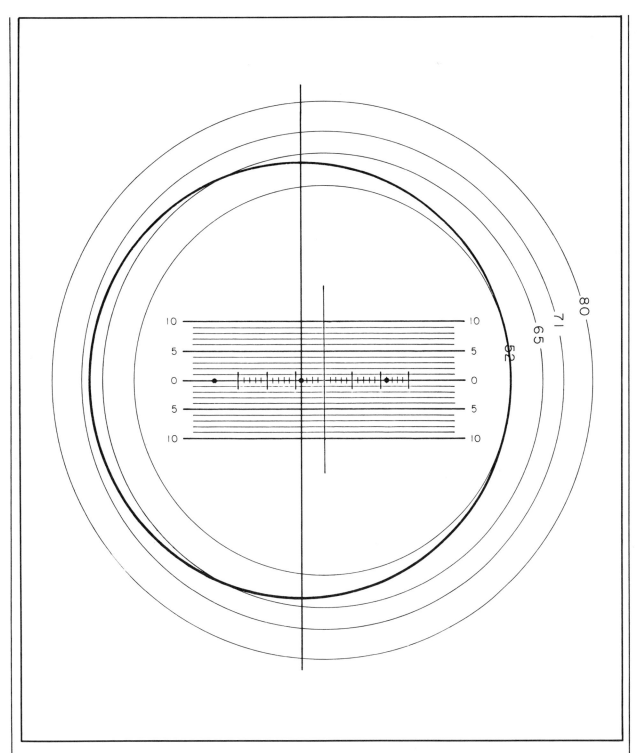

Figure 3–16. *It can be seen from the figure that if the frame to be used has an effective diameter greater than 52 mm, the 63 mm lens blank will not be large enough when decentered as shown.*

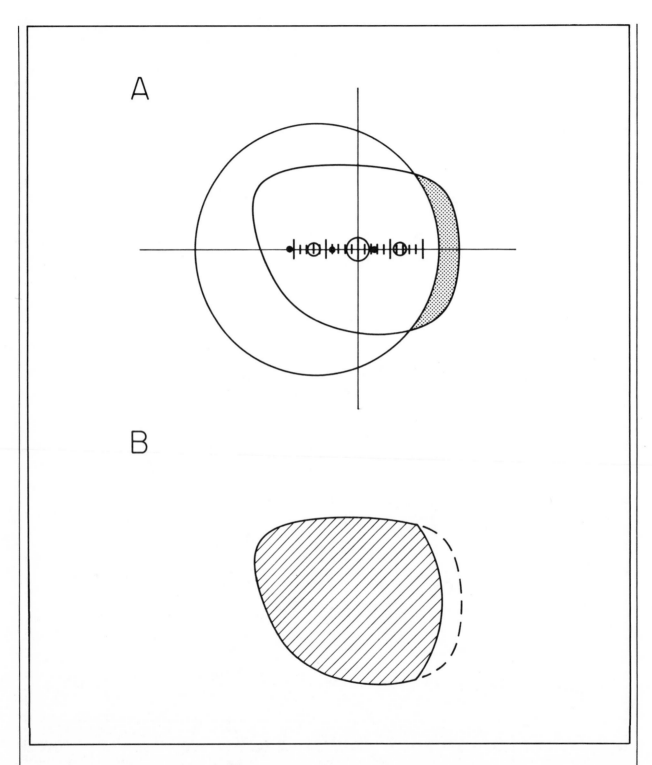

Figure 3–17. *When the on-size pattern superimposed on the correctly positioned lens is not completely enclosed by that lens as in A, the edged lens will not cut out and will have an air space, as shown in B.*

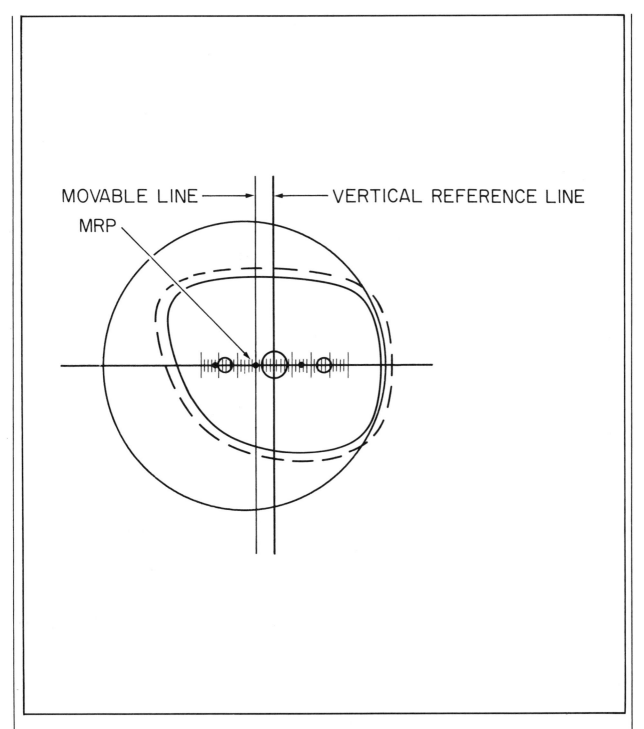

MOVABLE LINE ⟶ ⟵ VERTICAL REFERENCE LINE

MRP

Figure 3–18. *Centration devices using a shadow projection of the pattern work best when the pattern size equals the frame eyesize. When a pattern is smaller than the frame's eyesize, compensation must be made by visualizing if the lens will cut out. In this figure, the dotted line represents the "visualized" increase in pattern size that must be estimated to determine if lens blank size is sufficient. As shown here, it is not.*

47

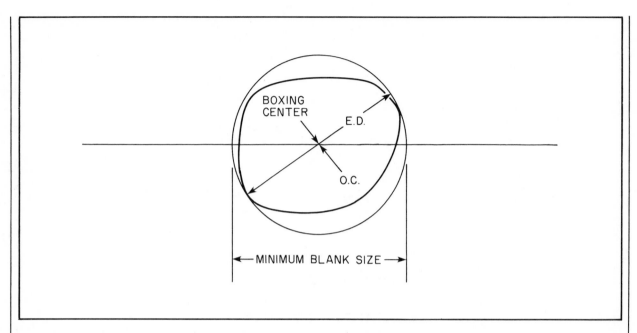

Figure 3–19. *When there is no decentration, minimum blank size equals effective diameter. (No allowance for lens chippage is shown.)*

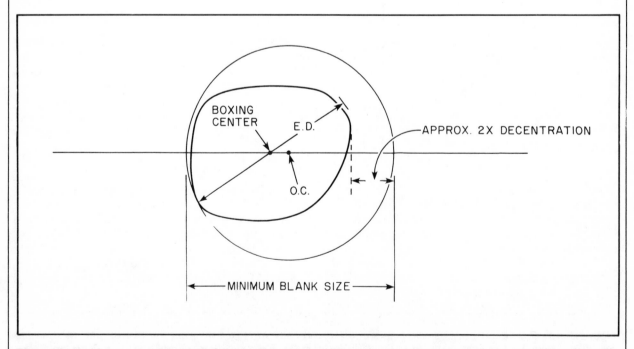

Figure 3–20. *For each millimeter of decentration, two millimeters of additional blank size must be added to the effective diameter to determine the minimum blank size. (No allowance for lens chippage is shown.)*

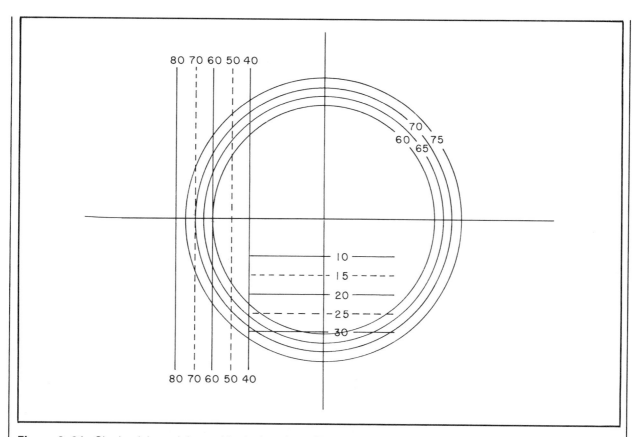

Figure 3–21. Single vision minimum blank size chart. *The blank size chart shown is used as follows: (1) Place the frame front face down on the chart with the right lens opening over the simulated lens circles. (2) Center the frame bridge over the correct binocular distance PD as indicated by the scale on the left. (3) Ensure vertical centration. This is done by positioning the lowest point on the inside groove of the lower eyewire on the lower chart scale. The correct level is one-half the B dimension of the frame. (If a vertical positioning for the optical center of the lens is specified, use this height instead.) (4) Note which diameter lens circle will just enclose the lens opening of the frame* including *the eyewire groove. This is the minimum blank size required for a nonprismatic, single vision lens.*

Minimum Blank Size

The smallest lens blank that can be used for a given prescription lens and frame combination is called the *minimum blank size* (MBS). The MBS depends upon:
1. the effective diameter of the frame, and
2. the amount of decentration of the OC away from the boxing center.

If there were no decentration and the lens OC were positioned exactly at the boxing center, the minimum blank size would be equal to the effective diameter plus 2 to 4 mm extra to allow for possible edge chipping (see Figure 3–19).

When 1 mm of decentration inward occurs, the lens must be 1 millimeter larger temporally. Yet since uncut lens blanks increase equally in all directions, the overall lens size must increase 2 mm. Therefore, for every millimeter of decentration, the blank size must increase 2 mm, as Figure 3–20 indicates.

In addition, it is advisable to allow an extra 2 to 4 mm for the possibility of a lens chipping.

Written mathematically, minimum blank size is

$$MBS = ED + 2(\text{decentration}) + 2.$$

There are blank size charts and devices available that allow the frame to be used directly in the determination of lens blank size. One such chart is shown in Figure 3–21.

"Pushing" the PD

When the situation arises where it is evident that a lens blank is only slightly too small, there is a temptation to move the lens blank outward slightly, "pushing" the PD to a larger value than was ordered. In so doing, the smaller, less expensive lens blank may be used, but because the lens MRP will be decentered from its intended position before the eye, unwanted prism can be induced. The amount of prism that will be induced by deviating from the ordered PD varies considerably with the power of the lens being used and depends upon the mathematical relationship known as Prentice's rule. As mentioned in Chapter 2, Prentice's rule states that the amount of prism (Δ) induced by decentration of a lens is equal to the number of centimeters (c) the lens is moved times the power of the lens (F). In equation form this appears as

$$\Delta = cF.$$

This means that the stronger the power of the spectacle lens (F), the more unwanted prism will be induced for the same amount of lens decentration (c). Once this relationship is understood, it is relatively easy to estimate the amount of prism induced by a given amount of lens decentration.

Example 1.

Suppose a lens blank lacks 2 mm of being large enough to cut out. The lens power is a $-5.00D$ sphere. If the PD is "pushed" 2 mm out for this lens, how much prism is induced?

Solution:

Since $\Delta = cF$,
we know F = 5.00D.
Since c is measured in centimeters we know
2 mm = 0.2 cm.
Therefore, $\Delta = (.2) (5.00)$
$$\Delta = 1.00.$$

The base direction will be base in for this eye, as is evident when seen in cross section (see Figure 3–22). Base-in prism forces the eyes of the wearer to turn in an outward direction in order to keep from seeing double. Were glasses with great amounts of unwanted prism dispensed, the best result would be a headache for the wearer and rejection of the glasses. The worst result would be for the wearer to gradually become accustomed to the prism, which would contribute to either an outward deviation of the

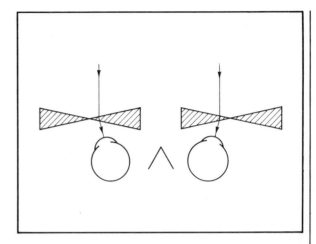

Figure 3–22. *Errors in optical center placement cause objects to appear displaced from their actual location. To compensate, the eyes must turn inward or outward; otherwise the wearer will experience double vision.*

eyes, or suppression of one eye with a resultant drop in its visual acuity. The degree of difficulty encountered will depend upon the amount of prism induced and the visual condition of the wearer.

Example 2.

Suppose a lens blank having a power of $-0.25D$ is 2 mm smaller than necessary to cut out. What would the consequences be of "pushing" the PD in this instance?

Solution:

Calculations are done in the same manner as previously.

$$\Delta = cF,$$
$$= (0.2) (0.25)$$
$$= 0.05.$$

The consequences here are practically negligible for pushing the PD by 2 mm.

Example 3.

A lens blank is marked for the following prescription:
$+5.00 - 1.00 \times 90$
How much prism is induced by pushing the PD 2 millimeters outward?

Solution:

When a lens contains a cylinder, the amount of prism induced depends upon the orientation of the

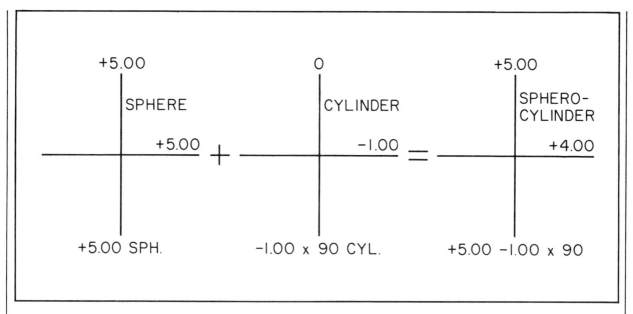

Figure 3–23. *The value of a lens in a given meridian can often be better visualized through the use of a power cross system.*

cylinder axis in relation to the direction of decentration of the lens. In this case the lens is being decentered in the horizontal meridian, so the power of the lens in the horizontal meridian is used for calculations.

Because the cylinder power is at right angles to the axis of the cylinder, the power (F) used in Prentice's rule is +4.00D (see Figure 3–23).

The prism induced by pushing the PD for this lens blank will be

$$\Delta = cF$$
$$= (0.2)\,(4)$$
$$= 0.80$$

which means 0.80∆ of prism base out will be induced.

Keep in mind that whenever a cylinder or spherocylinder lens having an oblique axis direction is decentered horizontally, a certain amount of vertical prism will always be induced. The amount of vertical prism induced increases as (1) the cylinder power increases, and (2) as the cylinder axis approaches the 45- or 135-degree position. In other words, moving an oblique spherocylinder horizontally would require a compensating vertical movement in order to counteract the vertical prismatic effect being induced.

The amount of vertical compensation depends upon the cylinder power and axis direction. In short, when oblique cylinder is present, pushing the PD horizontally will result in some degree of vertical prism.

How Much Accuracy Is Required?
Accuracy required for the location of the OC may be specified either in millimeters of deviation from the ordered PD, or in terms of the amount of prism induced by the incorrectly located OC, or both.

Low-powered lenses can have their OC off location by a relatively large amount before the prismatic effect becomes significantly detrimental to the wearer. However, as lens power increases, even small location deviations can cause a major prismatic effect. American and British Standards for prismatic effect or OC accuracy may be found in the Appendices at the back of the book. Note that published standards are recommendations only—the practitioner may demand higher or accept lower standards. The supplying laboratory may remind an account of the generally accepted standards, but should not attempt to hide behind them, as more precision in certain specified parameters is not an impossible task. If the practitioner and supplying laboratory cannot come to an acceptable agreement, then other sources of supply should be sought out. Wearers of low refractive powers are often more sensitive to deviations

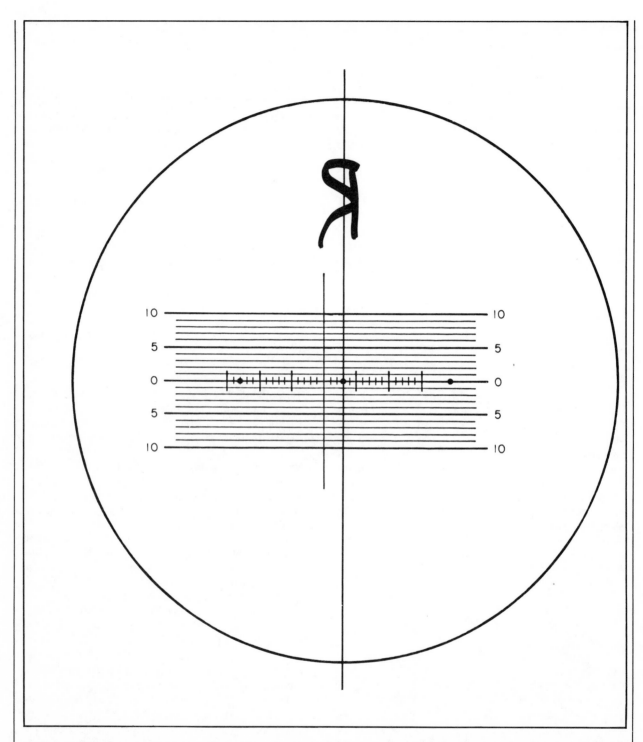

Figure 3–24. *Here the right lens is positioned convex side up. It has been decentered 3 mm inward and can now be blocked directly while still in the centering device. The nose or bridge of the frame can be visualized as if on the righthand side of the drawing.*

from the absolutes required than wearers of high prescriptions, making higher standards well within reason in certain circumstances.

Because these standards are recommendations only, the tendency may exist for a laboratory to supply an account with prescription materials that fall outside the normally accepted standards because no one raises an objection. Keep in mind that the laboratory supplying prescribed materials has an ethical responsibility to supply materials according to standard. Slackness on the part of the account to check for accuracy does not release the supplier from this responsibility. If anything, it places a responsibility more directly upon the laboratory. Ophthalmic frames and lenses cannot be regarded as a commodity for which the consumer is the ultimate judge of acceptability. The account who will accept materials that fall outside of normally accepted standards does not suffer from incorrect power or unpre-

scribed prism. The wearer who must trust in the judiciousness of those supplying his or her needs is the one who bears the consequences.

Centering Devices with Lens Blocking Capability
Many centering devices are capable of directly blocking the lenses for edging by using one or more of the currently available blocking systems. When this option is utilized, the lens must generally be centered while in the face-up position in order to permit placement of the block on the front surface.

Decentration rules naturally remain the same. The only difference is in the direction in which the lens is decentered. For example, as formally described, when a right lens is placed face down, in order to decenter inward it is moved to the left. Now, however, since the lens is face up it must be moved to the right, as the imaginary position of the wearer's nose is to the right (see Figure 3–24).

PROFICIENCY TEST QUESTIONS

1. How much decentration, and in which direction, is required for each of the following? (50 □ 20 means the 50 mm eyesize is a boxing system eyesize with a 20 mm bridge size.)
   a. PD 66, 50 □ 20
   b. PD 60, 50 □ 18
   c. PD 59, 44 □ 16

2. How much decentration per lens is required to correctly mark these lenses for edging?
   R: $+1.00 -1.00 \times 70$
   L: $-1.00 -1.00 \times 100$
   A = 52
   B = 49
   DBL = 16
   PD = 70
   a. 1 mm in
   b. 1 mm out
   c. 1.5 mm in
   d. 2.0 mm in
   e. None of the above is correct.

3. How much decentration per lens is required for an Rx having the following specifications?
   A = 52
   B = 43
   C = 50
   Boxing DBL = 18
   R monocular PD = 32
   L monocular PD = 33.5

4. How much decentration per lens is required for the following Rx if it is to be used for reading glasses only?
   R: $+3.25 -0.50 \times 90$
   L: $+3.00 -0.25 \times 90$
   A = 52
   B = 47
   ED = 57
   DBL = 20
   PD = 65/61
   a. 6 mm
   b. 4 mm
   c. 4.5 mm
   d. 3.5 mm
   e. 5.5 mm

5. Which of the following best defines *effective diameter*?
   a. The longest measure of a lens, whether that measure is horizontal or across a long diagonal

   b. Measured from the boxing center to the farthest corner times 2
   c. The eyesize of the frame plus twice the decentration

6. For the following frame and wearer PD, what is the minimum blank size required if 2 mm is allowed for lens chipping?
   A = 49
   B = 40
   C = 47
   ED = 54
   DBL = 20
   PD = 61
   a. 57
   b. 66
   c. 59
   d. 64
   e. None of the above is correct.

7. What decentration per lens is required for the following single vision Rx?
   $-1.25 -0.75 \times 15$
   $-1.00 -1.00 \times 162$
   height of OC's: 26 mm
   PD = 66
   A = 53
   B = 48
   ED = 57
   DBL = 17

8. How far away from the boxing center of the edged lens would the optical center be for the following lens? (Since the prismatic effect was achieved by surfacing the lenses, rather than by decentering a standard, uncut lens blank, the distance between these two points may not be directly measurable.)
   $-0.50D$ sph 3.5Δ base out
   A = 48
   B = 43
   ED = 53
   DBL = 18
   PD = 62
   a. 1.75 mm
   b. 17.5 mm
   c. 14.3 mm
   d. 72 mm
   e. None of the above is correct.

9. For the following Rx lens, how far from the marked cross on the uncut lens (i.e., the location of the geometrical center of the edged lens) will the optical center be?

+4.00D sph 2Δ base out

$$A = 50$$
$$B = 48$$
$$ED = 56$$
$$DBL = 18$$
$$PD = 60$$

10. A right lens has a power of $+5.00 -2.00 \times 30$. The frame chosen has dimensions of 52 □ 20. The patient's PD is 66. Assume that the uncut lens blank is facing up (*convex side up*). The OC is at the geometric center of the blank. Where on the lens would the mark made by the lens marking device (————┼————) be?
    a. 6 mm to the right of the geometric center of the lens blank.
    b. 6 mm to the left of the geometric center of the lens blank.
    c. 3 mm to the right of the geometric center of the lens blank.
    d. 3 mm to the left of the geometric center of the lens blank.
    e. None of the above is correct.

11. A left lens has a power of $-4.00 -1.00 \times 180$. The frame chosen has dimensions of 50 □ 18. The patient's PD is 60 mm. The prescription calls for 1.0Δ base-down prism for the left eye. The OC is at the geometric center of the lens blank. Assume that the uncut lens blank is *convex side down* (facing down). In relation to the mark made by the lens marking device at its correct position, how far horizontally and vertically is the center of the cross from the OC of the lens?

12. If the PD were "pushed" outward 1.5 mm per lens, what would the total horizontal prismatic effect (right and left lenses combined) be for each of the following prescriptions?
    a. R: +2.00D sphere
       L: +2.00D sphere
    b. R: $-4.00 -1.00 \times 90$
       L: $-4.00 -1.00 \times 90$
    c. $+5.25 -1.00 \times 180$
       $+6.25 -1.00 \times 180$

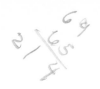

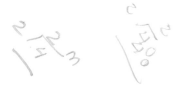

Chapter 4

Centration of Multifocal Lenses

During the centration process for multifocal lenses there are two important reference areas.

1. The multifocal segment area. Reference points here are (a) the highest point of the segment (seg top) and (b) either the geometrical center of the seg (mid point of the segment diameter) or symmetric points on the left and right sides of the segment.
2. The three dots denoting the MRP of the lens and the 180-degree cutting line.

These two areas should interrelate. If proper surfacing procedures have been followed one reference area will almost automatically fall into position upon correct centering of the other.

SEGMENT PLACEMENT

In the process of positioning a multifocal lens blank, the segment portion has a specific location in reference to the geometrical or boxing center of the edged lens. Unfortunately the information given in the prescription uses other points of reference instead. In centration for edging, these must be refigured in relationship to the boxing (geometrical) center. The parameters that must be refigured are the seg height and the near PD. Both parameter calculation processes have been introduced previously.

Seg Height

The seg height must be specified as seg drop or seg raise. In its true sense, *seg drop* is the vertical distance from the major reference point to the level of the seg top when the seg top is the lower of the two. In U.S. optical laboratory practice, however, seg drop is the vertical distance from the datum line to the seg top. (Fortunately, the MRP almost always falls on the datum line anyway.) If the seg top is higher than the datum line, laboratory practitioners refer to this measure as the *seg raise.*

In order to convert from seg height to seg drop, the same procedure is used as was described for calculating vertical positioning of the major reference point. First the vertical dimension of the frame's lens opening must be known (B). Half this measure is then subtracted from the seg height, giving the seg drop when negative, or seg raise when positive. That is,

$$\text{seg height} - \frac{B}{2} = \text{seg drop (or raise)}.$$

For example, for a frame with these dimensions:

$$A \text{ (eyesize)} = 52 \text{ mm}$$
$$B = 40 \text{ mm}$$
$$DBL = 20 \text{ mm}$$

and a seg height of 18 mm, what is the seg drop?

Figure 4–1 shows that only the vertical frame measure is important for seg drop, so

$$\text{seg drop} = \text{seg height} - \frac{B}{2}$$
$$= 18 - \frac{40}{2}$$
$$= -2 \text{ mm}[1]$$

Set Inset

The near segment is inset from the position of the major reference point to allow for the inward turning (convergence) of the eyes while reading or working at a short distance. This is known as *seg inset*[2] and may be defined as half the distance between distance and near PD's.

$$\text{seg inset} = \frac{\text{distance PD} - \text{near PD}}{2}.$$

Thus in the instance where the distance PD is 69 and the near PD 65, the seg inset would be 2 mm per lens.

---

[1]Since seg drop is measured downward from the point of origin, it is technically a negative number.

[2]The British refer to this measure as *geometrical inset* (g in).

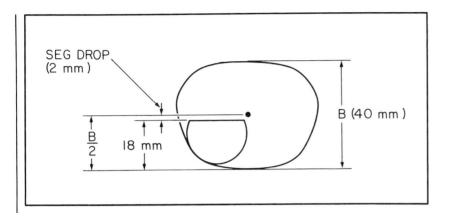

SEG DROP
(2 mm)

$\frac{B}{2}$

18 mm

B (40 mm)

Figure 4–1. *The vertical position of the segment top can be expressed either as segment drop or segment height.*

Total Inset

Lateral segment positioning is most often specified on the prescription as "near PD," which is interpreted as being the distance the two segment centers are separated, one from the other, when the finished lenses are mounted in the frame. To specify lateral segment placement for edging purposes the correct position for the two segments is calculated in exactly the same manner as was done for the MRP. The amount of near segment displacement is actually a total of the distance decentration for the MRP, plus the additional segment inset in a nasalward direction (seg inset). Hence, the amount that the seg center is displaced from the boxing or geometrical center of the edged lens is known as *total seg inset* or simply *total inset* (see Figure 4–2).

$$\text{Total inset} = \frac{A + DBL - \text{near PD}}{2}.$$

Example:

A frame has these dimensions:

$$A = 52 \text{ mm}$$
$$B = 40 \text{ mm}$$
$$DBL = 20 \text{ mm}$$
$$\text{wearer's PD} = 66/62$$

What is the total inset?

Solution:

$$\text{Total inset} = \frac{A + DBL - \text{near PD}}{2}$$
$$= \frac{52 + 20 - 62}{2}$$
$$= \frac{10}{2} = 5 \text{ mm.}$$

POSITIONING OF FLAT TOP MULTIFOCALS

In order to better understand the mechanics of multifocal lens positioning, the process can be initially described for hand marking with the aid of graph paper. Again, intersecting horizontal and vertical lines will be centrally drawn on the graph paper with the intersection denoting the boxing center of the edged lens.

Since total inset is the lateral distance of the seg center from the boxing or geometrical center of the edged lens, the seg center of the lens must be marked. This can be done by measuring the widest part of the seg, finding the midpoint, and dotting it. With practice this can be done visually, without using a ruler.

Now the lens is placed face down on the graph paper and moved laterally until the centrally placed segment dot is displaced from the intersection by an amount equal to the total inset. With the seg center at the correct total inset, the seg top may be moved up or down to the correct distance above or below the horizontal reference line.[3] The amount above or below corresponds to the seg raise or drop. When this positioning is complete, the seg will be at the correct height and inset. As a result the previously spotted MRP should also be properly inset and on the horizontal reference line.

---

[3]This horizontal reference line indicates the position of the datum line on the edged lens if the pattern is made according to accepted practices.

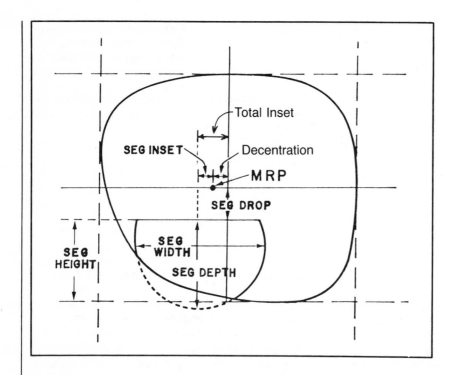

Figure 4–2. *Decentration is sometimes referred to as* inset. *This must not be confused with* seg inset *or* total inset. *As can be seen here, these are different measures.*

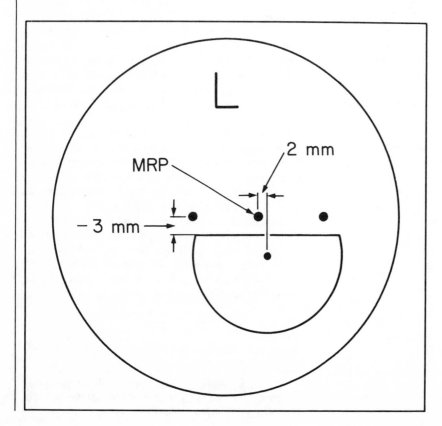

Figure 4–3. *The back view of the left lens shows the relationship between MRP and segment positions. Note that the MRP will not necessarily fall in the center of the lens.*

Example:

If a lens has been ordered with the following specifications:

R: +1.00 − 0.75 × 175
L: +1.00 − 0.75 × 005   PD 67/63
add +2.00
Flat top 28 bifocal, seg height 18 mm
Frame A = 55
B = 42
DBL = 18

How would the left lens be marked for eventual edging?

Solution:

The surfacing process has already positioned the major reference point and axis orientation relative to the segment. With the axis set for 5 degrees, the major reference point and the 180-degree reference dots have been marked on the lens. As in Figure 4–3, these three dots should be parallel to the top of the segment.

The lens is placed on the reference grid. The seg center must be inset.

As previously described,

$$\text{total inset} = \frac{A + DBL - \text{near PD}}{2} \text{.}^{[4]}$$

Therefore, in this example,

$$\text{total inset} = \frac{55 + 18 - 63}{2} \text{,}$$

$$= 5 \text{ mm.}$$

The vertical position of the seg line can be simultaneously positioned and is calculated as follows:

$$\text{seg drop} = \text{seg height} - \frac{B}{2} \text{,}$$

$$= 18 - \frac{42}{2} \text{,}$$

$$= -3 \text{ mm.}$$

---

[4]Remember that, expressed another way, total inset for the seg is equal to the distance decentration per lens (inset) plus seg inset (half of the difference between distance and near PD).

Figure 4–4 shows that the seg center is moved 5 mm to the right and the seg top 3 mm down. Because of exactness in surfacing, the MRP has been simultaneously inset 3 mm with the 180-degree line on the horizontal datum line. It should be evident that in this case centration could have been accomplished using only the three dots marked by the Lensometer.

To mark the lens by hand, four marks would be placed on the lens—one at each position where the two horizontal and vertical reference lines neared the lens edge, as in Figure 4–4. From these the standard cross could be marked on the lens using a lens marker and flexible ruler.

Use of a Centering Device for Flat Tops

The principle behind lens layout for marking remains the same when a lens centering device or marker is used, but the process itself is simplified considerably.

In order to better explain the process, consider the following.

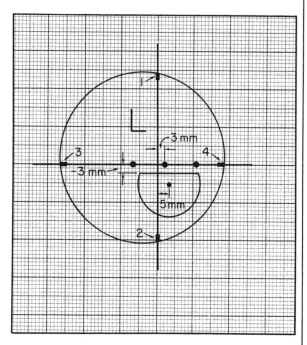

Figure 4–4. *The center of the seg may be used for horizontal reference and the seg top for vertical reference. The four marks at the edge of the lens become reference points for placing the standard cross mark on the lens surface.*

Example:

If a prescription reads as follows:

R: −2.50 − 1.75 × 10   PD 63/60
L: −2.75 − 1.50 × 171

add +1.25

Flat top 25 bifocal, seg height 15 mm
Frame: A = 50
B = 38
DBL = 18

How would the right lens be centered and marked for edging?

Solution:

Even though the lens has been previously dotted, ignore these dots until the lens has been centered with reference to the seg. After this has been completed, check the location of the dots for accuracy.

Before centration can occur, determination of seg drop (or raise) and total inset must first occur.

In this case,

$$\text{seg drop} = \text{seg height} - \frac{B}{2}$$
$$= 15 - \frac{38}{2}$$
$$= -4 \text{ mm.}$$

$$\text{total inset} = \frac{A + DBL - \text{near PD}}{2}$$
$$= \frac{50 + 18 - 60}{2}$$
$$= 4 \text{ mm.}$$

Assume that the lens is to be marked and later blocked. Then assume that the lens will be placed face down in the marker. Because the right lens is to be placed face down for marking, the nasal, segment side will be to the left. To preset the marking device, the movable vertical line is positioned 4 mm to the left of center. It is not necessary to mark the center of the segment, as boundary lines spaced equally to the left and right of the movable vertical line serve to border the segment on either side. Thus when the segment is symmetrically enclosed by bordering lines corresponding to its width, as in Figure 4–5, it may be moved to the correct height and checked for marking.

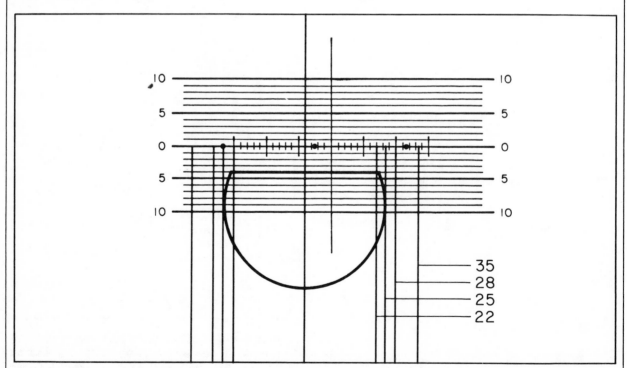

Figure 4–5. *This right lens, placed convex side down, has a 2.5 mm distance decentration, a 1.5 mm seg inset, a 4 mm total inset, and a seg drop of 4 mm.*

If there is a discrepancy, a decision must be made as to whether the lens will still fill the prescription as specified.

Reject or Accept

Up to now, whenever the multifocal segment has been positioned correctly, the inset for the MRP has also been correct, implying that the PD will be as specified by the practitioner. Since it cannot be anticipated that the two will always agree, certain guidelines for acceptability need to be established. Each time before marking the lens, the operator must ask the following.

1. Is the height of the major reference point standard or as specified?
2. Is the inset for the major reference point correct?
3. Is the axis of the cylinder oriented as it should be?

Incorrect Height of the MRP

Suppose after centering a lens with a flat top bifocal segment it is discovered that the MRP is 2 mm above the horizontal datum line location (as the example in Figure 4–6 indicates). In some cases this may be considered inconsequential—even normal. But in other instances the lens will almost certainly cause the prescription to be unsuitable and should be rejected or returned before more production time is wasted. Assuming the MRP to be properly marked, there are two factors to consider in making this decision.

First, determine if the second lens in the pair is identically flawed. If the second lens in the pair also has its MRP 2 mm above the datum line, then no differential vertical prism will result between the two eyes. In fact, if no vertical MRP height was specified, then with both MRP's at the same vertical height

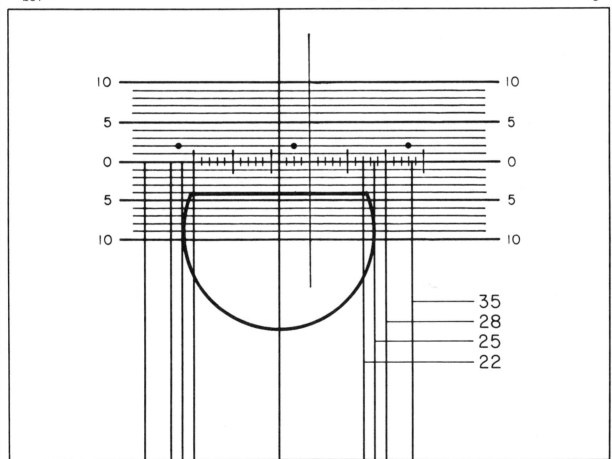

Figure 4–6. *There is but one error in this figure: The inset is correct; the axis should also be correct, since the 180-degree line marked by the Lensometer is parallel to the horizontal; but the MRP will fall above the datum if fabricated.*

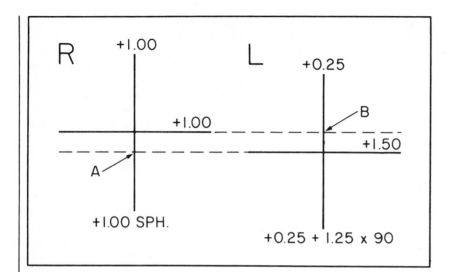

Figure 4–7. *Evaluated in terms of point A, the vertical prism would be 0.30Δ base up. In terms of point B, however, the prismatic effect is only 0.075Δ base down.*

(within reasonable limits) no error has occurred.[5]

Second, consider what powers the two lenses have in their 90 degree meridians. When the lens is finished, any unwanted vertical prismatic effect is measured as the difference in prismatic effect between the two lenses, finding the OC of the stronger lens and sliding the glasses across the Lensometer table to compare the prismatic effect induced by the weaker lens through any difference in vertical height. Therefore, the power of the weaker lens in the 90 degree meridian is important.

Example:

The following prescription is to be fabricated:

R: +1.00
L: +0.25 + 1.25 × 90
   +2.00 add

In order to end up with the correct bifocal heights, the right lens MRP is found to be 3 mm above the future datum line, while left lens MRP is right on the datum line. Will the lens pair prove suitable after edging?

Solution:

The powers of both lenses in their 90-degree meridians are evaluated. This may be visualized as in Figure 4–7. As can be seen, two different results would be obtained depending upon whether point *A*

---

[5]This should emphasize the importance of care in measuring lens parameters for the duplication or replacement of a single lens in a pair of lenses.

on the right lens or point *B* on the left were considered. Prentice's rule is used to evaluate the prismatic effect on the decentered point of the lens.

For the weaker lens,

$$\Delta = cF,$$

and the reference point on that lens is 3 mm (.3 cm) away from its center, then

$$c = .3 \text{ cm}.$$

Because a + 1.25 cylinder with axis 90 has no power in the axis meridian, then the only power manifested in the vertical meridian is the +0.25 power of the sphere.

$$\Delta = (.3)(0.25)$$
$$= .075\Delta.$$

This is sufficiently below the maximum allowable tolerances to make the lens pair acceptable and not cause discomfort for the wearer.

Methodology in evaluation of vertical prism tolerance should not be considered license to move OC's up or down simply to enable a lens to be cut out for a particular frame shape. There are certain optical consequences that can result from moving the OC away from its normal placement, even if both lenses are moved in unison.

Incorrect MRP Inset.

As previously stated, the location of the MRP in relationship to the segment has been ground by the surfacing lab. In other words, if the distance PD is 65 and the near PD 62, then the MRP should already be 1.5 mm outward from the vertical plane running through the seg center. This is checked for accuracy after the lens has been centered by using the segment for reference. If the MRP is found to be inaccurately placed, then the significance of the error must be evaluated and methods of correcting the difficulty considered.

Four choices are available in such a case where *either* distance PD *or* near PD will be right, but not both. They are:

1. Reject the lens and have it reground.
2. Elect to have a correct *near* PD, but an incorrect distance PD. (This choice is only possible if the resulting horizontal prism will be within tolerance.)
3. Elect to have a correct *distance* PD, but an incorrect near PD.
4. Elect to position the lens midway between near and distance, altering both PD's slightly, if the

prismatic effects resulting from this choice are insignificant.

There are several factors that affect these decisions. These can most easily be seen by considering some specific instances. (See also Table 4–1.)

Consider the following prescription.

R: +5.50 sphere   PD 69/65
L: +5.50 sphere
+2.00 add
Flat Top 28 seg: seg height 19 mm
Frame Dimensions: A = 53
B = 42
DBL = 20

The left lens is laid out for marking, as is shown in Figure 4–8. Although the seg height and total seg

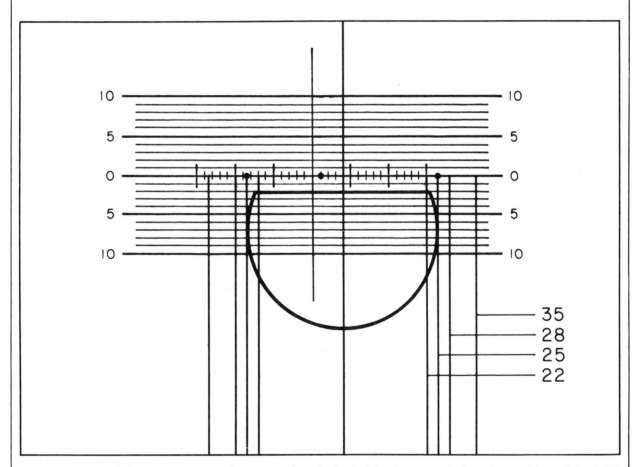

Figure 4–8. *After the near segment is centered as indicated by the prescription, the position of the MRP should be checked to assume accuracy of the finished PD. In this instance, the required total inset is 4 mm, which is correct. Yet the MRP is incorrect, since a 2 mm decentration per lens is indicated and only 1 mm appears. Correcting the position of the MRP to achieve the correct distance PD will throw the near PD off.*

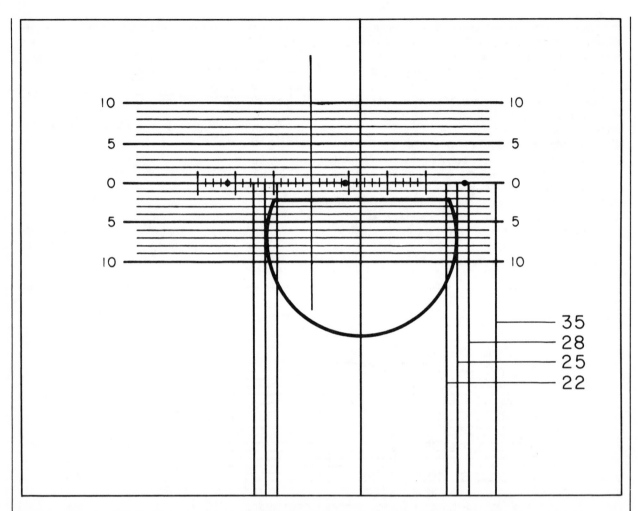

Figure 4–9. *After positioning a near segment, the spotted MRP location is checked for accuracy on this concave side up left lens. The inset (decentration per lens) calculated from the distance PD is 2 mm. It can be seen here that the seg inset, which should be 4.5 mm, is 2 mm. The inset, which should be 2 mm, is 4.5 mm.*

inset is correctly positioned so that the lens will cut out with the near PD correct, the MRP is incorrectly positioned. The inset for the MRP must be

$$\text{inset} = \frac{A + DBL - PD}{2}$$
$$= \frac{53 + 20 - 69}{2}$$
$$= 2 \text{ mm per lens.}$$

The center dot, which indicates the lens MRP, must be inset 2 mm for the distance PD to equal 69 mm. Unfortunately there is only 1 mm of inset. If the paired lens is accurate, the distance PD will still be 70 instead of 69, and the near PD will be a correct 65 mm. Because of the power of the distance portion, the horizontal prism will be

$$\Delta = (.1)(5.5) = .55\Delta \text{ base out.}$$

However, if the near PD is decreased by 1 mm, this will decrease the distance PD back to the required 69 mm, eliminating the horizontal prism in the distance portion. Two optical effects will be produced at near. The first is to change the prismatic effect at near by 0.20Δ [$\Delta = (c) \cdot (F \text{ of add})$]. The second is to reduce slightly the temporal field of view at near for this lens—a point that becomes less significant with increased near segment sizes.

Suppose that the tolerances for the distance between seg centers (near PD) for multifocals specifies that the final product be within ± 2.5 mm of that actually ordered. This means that for a near PD of 65 mm, measures between 62.5 mm and 67.5 mm are considered acceptable.

Although an alternation in the near PD could be a reasonable choice if it did not cause significant degradation of optical quality, this may not always be the case.

In another example, a pair of glasses is ordered using the same frame as previously. The Rx, however, is somewhat different.

R: +0.25 + 0.50 × 180   PD 69/60
   +0.25 + 0.50 × 180
               add + 5.00

Flat top 22: seg height 19 mm
Frame dimensions: A = 53 mm
                 B = 42 mm
          DBL = 20 mm

In this instance, after correctly positioning the near segment of the left lens for a total inset of 6.5mm, it is discovered that instead of an inset of 2 mm for the MRP, the actual inset is 4.5 mm. (See Figure 4–9.) This is 2.5 mm greater than was ordered.

In evaluating what the best solution might be, the first factor for consideration is the prismatic effect induced.

Because the error occurs in the horizontal meridian alone, the power in that meridian is of importance. Were the lens to be edged as it presently appears in the marking device, the relative positions of the eye in comparison to the MRP would be as in Figure 4–10. Because the eye looks through

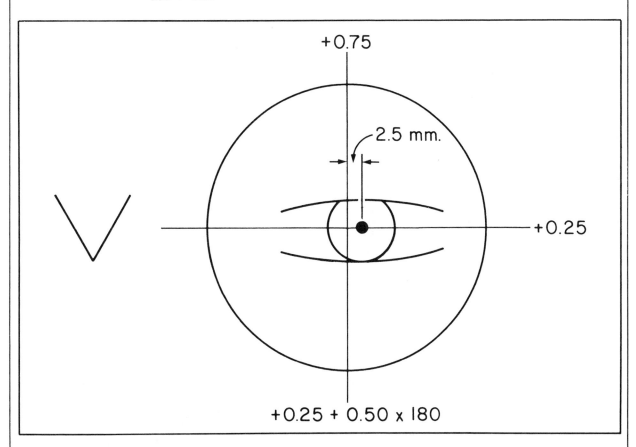

Figure 4–10. *Imagining or sketching out a power cross on an eye can help in understanding how prism is figured using Prentice's rule. Here it is seen that the horizontal meridian of the lens containing the +0.25D lens power is used for calculations.*

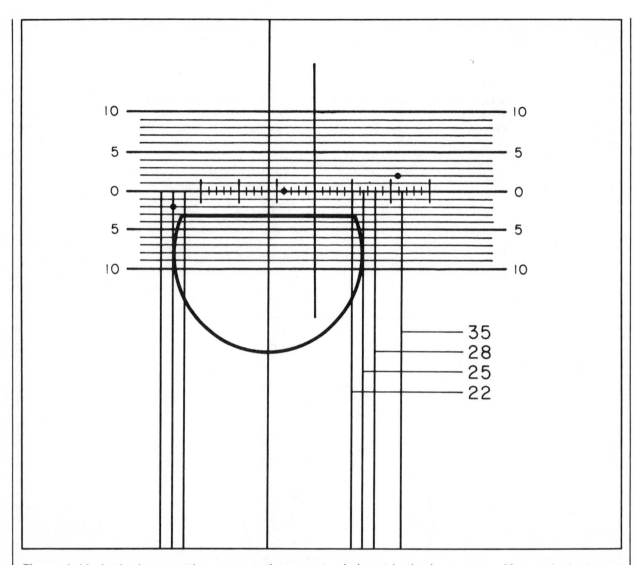

Figure 4–11. *In the lens spotting process, the correct axis is set in the Lensometer. Afterwards the lens is rotated until it conforms to the specified axis, then spotted along the 180-degree line. While centering this lens, it is discovered that when centration is "complete," the spotted 180-degree line is no longer on the 180. This indicates an axis error during surfacing.*

a point 2.5 mm away from the MRP, according to Prentice's rule the amount of unwanted prism that occurs is

$$\Delta = cF$$
$$= (0.25 \text{ cm}) (0.25 \text{D})$$
$$= 0.0625\Delta \text{ base in.}$$

The amount is of little significance as compared to the effect of displacing the near portion. Displacing the near portion changes the prismatic effect by

$$\Delta = (0.25 \text{ cm}) (5.00 \text{D})$$
$$= 1.25\Delta \text{ base out,}$$

and it also narrows the nasal field of view for an already small viewing area. The best choice is not to alter the MRP location.

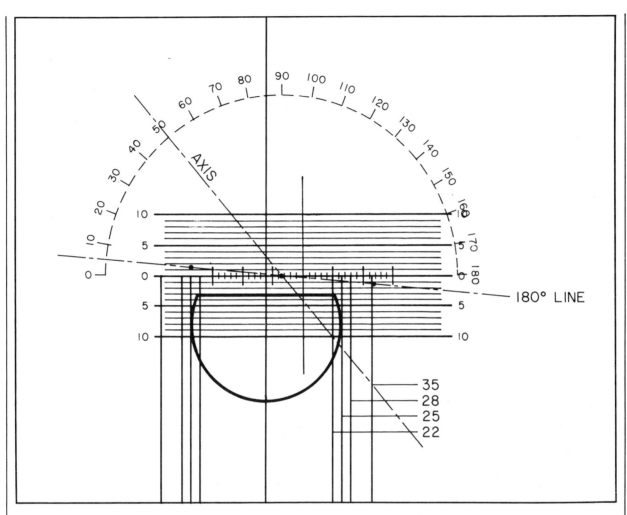

Figure 4–12. *The scale appears backwards because the concave surface of the lens is up. The lens is seen from the wearer's point of view. In the figure, the required cylinder axis is 45 degrees. The lens was oriented in the Lensometer during spotting—it correctly reads 45 degrees and the 180-degree line has been marked. If the 180-degree line is tilted in relationship to the seg top, the reason is that the cylinder was ground off axis, the amount in degrees being equal to the degree of tilt of the 180-degree line.*

As can be seen, the accurate spotting of lenses is of extreme importance—an inaccurately spotted lens can be extremely misleading. It is understood that when any doubt as to the accuracy of the original spotting exists, it should be double checked.

Tilting of the 180-Degree Line
Another error that can be manifested after a segment is properly positioned is a tilting of the previously spotted 180-degree line. Again, there are several factors that indicate how serious a problem this might be.

First of all, if the lens is a sphere and the central MRP dot is located at the proper vertical height and inset, there is no problem at all (as in Figure 4–11). A spherical lens is of equal power in all meridians, meaning that any rotational orientation will result in the same refractive power.

However, if the lens is a cylinder or spherocylinder the cylinder axis will only be correct if the 180-degree line is indeed at 180 degrees. For example, in Figure 4–12, a tilt of 5 degrees in the 180-degree line results in an error of the cylinder axis of 5 degrees as well. The amount of error considered to be within tolerance depends upon the power of the cylinder. (See Appendices 2 and 3). Because a flat top bifocal segment cannot be rotated to allow for correction of the cylinder axis, the 180-degree line must not be at an angle that exceeds accepted standards.

Positioning of Flat Top Trifocals

Keep in mind that there is essentially no difference between the basic procedure for centration of trifocals and that of bifocals. To avoid confusion, there are certain points to remember.

First, remember only the *top* line of the trifocal is used in segment positioning. (The lower line can be ignored.) Therefore, if a segment height is 19 mm, the uppermost line will be at 19 mm.

Secondly, it is much more likely for the top of the trifocal to be above the horizontal midline than in that of a bifocal, although a seg raise instead of a seg drop occurs with bifocals as well. In the case of a seg raise above the datum line, the major reference point of the distance portion will fall within the seg. Because of the slight prismatic effect exerted by the segment add power, spotting of the MRP may not have been entirely accurate, making dependence upon seg positioning for centration purposes preferable.

In the event of a seg raise, if there is no specification given by the practitioner for the vertical placement of the MRP, it may be the policy of the individual surfacing laboratory to automatically raise the MRP a certain amount above the seg top. For example, the policy of the laboratory may be to grind the MRP 2 mm higher than the seg top whenever the seg reaches the horizontal midline (datum line). If this is the case, the dot indicating MRP positioning should still have the correct horizontal inset, but will be vertically displaced by an amount equal to the seg raise above the datum line plus 2 mm. Both lenses in the pair will have MRP's of equal vertical height.

Table 4–1. Compensating for Small MRP Placement Errors	
Factors favoring maintaining distance PD, altering near PD	Factors favoring altering distance PD, maintaining near PD
1. A high-powered distance Rx (in 180-degree meridian)	1. A low-powered distance Rx (in 180-degree meridian)
2. A low near addition power	2. An especially high near addition power
3. A very wide segment	3. An especially small segment

CURVE TOP SEGMENT POSITIONING

Curve top segments are positioned in a manner nearly identical to that of flat top segments. The only difference is in the horizontal orientation: Segment height is judged from the highest point of the curved upper portion. Horizontal orientation is ensured by aligning both corners of the seg top with the same horizontal line. This procedure may be seen from the following problem.

Example:
Correctly center a right lens for the following order:

R: +1.00 + 1.75 × 78   PD 62/59
L: +0.75 + 2.00 x 109

add +2.25

Curve top 25 segment
Seg height 17 mm

Frame dimensions: A = 48
B = 39
DBL = 18

Solution:
Before placing the lens in the marking device, inset, total inset, and seg drop should be figured.

Inset will only be used to check for accuracy of MRP placement in surfacing. From this, the practitioner can then determine the probability of successfully remaining within standards of accepted tolerance.

$$\text{Inset} = \frac{A + DBL - \text{distance PD}}{2}$$
$$= \frac{48 + 18 - 62}{2}$$
$$= 2 \text{ mm per lens.}$$

Total inset will be used to preset the centering (i.e., marking) device and can be figured two ways:

$$(1) \text{ Total inset} = \frac{A + DBL - \text{near PD}}{2}$$
$$= \frac{48 + 18 - 59}{2}$$
$$= 3.5 \text{ mm per lens.}$$

(2) Total inset = inset (decentration per lens) + seg inset.

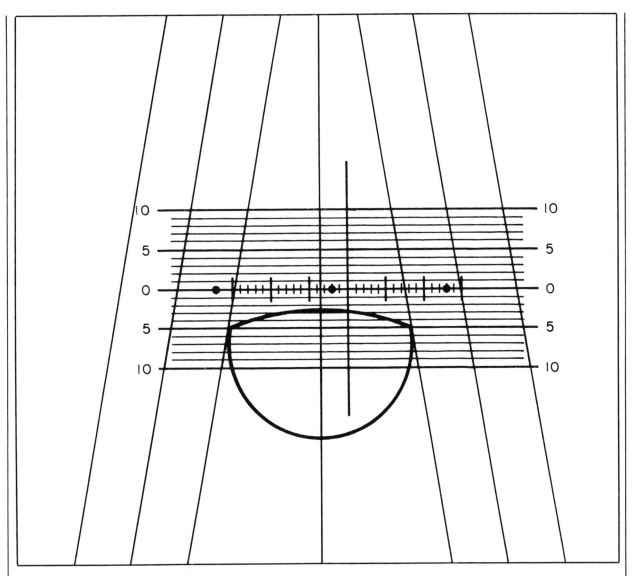

Figure 4–13. *For a curved top seg, the lateral corners of the curved upper segment border are equidistant from the horizontal reference line. They both must be at the same level.*

Recall that seg inset = $\dfrac{\text{distance PD} - \text{near PD}}{2}$.

Therefore if seg inset = $\dfrac{62 - 59}{2}$

$\qquad = 1.5$ mm/lens,

then total inset = 2 mm + 1.5 mm

$\qquad\qquad = 3.5$ mm per lens.

The movable vertical line in the marking device is moved 3.5 mm to the left. The line is moved to the left because the lens is placed face down in the unit and marked on the back side. (Were the lens to be placed convex side up—as would be the case when directly blocking the lens in the centering device— then the movable vertical line would be positioned to the right.)

Another style of instrument screen design is shown in Figure 4–13, where the multifocal segment is

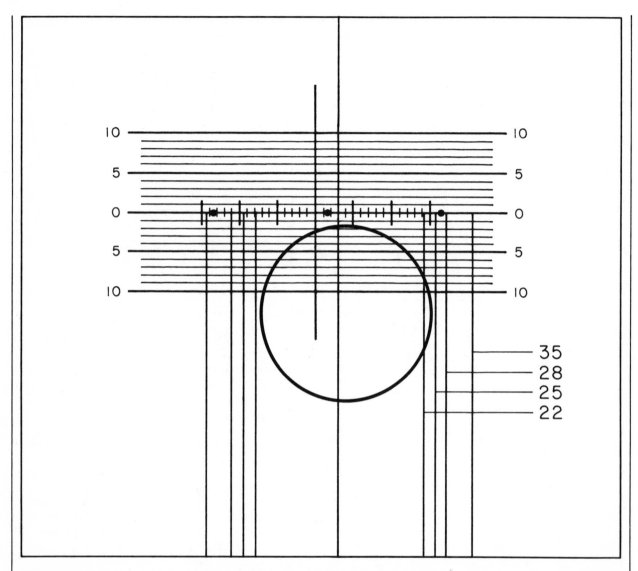

Figure 4–14. *If the dotted 180-degree line is used initially in centration of round segments with spherical distance portions, accurate segment placement almost always requires modification. As can be seen, although the instrument is set for the correct total inset, the segment is not centered between the appropriate bordering lines.*

bordered for centration by angled lines. The angled lines move up and down by means of a separate adjustment mechanism that does not affect the lateral positioning of the movable vertical inset line. By moving these angled lines up or down their separation at the plane of the bifocal segment increases or decreases. In this manner a segment of any size may be centered.

The grounds for acceptance or rejection of a curve

top multifocal blank are the same as those for flat tops. The seg should not be tilted in an effort to compensate for an incorrect cylinder axis simply because the top is curved.

POSITIONING FOR ROUND SEGS

To position a round top seg it is not possible to rely solely upon the segment for positioning and only secondarily to check for accuracy of MRP and axis. This is because the round seg offers no fixed horizontal reference plane; for this reason the process begins somewhat differently.

The first step is to position the blank so that the previously dotted MRP falls at its calculated inset. This may be done with the aid of the vertical inset line. Once the MRP and 180-degree line are correctly set, the vertical inset line is moved again, this time to the total inset position. For spherocylinder lenses the round segment should now be at its correct height and inset.

For spherical lenses, however, it is quite likely that this will not be the case, since the 180-degree line could be dotted only arbitrarily ahead of time. In the case of spherical lenses with no prescribed prism, the only point of importance is the dotted OC.[6] Once this OC is correctly positioned, the lens may be rotated around the OC until the correct seg inset and/or the correct seg height is achieved.

For example, the right lens in the following prescription is centered using the three Lensometer-spotted dots for reference.

R: +3.00 sph   PD 65/62
L: +3.25 − 0.50 × 175

add +2.00

22 mm round segment
seg height = 18 mm

Frame dimensions: A = 50 mm
                    B = 40 mm
          DBL = 18 mm

The calculated inset is 1.5 mm per lens. This is correctly positioned as shown in Figure 4–14. Because the calculated total inset is 3 mm, the movable vertical reference line has been moved to the right 3 mm. For the centering process to be complete, the segment should be evenly bracketed by the bordering lines within the instrument. In Figure 4–14 this is not the case, nor is the required 2 mm of seg drop evident. These can both be corrected by rotating the lens around its OC until the correct measures are obtained; the proper position is shown in Figure 4–15. Because there is no axis, the position of the two outer dots is of no consequence.

If the left lens were the lens in consideration for the above example, it should be evident that rotation

---

[6]For lenses having no prescribed prism, recall that the optical center and the major reference point are one and the same point.

around the OC will also result in the lens being off axis when edged.

When a lens protractor is being used to mark the round seg lens for edging, the lens is most easily oriented when the center of the seg is dotted. It is sometimes helpful to border the seg with dots so that it becomes more easily visible, especially since a lens protractor has no back lighting. These dots are applied, as shown in Figure 4–16, by viewing a well-lighted background through the lens and using an orange stick dipped in marking ink (or an appropriate marking pen that will not stain plastic lenses).

With the OC of the distance portion at the correct inset, the lens may be rotated until the central dot on the segment achieves the desired total inset, with the segment top at the correct drop position (see Figure 4–17).

With the exception of the option available for rotating of spherical blanks, the grounds for acceptance or rejection of the lens blank remain the same as with previously introduced multifocals.

POSITIONING FOR FRANKLIN STYLE LENSES

The Franklin style lens is made from one piece of lens material. The entire lower half of the lens is devoted to near vision and is divided from the upper half by a horizontal ledge running the entire width of the lens.

Because there are no lateral borders on a Franklin style segment, inset is accomplished by use of the dotted MRP location. The physical border of the segment is only used for seg height. Seg inset, when specified, must be accomplished during the surfacing process and may not always be possible, depending upon constraints produced by the size of the lens blank.

Some surfacing laboratories place the MRP directly on the segment line, although this is not necessary for optical reasons nor always required by blank size restraints.

The step-by-step procedure for Franklin style lens centration is:

1. Set the movable vertical reference line for the proper inset.
2. Place the marked MRP on this line.
3. Move the lens up or down until the segment line is at the correct height.
4. Check to be sure that the segment line is horizontal. (If the lens is spherocylindrical, the three Lensometer dots must also be parallel to the horizontal.)
5. Mark the lens.

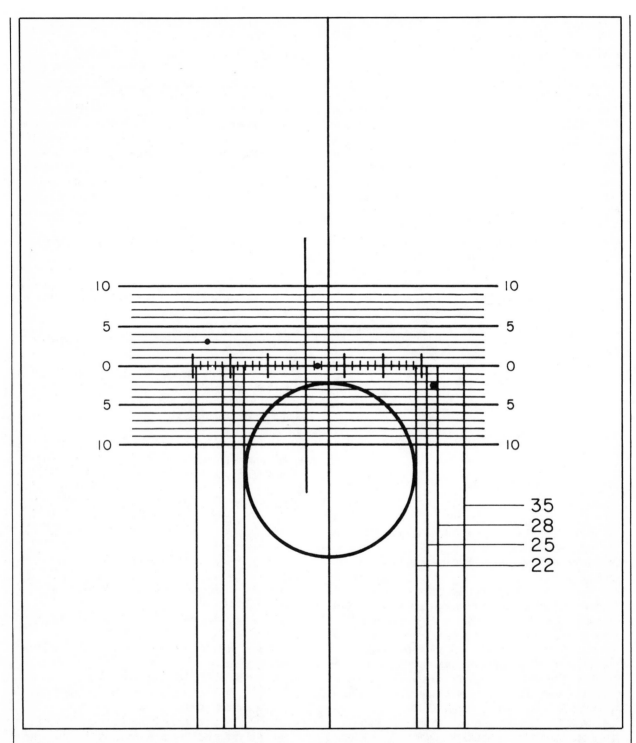

Figure 4–15. *Rotation of a round segment is mandated when the distance portion is spherical. When the distance power is spherical and the lens has no prism, the only dot of importance is the middle one designating the optical center of the lens.*

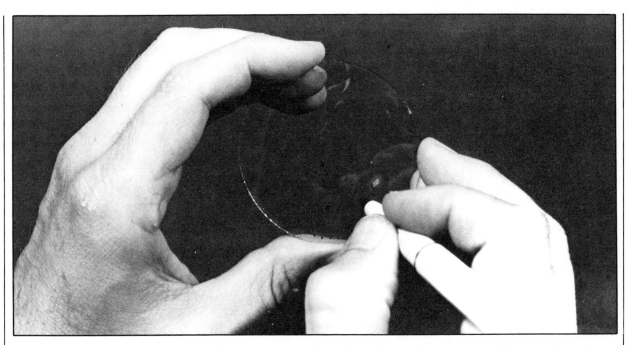

Figure 4–16. *Illuminated centering devices make hand marking of lenses unnecessary. When hand marking a spherical lens with a round seg, the most important points to have marked are the distance optical center and the geometric center of the segment.*

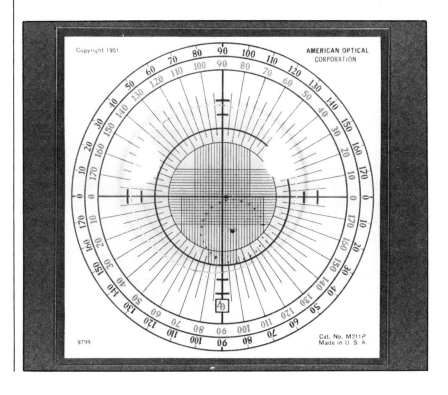

Figure 4–17. *Centration for multifocals using a lens protractor is different from a centration device in that there is no movable vertical line. This also eliminates the convenient segment bordering lines, making it necessary to mark the segment center. When marked, the segment center is placed at the total inset, seg top is placed at the correct drop (or raise) and the MRP is checked for accuracy of placement.*

POSITIONING FOR DOUBLE SEGMENT LENSES

Double segment lenses not only have a near addition in the lower half of the lens, but also a second seg area in the upper half of the lens. This allows freedom for wearers to work comfortably and clearly see near objects if they gaze upward.

Styles of segments used for double segment lenses parallel those used for conventional bifocal or trifocal lenses; the most common are flat top, small round, and Franklin style. Upper and lower segments are separated by a standard distance. Because this separation is always standard (as predetermined in the original manufacturing process), both segments are positioned by specifying the location of the lower seg. Lower seg specifications are given in exactly the same manner as for the regular bifocal. Therefore, lens centration procedures are identical to those previously described. The upper seg positions itself automatically.

If the opportunity exists to check how the blank will cut out by superimposition of the image of the lens pattern during centration, it is helpful to note the location of the upper seg in reference to the top of the edged lens. If there is less than 5 mm of upper seg showing below the upper rim of the frame, it is quite likely that an error was made in fitting. The practitioner should be consulted to verify accuracy before proceeding.

POSITIONING FOR BLENDED BIFOCALS

Blended bifocals are those having two sections of refractive power—distance and near—but in order to make the bifocal demarcation line invisible, the line is blurred out or blended. Because the demarcation line is blurred out, different methods of lens centration must be used.

Using the Seg Center
Because all presently available blended bifocals are round, the procedure followed parallels that previously listed for conventional, round bifocal segments. Some blended bifocals come with the center of the segment marked. This mark is usually not water soluble, and after edging it should be removed with acetone. As the size of the blended segment is known, this central seg dot is exactly half the seg diameter from the seg top. Therefore the seg may be positioned using only this single dot and the distance OC.

Example:
A blended bifocal having a seg diameter of 25 mm calls for an inset of 3 mm and a seg inset of 2 mm. The seg drop required is 2 mm. If the lens in question is a right lens and is spherical in power, how would the lens be centered for marking?

Solution:
This distance OC (or MRP) is used to position the distance portion at its 3-mm inset. The central seg dot may then be rotated until it reaches its correct position. The lateral position of the dot is an additional 2 mm in from the OC, as shown in Figure 4–18. It must also occupy a given position below the horizontal reference line. Since the seg dot is in the center of the seg, it will be half the seg diameter below the seg "line." This blended seg "line" must also fall 2 mm below the horizontal reference line. Therefore the vertical position of the seg center will be

$$\frac{\text{seg diameter}}{2} - \text{seg drop}^7$$

below the horizontal reference line. In this instance the vertical position will be

$$\frac{25}{2} - (-2) = 14.5 \text{ mm}$$

below.

Were the lens in the example marked with a circle of dots that fell on *the border* of the circular blended zone, it could be laid out in a manner identical to that of a conventional round segment.

Using the Seg Border
As mentioned previously, some blended bifocal lenses come with the circumference of the seg dotted. When marking such a lens on a centering device, the seg may be positioned using the bordering dots for reference. These dots are most generally in the middle or toward the outside edge of this blurred out or blended zone (see Figure 4–19).

If, by chance, all markings have been removed, they may be reapplied by holding the lens up in front of a textured, illuminated background. The blurred outline of the segment immediately becomes visible and the seg center and/or blended zone may be hand dotted.

---

[7]Recall that "seg drop" is a negative number.

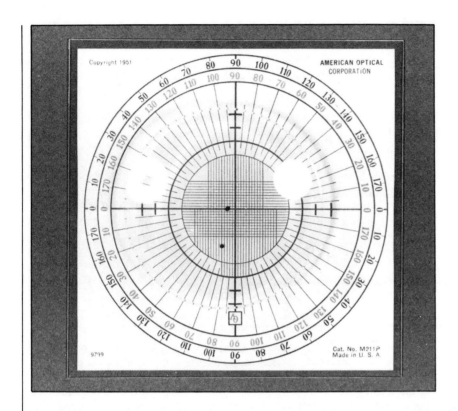

Figure 4–18. The center of a blended bifocal may be marked in a manner similar to that of a round bifocal. In the figure, this right lens is placed convex side down with a 3-mm inset (distance decentration) and a 2-mm seg inset, resulting in the 5-mm total inset, noted by the lower dot in the middle of the invisible seg.

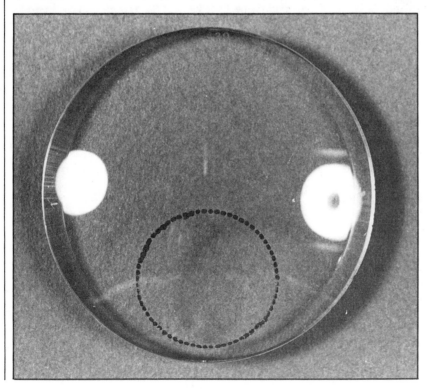

Figure 4–19. This factory-marked blended bifocal outlines the segment around the outermost borders of the blended zone. The optically usable portion of the segment is of a smaller diameter than the circle shown.

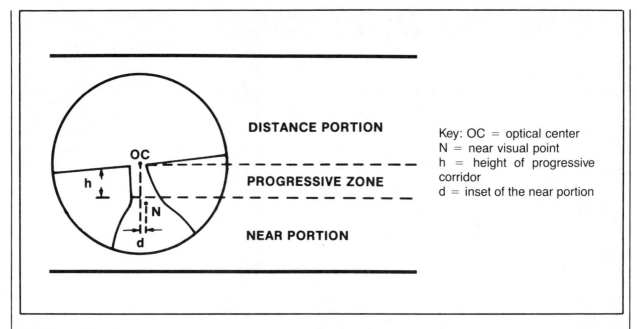

Figure 4–20. *Progressive addition lenses leave the upper distance portion of the lens relatively undisturbed. The power begins to change at the OC or MRP and increases in plus along a central corridor. The spin off of a gradually increasing power in combination with the nonvisible near section is a peripherally aberrated area. This area varies in optical usefulness to the wearer, depending upon the width of the progressive corridor and the power of the add. In the figure an oversimplified schematic of one lens philosophy is shown. (Brooks and Borish,* System for Ophthalmic Dispenisng, *Chicago: Professional Press, 1979, p. 268. Used by permission.)*

POSITIONING FOR PROGRESSIVE ADDITION LENSES

Progressive addition lenses are similar to blended bifocals in that neither blendeds nor progressives have segments that are visible to the casual observer. After this point, however, the lenses exhibit considerable differences in basic design. The *progressive addition lens* attempts a gradual increase in power from distance to near portions of the lens so that the wearer may see an object clearly at any distance by a slight repositioning of the head. This is in contrast to the bifocal, which focuses light for two distances only.

As Figure 4–20 shows, in most instances the power of the lens begins changing at the major reference point of the lens and continues to increase in plus power until the full add power is reached some 10 to 14 mm below the MRP.

Because of the gradualness of the power change and the lack of any distinct reference points on the lens, there is no such thing as a seg height with a progressive addition lens. Instead, the dispenser fitting the lenses measures in terms of either the MRP, or a "fitting cross." This fitting cross is to be positioned exactly in front of the wearer's pupil and the corresponding lens point is visibly marked on the lens with ink or a decal when it comes from the surface laboratory. (If these marks are removed, they can be reconstructed using etched reference marks on the front surface of the lens.)

The fitting cross is always a given number of millimeters above the MRP, depending upon manufacturer. This distance is equal to how far the lens designer believes the MRP should fall below the pupil. (Recall that with progressive addition lenses, the MRP marks the beginning of the progressive section of the lens.)

In simplest terms, the centration of progressive add lenses is done as if the lens were a single vision lens. The only difference is that for the progressive add lens, both horizontal *and* vertical positions of the MRP are always specified.

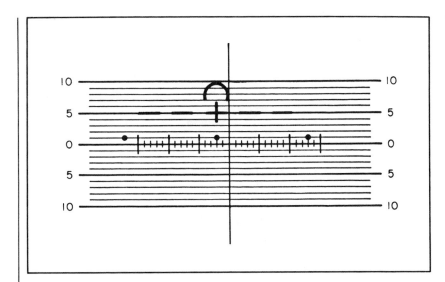

Figure 4–21. *Progressive lenses using a fitting cross system require that the fitting cross be used for reference in centration instead of the MRP. In the example shown, a 5-mm raise and a 2-mm inset are required. The near portion should automatically fall into place.*

Example:

	PD
R: +3.00 − 1.00 × 70	R 33
L: +3.00 − 1.00 × 110	L 31

add +1.50

Vertical fitting cross heights R: 25
                                L: 23

Frame dimensions: A = 50
                            B = 40
                  DBL = 20

How will the right lens appear when correctly centered for marking?

Solution:

Inset per lens must be calculated using monocular PD's. PD's are specified monocularly because the progressive corridor must begin directly below the eye. If the corridor is not exactly centered, the eye will enter the aberrated area to either side of the corridor when changing gaze positions to look at a closer object. For monocular PD's

$$\text{inset} = \frac{A + DBL}{2} - \text{monocular PD}$$

$$= \frac{50 + 20}{2} - 33$$

$$= 2 \text{ mm.}$$

The inset for the right lens is 2 mm (while the calculated inset for the left is 4 mm).

Most progressive addition lenses have a standard "seg" inset. The amount of seg inset may be constant or increase slightly with higher adds. Because seg inset is usually not possible to specify for progressives, no near PD was specified in the example under consideration. (However, some progressive add lenses *are* designed to allow some variation in "seg" inset. When this is the case, achieve variation by rotation of spherical lenses in the manner described for lenses having round segments. Spherocylinders must be rotated before surfacing.)

After horizontal lens positioning has been determined, calculate the vertical position of the lens. For the right lens the fitting cross raise or drop above or below the datum line is calculated as follows:

$$\text{raise or drop} = \text{fitting cross height} - \frac{B}{2}$$

$$= 25 - \frac{40}{2}$$

therefore raise = +5 mm.

The right lens appears correctly positioned on the centration device as shown in Figure 4–21.

It will be noted that the left lens has a raise of 3 mm instead of 5. If verification is done without considering the resulting unequal MRP heights, it will be assumed that an error has been made because of the vertical prism that will be manifested.

PROFICIENCY TEST QUESTIONS

1. If the seg height is 20 mm, what is the seg drop or raise with reference to the datum line for a frame with the following dimensions?

$$A = 42$$
$$B = 38$$
$$C = 37$$
$$DBL = 16$$
$$ED = 43$$

   a. 0
   b. −1 mm (drop)
   c. 1 mm (raise)
   d. −2 mm (drop)
   e. 2 mm (raise)

2. A frame has the following dimensions:

$$A = 50$$
$$B = 44$$
$$C = 39.5$$
$$DBL = 20$$
$$ED = 55$$

   Given a wearer with a PD of 66/62, for which of the following is "4 mm per lens" the correct measure?

   a. seg drop
   b. seg inset
   c. total seg inset
   d. decentration per lens (inset)

3. What is the seg inset for the following frame and PD measures?

$$A = 51$$
$$B = 44$$
$$C = 48 \quad PD = 64/61$$
$$DBL = 17$$
$$ED = 55$$

   a. 1.5 mm
   b. 2 mm
   c. 3 mm
   d. 4 mm
   e. 8 mm

4. For a flat top 25 lens, how far vertically and laterally will the MRP of each lens be from the center of its seg top line? The lens and frame have the following parameters:

   R: $+2.00 - 0.25 \times 15 \quad 2\Delta$ BO
   L: $+4.25 - 0.25 \times 165 \quad 2\Delta$ BO
   add $+1.50$

$$A = 52$$
$$B = 47$$
$$C = 50.5$$

$$DBL = 17 \qquad PD = 64/61$$
$$ED = 57 \qquad \text{seg height} = 21$$

5. A bifocal prescription is received from surfacing with the right MRP 4 mm above the seg line and the left lens MRP 2.5 mm above the seg line. For the Rx listed here, how much vertical prism could be manifested, assuming equal seg heights?

   R: $+2.75 - 1.00 \times 180$
   L: $+0.50$ sph

   a. 0.26Δ
   b. 0.08Δ
   c. 0.19Δ
   d. 0.13Δ
   e. 0.41Δ

6. If a 2.5 mm variation in near PD is considered to be within accepted standards, what are the largest and smallest near PD's that fall within these standards for a wearer with a PD = 59/56?

   a. 61.5–56.5
   b. 61.5–53.5
   c. 58.5–53.5
   d. The correct answer depends upon the distance power.

7. A prescription calls for a seg inset of 2 mm (per lens). During centration it is noticed that the lateral distance from the seg center to the distance OC is actually 4 mm for each lens. How much lateral prism will be induced in the distance portion if the near PD is set correctly? The distance Rx is

   R: $+5.00 - 1.00 \times 180$
   L: $+5.00 - 1.50 \times 180$

   a. 1.4Δ
   b. 1.5Δ
   c. 1.6Δ
   d. 2.0Δ
   e. None of the above is correct.

8. For the prescription described in question 7, what will the base direction of the induced prism be?

   a. Left
   b. Right
   c. In
   d. Out
   e. Down

9. During centration of a flat top bifocal it is noticed that the spots made by the Lensometer are tilted

10 degrees in reference to the seg line. The central dot is correctly placed. When would this be of no consequence?
a. It would always be of consequence.
b. In the case of a plano cylinder
c. When oblique prism is prescribed
d. When the decentration is small
e. When the lens is spherical

10. A flat top, 7×25 trifocal calls for a seg height of 23 mm. If the frame B dimension is 46, what would the seg drop (or raise) be for correct centration?
a. 0
b. -7 mm (drop)
c. 7 mm (raise)
d. -2 mm (drop)
e. 2 mm (raise)

11. A bifocal for the right eye is placed convex side up on the centration device so it may be blocked directly. If A = 47, DBL = 16 and PD = 61/57, where is the center of the segment in reference to the center (origin) of the grid?
a. To the left
b. To the right
c. Exactly in the middle

12. Which lenses from the following group could not be centered correctly using only the segment?
a. Curve top bifocals
b. Round seg bifocals
c. Flat top bifocals
d. Executive (Franklin style) bifocals
e. Progressive add lenses

13. To center an occupational double seg exactly as indicated on the order during the layout process,
a. center first the lower segment and mark the lens, then center the upper seg and remark. The lens is blocked exactly between the two marks.
b. center the first upper segment and note whether the lower segment occupies the prescribed location before marking.
c. center the lower seg as indicated and ignore the upper seg.

14. In lens layout, a blended bifocal lens is centered in a manner most similar to
a. a progressive addition lens.
b. a trifocal lens.
c. a flat top segment lens.

d. a round segment lens.
e. a curve-top segment lens.

15. For those progressive addition lenses using a fitting cross system, which reference point is used during centration for lens layout?
a. The fitting cross
b. The major reference point
c. The center of the near progressive zone

16. T or F   In most simple terms, the centration of progressive add lenses is done as if the lens were a single vision lens.

17. A progressive lens not using a fitting cross system is to be marked for edging. The frame and PD dimensions are as follows:

		PD	height of MRP's
A = 51			
B = 47	R:	31	26
C = 50	L:	33	25
DBL = 17			
ED = 59			

What raise or drop and what inset is required for each lens?

18. For the following Rx, how far in is the segment positioned for blocking the lens? How is the seg positioned vertically?

$$R: -1.75 -1.00 \times 180$$
$$L: -1.50 -1.25 \times 180$$
$$A = 46$$
$$B = 42$$
$$ED = 50$$
$$DBL = 16$$
$$PD = 59/56$$
$$\text{seg height} = 18$$

19. When a seg inset is incorrect after surfacing and it is decided that the lens is nevertheless within normal limits of quality, which factor(s) would favor altering the near PD and maintaining distance PD?
a. An especially small segment
b. A low near addition power
c. A high-powered distance Rx in the 180 meridian

20. Which bifocal(s) can be marked for blocking without having been spotted?
a. Executive bifocals
b. Flat top bifocals
c. Round seg bifocals
d. Curve top bifocals

21. Which of the lenses listed below *may* be rotated slightly around the distance OC in order to alter the seg inset before edging the lens?
    a. − 2.00D sph, FT-25 seg
    b. − 2.00 − 1.00 × 15, kryptok (22 mm round) seg
    c. + 3.25D sph, panoptik seg
    d. + 1.25 − 0.25 × 30, executive or Franklin style seg
    e. − 7.25D sph, ultex A seg (38 mm semi-circular seg)

Chapter 5

Blocking of Lenses

In order for a lens to be edged to its proper shape it must be clamped in the lens edger so that the axis will be properly oriented, the decentration correct, and the segment in the right position (in other words, in such a manner that all parameters which were so carefully attended to during the centration process will remain as specified). This process of preparing the lens so that it will remain correctly oriented while being edged is referred to as *blocking*.

There are four basic methods for blocking a lens for edging.

These methods are

1. *Pressure blocking:* The lens is held in place between felt pads.
2. *Suction blocking:* A small suction cup is pressed onto the lens.
3. *Metal alloy blocking:* A low melting temperature metal alloy is molded onto the protected surface of the lens.
4. *Adhesive pad blocking:* A thin pad which is adhesive on both sides is applied to the lens and a holding block applied to the pad.

Each method has been used extensively and offers certain advantages.

PRESSURE BLOCKING

Perhaps the most basic blocking method is that of pressure blocking, usually accomplished by squeezing the lens between two felt pads in the edger. It is, to be certain, totally impractical to simply hand position the lens between the felt pads and expect the edged lens parameters to be accurate. Instead the lens is prepositioned in a centering fork. In order to carry this out, a felt pad attached to an adaptor is placed in the centering fork. Then the previously marked lens is positioned on the felt pad, concave side up with the top of the lens toward the handle. The marked 180-degree cutting line on the lens must be horizontally aligned with the etched reference lines of the centering fork. In addition, the center of the marked cross must be directly over the hole in the center of the pad. (There are specially designed sighting systems into which the fork may be placed to make alignment easier and reduce the possibility of parallax error.)

With the lens properly aligned in the centering fork, the adapter is slipped into the accepting portion of the edger. The second felt pad may then be pressed into place and tightened. Now the centering fork may be removed as the lens is clamped in at the correctly centered cutting line orientation.

In order to achieve the best results using this pressure blocking system, replace the felt pads periodically before they become worn. These pads should also be wet thoroughly prior to edging lenses by cycling the edger without a lens in place. This prevents the pressure-blocked lens from slipping during edging, which would otherwise result in off-axis lenses.

Currently the felt pad system of blocking is more generally used as a backup system. Besides the danger of lens slippage, such a system does not allow for periodic removal of a lens from the edger in order to check for size, since once the lens is removed it is practically impossible to put back in the edger in its exact previous position.

BLOCKING WITH SUCTION

Another method of holding the lens in place is by means of a small suction cup. This suction cup is constructed with an adapter on the back surface that allows it to fit into the spindle assembly within the lens edger.

The advantage of a suction cup system is that it may be used with no preparation. Although it is not often used for mass production purposes, it lends itself to smaller facilities where lenses are edged on a more periodic basis. In Europe, where most of the

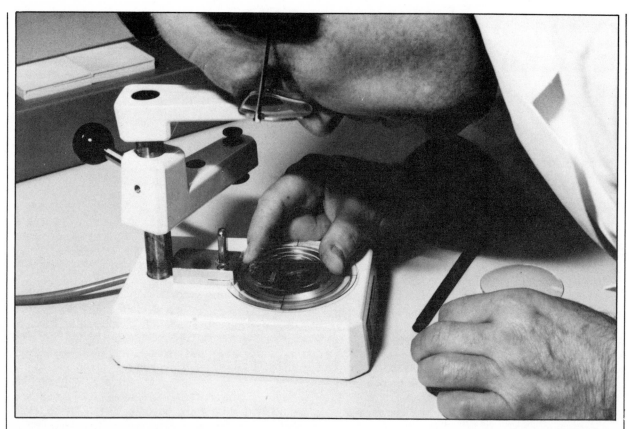

Figure 5–1. *The centration process that precedes suction blocking on a centering device is identical to that process used when simply marking the lens. In this case the lens is placed convex side up.*

edging is done on location at the dispensary, this system is more widely used than in the United States.

Figure 5–1 shows that suction blocking may be more expediently used in combination with a centration device, allowing centering and blocking functions to be performed at the same time. Then, instead of marking the lens, an arm containing the suction cup is swung into position and pressed against the lens (see Figure 5–2). Once the cup is so attached, as in Figure 5–3, the lens is ready for edging.

The holding surface of the suction cup must be kept free of oil or foreign substances. Suction cups must be applied dry to a dry lens in order to prevent slippage and a corkscrewing effect. These cups may be reused often, but should be regularly inspected for cracks in the rubber caused by drying. Once the surface begins to show signs of cracking, the

chances of a lens slipping in the edging process are greatly increased.

METAL ALLOY BLOCKING

Another system that has enjoyed widespread usage is a metal alloy blocking system. In this system a metal alloy with a low melting point is heated until fluid, then poured into a mold positioned on the lens. The metal cools, forming a small metal block that adheres to the lens. The lens may then be mounted in the edger. Metal blocking has certain distinct advantages and disadvantages that must be considered in choosing the blocking system to meet the need of each laboratory.

The Alloy

The metal alloy itself is available in three different melting temperatures. These are 117°F, 136°F, and

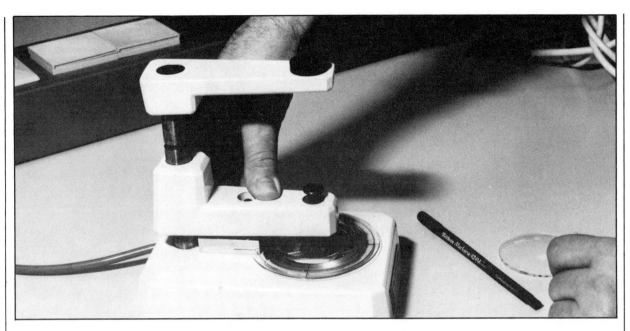

Figure 5–2. *The suction cup is pressed onto the convex side of the lens surface.*

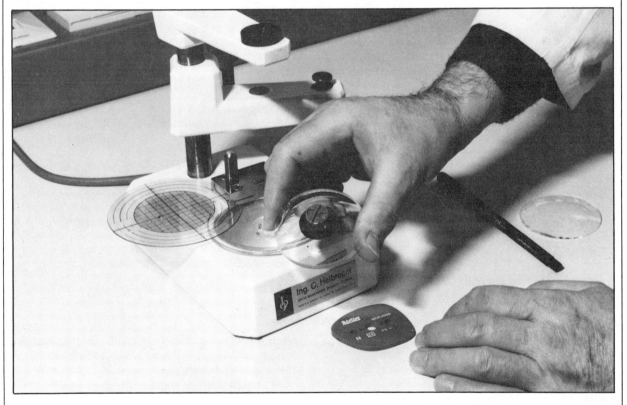

Figure 5–3. *The adapter attached to the suction cup may vary in its configuration, depending upon the edger manufacturer's design.*

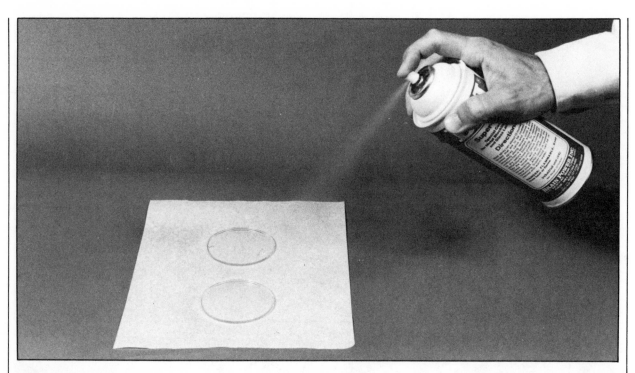

Figure 5–4. *Drying time for a spray-coated lens will vary, depending upon humidity. High humidity not only slows drying, but can cause occasional problems because metal alloy blocks lose adherence to the lens during processing.*

158°F. The *lowest temperature alloy* is often used when only plastic lenses are being blocked. It is more advantageous because it does not warp the lenses with excessive heat. Its principle disadvantage is the increased time required for the alloy to solidify once poured into the mold. The alloy cools more slowly since the mold is closer in temperature to the alloy, resulting in a slower heat exchange.

The *158°F alloy* is used when only glass lenses are being blocked. It hardens rapidly, but warps a plastic lens.

The alloy most often used in blocking for edging is the 136° alloy. Because of the small size of the block, for "finish" blocking (i.e., blocking for edging) the 136°F alloy proves suitable for plastic, although when blocking for surfacing the large size of the block required makes a lower temperature alloy more advantageous.

Precoating of Lenses

Unfortunately, metal alloy will not adhere directly to the lens surface tightly enough to withstand the edging process. Therefore the surface must first be precoated. The coating may be applied to the front surface of the lens in the form of a spray (see Figure 5–4) or with a brush or daub-on applicator as shown in (Figure 5–5).

Spraying the lens surface is a fast process, but requires that the lenses be removed from their trays and placed in an area designated for this purpose. As with any spray system, unless a fume hood exhaust system is used, if the laboratory has poor ventilation the residual spray remaining in the air can be irritating.

Although a brush-on application system allows the lenses to remain in the trays, they must nevertheless have a certain amount of ventilation to allow sufficient drying.

Therefore, if trays are stacked, each tray should be placed crosswise on the one below in alternate directions. Each lens must be dry to the touch before blocking. Drying time is not less than half an hour, and it can be longer depending upon air circulation and humidity. In locations where humidity is high, a heat lamp may be used to aid in drying.

The spray used in "finish blocking" (blocking for

84

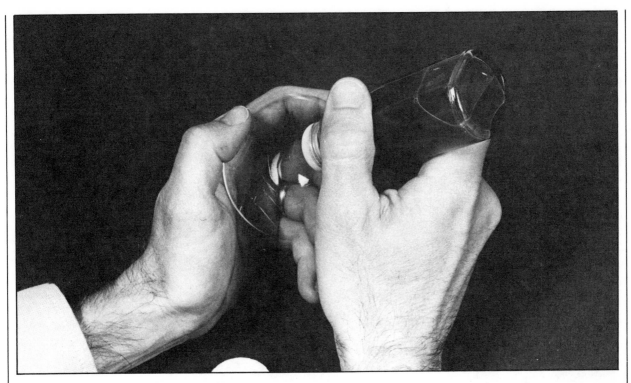

Figure 5–5. *Lens coating liquid applied with a sponge tip applicator is daubed onto the lens surface only in the area where the block will be applied. Application with a brush is also commonly used.*

edging) is clear, in order to allow for ease in seeing lens markings during the blocking process. (When liquid coatings are used for "surface blocking," they are often a dark color.)

The Blocking Unit

The metal alloy blocking unit consists basically of a pot for heating the alloy to a liquid state, and a mold to form the molten material into the desired shape of the block. There are many variations to choose from, beginning with units that are very simple, such as a small pot with a handle from which alloy may be hand poured, all the way up to the more complex models with a timed, measured flow release that responds to the push of a button.

The unit should be thermostatically regulated so that alloy temperature may be monitored. (See Figure 5–6). The alloy must be kept hot enough so that it does not solidify before the block properly forms, but not so hot as to cause a long waiting period before the lens may be removed from the blocker. Suggested temperatures are

130°F for 117°F alloy
150°F for 136°F alloy
180°F for 158°F alloy.

Although the temperature may be regulated, before readjusting the temperature control, be certain that sufficient time has elapsed for the unit to warm up. Thereafter adjustments should only be made in small increments, allowing a suitable length of time for the temperature to change throughout the pot and all alloy it contains.

Simultaneously adding a large number of recycled blocks to the molten alloy can substantially reduce alloy temperature. If sufficient time for reheating is not allowed before continuing to block lenses, laboratory staff may get the false impression that the unit is not turned up sufficiently.

The Alloy Blocking Process

As expected, the metal alloy blocking process begins with aligning the lens on a holding device so that the block will be applied at the correct location.

85

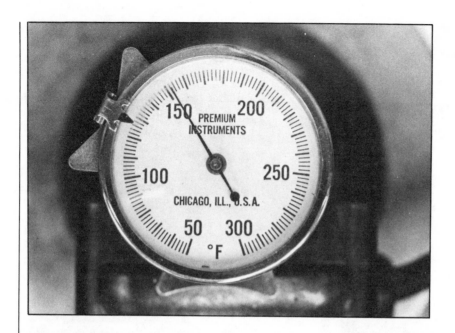

Figure 5–6. *Using a dial thermometer takes the estimation out of maintaining optimum alloy temperature. In an effort to bring the unit into operation quickly, some technicians keep the alloy temperature too high. This results in longer metal solidification time and subjects plastic lenses to inadvisably high temperatures.*

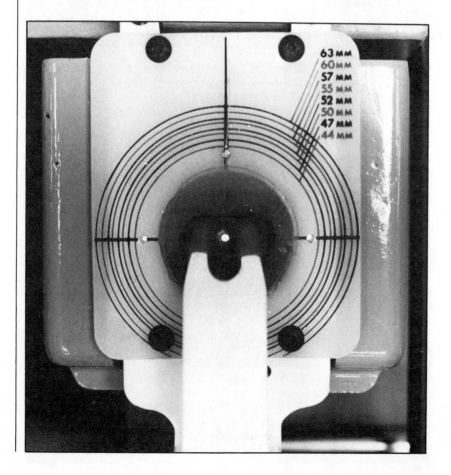

Figure 5–7. *If all three transilluminated holes do not show visible light simultaneously, the operator is not exactly in front of the unit. This results in parallax, causing the lens to be blocked slightly off center.*

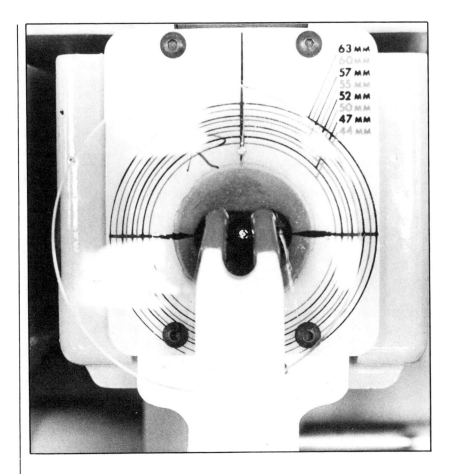

Figure 5–8. *Concentric rings on some blocking units provide yet another method of checking as to whether or not the uncut lens is large enough for the shape to be edged. In this instance the lens falls just short of completely enclosing the 57-mm ring.*

A centering fork may be utilized in a manner similar to that described for felt pad blocking. Such a centering fork often contains three drilled holes on a scribed 180-degree line that allows light to pass through. This facilitates easier alignment. As Figure 5–7 shows, when the centering fork is mounted to the blocking unit, it is often transilluminated so that the three guide holes are even more visible.

On the centering fork or mounting area of the unit, the lens is positioned convex side down. Concentric rings radiating out from the middle of the centering area where the block mold is located aid in determining whether a lens will be large enough for the frame. If the lens does not completely encircle the ring corresponding to the eyesize of the frame indicated, it is certain that the lens will not cut out. To be completely sure that the lens will be large enough, a circle equal to the effective diameter of the frame must be enclosed.

Example:

In Figure 5–8 the marked lens has been positioned for blocking. If the frame to be used has an eyesize of 57 mm and an effective diameter of 60, will the lens be sufficiently large to allow the shape to be cut out?

Solution:

It can be seen from the figure that the lens does not enclose the 57-mm ring. Therefore it is certain that the lens will not cut out. If edged, there will be an air space somewhere between the lens edge and frame rim. It should be noted that had the lens encircled a 57-mm ring, but not a 60-mm ring, there would still be no absolute guarantee that the lens would cut out. Whether it actually would cut out or not depends upon the location of the longest corner of the frame's lens shape (i.e., the angle that the longest radius creates with the datum line).

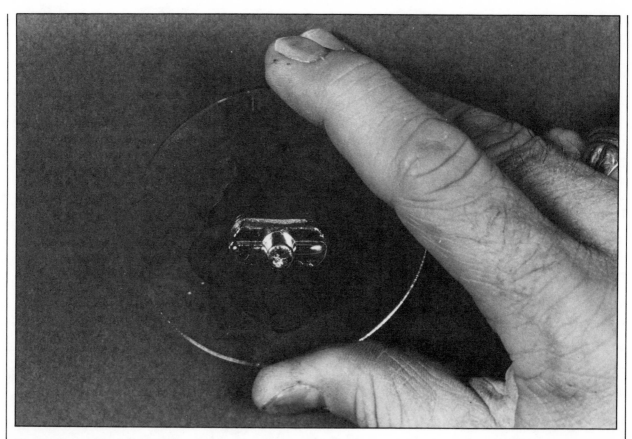

Figure 5–9. *The shape of the metal block can be molded to any one of several different chucking systems.*

Dispensing of alloy should not be attempted before the metal is fluid and has reached the recommended temperature. This is especially true with automatic units, because clogging of the unit can occur. Once the correct temperature has been reached, it is best to activate an automatic dispensing mechanism several times before actually using it, catching the dispensed alloy in a small container. This ensures that the valve is free of hardened alloy, giving a smooth flow and hence a more even measure. This procedure also helps prevent unwanted leakage of alloy.

Once the alloy has entered the mold it should be given a short period of time to harden before the lens is removed from the centering fork. For this reason some units have two centering forks, so that a second lens may be in preparation while the alloy is hardening on the first (see Figure 5–9).

If an excess of fluid alloy is introduced, causing it to mushroom out of the mold, before it hardens the excess alloy should be wiped away with the finger. If this is not done in time the block must be removed by breaking the hardened overflow away.

There are some centering devices that may be adapted to allow the lens to be metal blocked before removing it from the centering unit.

ADHESIVE PAD BLOCKING

Another method for blocking lenses utilizes adhesive pads.[1] A block made of metal or plastic is fastened to the lens by means of an adhesive pad (Figure 5–10) on the order of double-sided tape.

The Blocks
Blocks vary according to manufacturer. The block

---

[1]Adhesive pad blocking is sometimes referred to as *LEAP blocking*. The product of 3M Company used for this purpose is known as the 3M LEAP System.

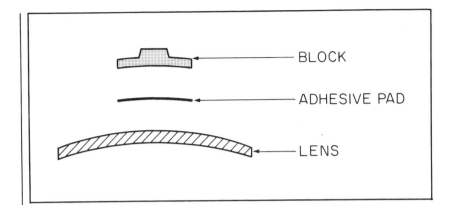

BLOCK

ADHESIVE PAD

LENS

Figure 5–10. Adhesive pad blocking consists of a block applied to the lens by means of double-sided tape.

backs come in a variety of contours to adapt to the chuck of the edger being used. When the block is made of metal or a nonflexible, hard plastic, the side contacting the adhesive pad must approximate the front curve of the lens. Blocks can be classified as low, regular, and high base, depending upon the steepness of curvature.

Some suppliers furnish a block made of flexible plastic material. This type of block may be used on a lens of any base curve regardless of steepness, since the flange of the block is designed to take on the curvature of the lens.

The Basic Pad Blocking Process
The lens and block should be thoroughly cleaned before use to prevent slippage during edging. Methods of cleaning vary. Some practitioners find that little cleaning of the blocks is necessary, while others soak recycled metal blocks in a container of acetone to remove all grease and oils before reusing. If slippage does occur, the first thing to check for would be the use of an incorrect base block. After that, one would suspect incomplete cleaning as a cause. If more thorough cleaning does not alleviate the situation, it may indicate that the roll of adhesive pads has been exposed to excess heat or humidity.

If lenses slip on adhesive pad blocks, check to determine whether
1. the block is correct for the lens base curve.
2. the lenses are clean.
3. each block is free from foreign material.
4. the pad has been exposed to humidity or high temperatures.

In preparation for blocking, a pad is peeled from the roll and placed over the marked cross on the lens so that the central hole leaves the cross intersection exposed (see Figure 5–11). The appropriate base block is then chosen and placed in the blocker as Figure 5–12 shows.

One of the most simply made blocking units consists of a holder for the block and three parallax lights. The central light shines through a hole in the middle of the block with the remaining two lights on either side along the 180-degree line. After peeling the protective paper off the pad to expose the second adhesive surface, the lens is centered on the blocker.

To center properly, sight from above until the marked cross intersection on the lens is exactly over the light coming through the center of the block and both light pinpoints to either side are aligned with the 180-degree line on the lens, as in Figure 5–13. All three lights must be visible simultaneously. If they are not, the operator's eye is not directly above the center of the point in question, which could result in an off-centered lens.

Once the operator is assured that the alignment is correct, the lens is pressed firmly against the block, bonding the block to the lens.

Adhesive Pad Blocking with a Marker/Blocker
Centration devices that allow an immediate blocking of the lens are often referred to as marker/blockers. In most cases they can be used to either mark the lens with an inked stamp, or, with a simple, reversible adjustment, block the lenses directly. The ease with which an adhesive pad system adapts to direct blocking in this manner has caused an increase in the use of the marker/blocker combination.

As previously mentioned, when a lens is to be

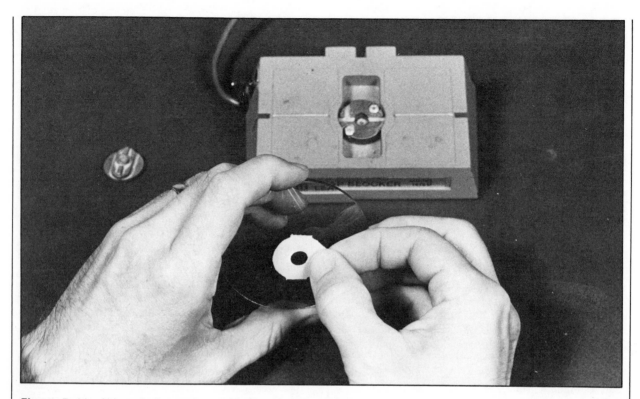

Figure 5–11. *Although the recommended procedure is the application of the adhesive pad to the lens first, many technicians prefer to first apply the pad to the block. Thus quite a number of blocks can be padded during opportune times, speeding the process during actual production.*

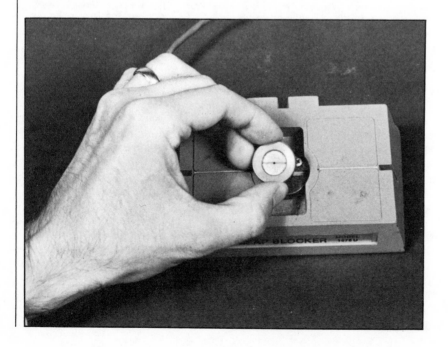

Figure 5–12. *The block chosen and placed in the unit in preparation for blocking should approximate the base curve of the lens.*

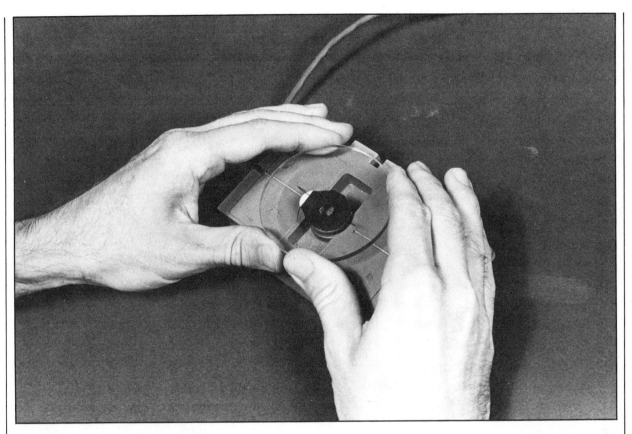

Figure 5–13. *The marked cross on the lens is exactly centered over the pinpoint of light emitting through the small hole in the block. As in any procedure of this sort, parallax must be avoided by positioning the eye directly in front of the block center.*

directly blocked on the centration device it must be centered with the front surface up. This reverses the direction of inset.

Example:

When centering a left lens face up in the marker/blocker, if a 3-mm inset is required, in which direction should the lens be moved?

Solution:

It is helpful to visualize the lens as if already mounted in a pair of glasses. The glasses are "looking up at" the operator. As the word *inset* implies *in* toward the nose, and since the lens is a left lens, the bridge of the imaginary pair of glasses is to the operator's left. Therefore the lens is decentered 3 mm to the left. (Had the lens been placed face down for marking, decentration would have been to the right.) After centration is complete, the adhesive pad is placed on the block instead of on the lens. The block is then mounted on a movable arm that may be manually or automatically swung into place over the lens and pressed onto the lens surface. (See Figure 5–14.)

An Optional Coating

Note that the only blocking system requiring a lens coating is the metal blocking system. All other blocking systems allow for direct mounting to the uncoated lens surface. One of the advantageous side effects to a coating, however, is the surface protection it affords plastic lenses.

In order to insure against lens scratching, which may occur during the edging process, some practi-

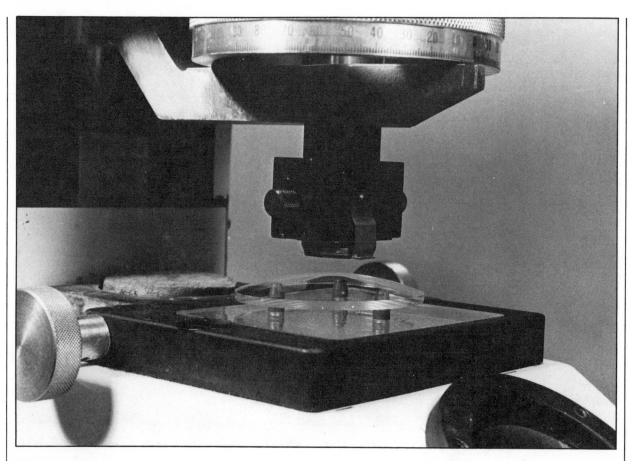

Figure 5–14. *By centering the lens convex side up in the centration device, a pretaped lens block can be lowered directly onto the lens. This eliminates one step in the production process.*

tioners elect to use a protective coating[2] on plastic lenses; as Figure 5–15 shows, this coating may be applied around the block on both front and back surfaces. The coating provides an additional value to practitioners who edge both glass and plastic lenses in the same edger, because the coating helps to protect lenses from glass debris found in the edger coolant.

A protective tape, such as the 3M Surface Saver system developed for the surfacing laboratory, works well as a protectant on all but coated polycarbonate lenses. On polycarbonate, the scratch resistant coating tends to pull off when the tape is removed. A compressed air-powered applicator is required to use the tape.

BLOCKING POLYCARBONATE

Blocking of polycarbonate lenses may be done using a *low-temperature alloy*. If the temperature is not kept within recommended ranges, however, localized distortion of the lens surface can occur (as is the case with any plastic lens). Because of the thermoplastic[3] nature of the material, this method also can present problems if deblocking is done using heat.

Felt pad blocking with larger chucks and an air chucking system set to deliver approximately 80 PSI[4] works satisfactorily. When difficulty is experi-

[2]An example of this type of coating would be Kote-Guard, supplied by Coburn Optical Industries.

[3]Thermoplastic material will return to a soft or moldable state when subjected to heat, while thermosetting materials such as the CR-39, so often used for plastic lenses, will not.

[4]Jud Westgate, "Edging Tough Polycarbonate Is a Matter of Technique," *Optical Index,* Vol. 56, No. 1, Jan. 1981, pp. 37–42.

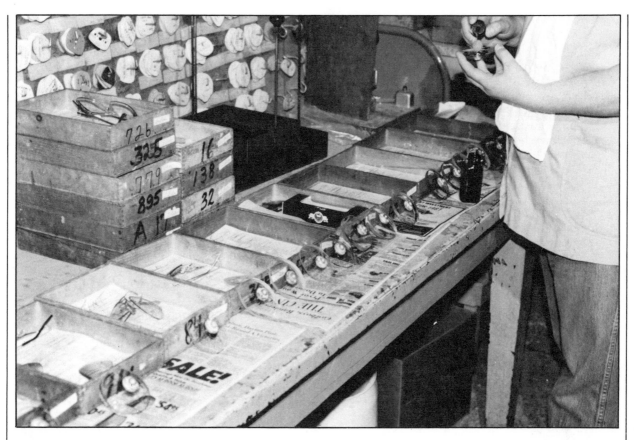

Figure 5–15. *Plastic lenses may be coated on both front and back surfaces to increase scratch resistance during edging; they are leaned up against their tray for drying purposes.*

enced, it is generally with high minus lenses, where the large amount of stock being removed produces enough drag to occasionally allow slippage of the lens. Any other disadvantages are inherent in any felt pad blocking system and were discussed previously.

The current method of choice for blocking polycarbonate is the *adhesive pad system.*

BLOCKING LAMINATE LENSES

Blocking of lenses made from more than one material is still done conventionally and any precautions would depend primarily upon the materials being used. For example, the Corlon[5] lens may be blocked using customary methods. The outer convex surface is the crown or photochromic glass. Exercise caution, however, if the lens is sprayed with a precoat material to be certain that the lens is concave side down on a flat surface, as the spray may otherwise damage the polyurethane back surface. (Marking of Corlon lenses should be done on the front surface to avoid staining the more absorbant rear surface.)

---

[5]Corlon is a trade name for Corning Glass Works combination glass and polyurethane lens.

PROFICIENCY TEST QUESTIONS

1. List advantages and disadvantages for each of the main blocking systems.

2. Which system(s) does/do not allow lenses to be removed from the edger to check for correct size, and then put back in the edger again?
   a. Pressure blocking
   b. Suction blocking
   c. Metal blocking
   d. Adhesive pad blocking

3. Which systems can be incorporated directly into a marker/blocker style system?
   a. Pressure blocking
   b. Suction blocking
   c. Metal blocking
   d. Adhesive pad blocking

4. T or F   Suction blocking can only be used with glass lenses.

5. Which system requires planning ahead before use?
   a. Pressure blocking
   b. Suction blocking
   c. Metal blocking
   d. Adhesive pad blocking

6. To obtain best results in suction blocking, water is applied to
   a. the lens surface.
   b. the suction cup.
   c. both the lens surface and the suction cup.
   d. neither the lens surface nor the suction cup.

7. The alloy type most suitable for finish blocking of both glass and plastic lenses has a melting point of
   a. 117°F.
   b. 136°F.
   c. 158°F.
   d. 212°F.

8. Coating of the lens surface is necessary for
   a. Pressure blocking.
   b. Suction blocking.
   c. Metal blocking.
   d. Adhesive pad blocking.

9. If alloy "mushrooms" out of the mold because of overfilling, it should

a. be left to harden.
b. be wiped away with an asbestos towel before it hardens.
c. be wiped away with the finger.

10. The recommended temperature for using 136-degree Lo-Melt Alloy when blocking is
    a. 136°F.
    b. 138°F.
    c. 150°F.
    d. 180°F.

11. A check system of concentric circles is used with a blocker or marker/blocker to determine if a lens will cut out for a given frame. Which size circle must be completely covered by the de-centered lens blank to be certain that the lens will cut out?
    a. A circle whose diameter equals eyesize (*A*) plus ½ DBL
    b. A circle whose diameter equals eyesize only
    c. A circle whose diameter equals eyesize plus twice the decentration per lens
    d. A circle whose diameter equals the effective diameter only

12. T or F   In metal blocking units, the level of alloy in the melting pot should not be allowed to drop too low before replenishing the alloy, as the impurities on the top surface may have a tendency to clog the feeder line.

13. To block according to the boxing system, the center of the block is *always* positioned
    a. on the MRP of the lens.
    b. on the lens OC.
    c. at the geometric center of the lens blank.
    d. on what will become the boxing center of the edged lens.
    e. The center of the block may sometimes be at any one of the above locations, but not *always* at any of them.

14. Were the datum system being used in conjunction with a pattern cut for the datum system, where would the center of the block be? (Give the *best* answer.)
    a. MRP
    b. Datum center
    c. Boxing center
    d. OC
    e. Geometric center of the lens blank

15. A right lens is being blocked on a marker/blocker with its convex surface up. If the lens requires inset, in which direction must it be moved?
    a. left
    b. right
    c. cannot say

16. The current method of choice for blocking polycarbonate prescription lenses is
    a. felt pad.
    b. suction cup.
    c. metal alloy.
    d. adhesive pad.

17. T or F   Thermoplastic materials will return to a soft or moldable state when subjected to heat.

18. A lens must be blocked for edging. Here are the raw data:
    OD −4.00 −1.00 × 90 1Δbase in
    PD = 68
    Frame eyesize = 52
    DBL = 22
    Blank size = 71 mm
    How far from the center of the lens block will the optical center of the lens be? Is the OC nasal or temporal to the block center?

19. For the above problem, how far from the optical center is the major reference point?

Chapter 6

Lens Shape Formation

Once a lens is properly marked, blocked, and ready for edging there must be a system for achieving the desired lens size and shape. The system presently used consists of a pattern that duplicates the shape of the frame area into which the lens is to be placed. This pattern, or *former* as it is sometimes called, is usually made from plastic, but occasionally of metal. The pattern is mounted onto the lens edger to serve as a guide in the grinding process.

PATTERN MEASUREMENTS AND TERMINOLOGY

As stated, patterns duplicate the desired lens shape for a specific frame. Just as their shape is critical for the correct duplication of lens shapes, so also is their size of utmost importance. Therefore, in order to maintain accuracy, a standard method of measuring patterns is essential.

To determine pattern size, a pattern must be positioned exactly in the same orientation as the frame shape when the frame is held horizontally—in other words, the pattern may not be rotated. The pattern shape is then boxed about by four tangent lines according to the same boxing system as used for frames and lenses. The perpendicular lines used for boxing in the pattern must be perfectly horizontal and vertical, and each side of the box must touch the pattern as shown in Figure 6–1. The pattern size for

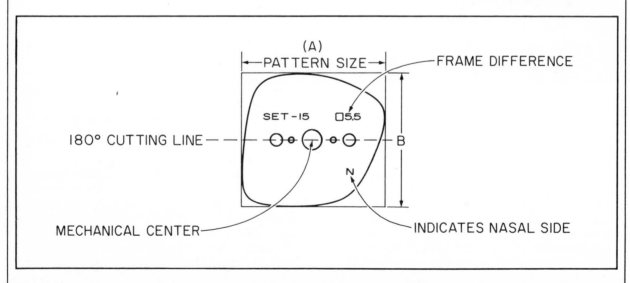

Figure 6–1. The same system of measurement as is used for frames and lenses is also used for patterns. It is always advisable to check pattern measurements, recalculating the set number for new patterns as they have been known to come erroneously marked.

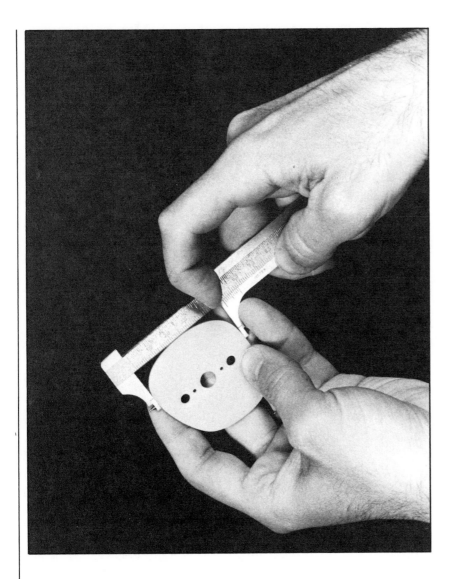

Figure 6–2. *Use extreme caution if measuring a pattern according to the boxing system with a slide gauge. Most gauges do not extend far enough to allow an accurate boxing measure. (Measuring according to the datum system is much easier with a slide gauge, as the gauge is held perpendicular to the plane of the pattern at the level of the datum line—essentially measuring the boxing C dimension.)*

the boxing system is the distance between the two vertical sides of the box, *not* the width of the pattern in the middle! (The width of the pattern along the middle is the correct method using British Standards.) Boxing pattern size corresponds to the frame eyesize or *A* dimension. The vertical dimension of the pattern is measured vertically between the top and bottom of the box and corresponds to the *B* dimension of the frame. In no case may *A* or *B* dimensions be measured holding the ruler at a tilt or if the pattern is in a rotated position. More accuracy in measurement may

be obtained by using some sort of eyesize gauge (as in Figure 6–2) if the side of the measuring portions are high enough to enclose the outermost portions on both left and right sides. This same gauge can be used to measure lenses and other objects. Even with such a hand-held gauge, the possibility of a slight rotation of the pattern occurs. Because of the critical size accuracy required (especially in edging for metal frames), even a few tenths of a millimeter can make a considerable difference. Because of the desire for exactness, many practitioners choose to

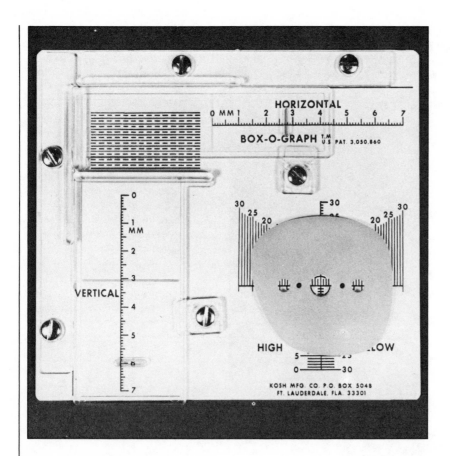

Figure 6–3. *A pattern may be measured on the Box-o-Graph by placing it over the centrally marked circles to assure horizontal and vertical alignment. The A dimension is the sum of the farthest left and right measures. If only A and B dimensions are needed (and not a check on the accuracy of central hole placement), the measures may be taken in the same manner as with lenses, placing the pattern in the upper lefthand corner of the Box-o-Graph. The pattern holes must nevertheless be perfectly horizontal. (Box-o-Graph supplied courtesy of Coburn Optical.)*

use a *Box-o-Graph*[1] for pattern and lens size measurements. The Box-o-Graph is shown in Figure 6–3. This allows a practitioner to be certain that no rotation has occurred.

Measuring Frame Difference

The difference between the horizontal and vertical dimensions of the pattern is the *pattern difference.* Pattern difference has the same numerical value as frame difference. As would be expected, the frame difference is the difference between frame *A* and *B* dimensions. Therefore, the term *frame difference* is used synonymously with *pattern difference.*

Expressed as a simple equation, this takes the form:

$$A - B = \text{frame difference.}$$

The frame difference number is often printed on

---

[1]Box-o-Graph is manufactured by Kosh Mfg. Co., Ft. Lauderdale, Florida.

the pattern and does not change, even when the pattern is used to cut out lenses of different sizes.

Initially it would appear that when eyesize changes for a given frame style, the frame difference should be slightly altered. Were the integrity of the lens shape exactly maintained, this would indeed be the case. However, it must be considered that because of the manner in which the edger operates, each time the size is set higher by one unit, one-half unit is added to the original pattern shape in every direction! (Figure 6–4 illustrates this.)

The point may be more easily visualized by using a theoretical rectangular lens as an example problem.

Example 1:

A pattern is rectangular, having an *A* dimension of 36.5 mm and a *B* dimension of 26.5 mm. The operation should simply enlarge the rectangle without distorting its shape. If the new horizontal measure A_1 is to be 46.5 mm, what should the vertical B_1 measure be?

Solution:

The solution to this problem is a proportionality problem and can be handled by simple algebra. In other words,

36.5 is to 26.5 as 46.5 is to B_1

or $\dfrac{36.5}{26.5} = \dfrac{46.5}{B_1}$,

which transposes to

$$(36.5)\,(B_1) = (46.5)\,(26.5);$$

therefore,

so

$$B_1 = \frac{(46.5)\,(26.5)}{36.5}$$

$$B_1 = 33.76 \text{ mm}.$$

This proportion is shown in Figure 6–5A.

Example 2:

Now suppose we take this same pattern ($A = 36.5$, $B = 26.5$) and put it on an edger. If we set the machine to cut a lens having an eyesize of 46.5, what will B_1 of the edged lens be?

Solution:

The newly cut lens will be 10 mm larger in the A dimension than the pattern. To each side 5 mm have been added. Since 5 mm will also be added above and 5 mm below the top and bottom edges of the pattern size, B_1 will be 10 mm larger, or 36.5 mm. Although this may look more nearly proportional when the two are superimposed as in Figure 6–5B, they are not the same shaped rectangles.

The phenomenon of nonproportionality that occurs is more evident the larger the pattern size is than the actual size of the lens to be ground. It is therefore advantageous to utilize a pattern as close in size to the finished lens as possible. Some manufacturers provide different patterns for different groups of eyesizes for this very reason. Others furnish one size pattern only and manufacture frames that differ slightly in proportionality from size to size. In this manner any sized lens edged with the pattern provided still fits the corresponding eyesize frame.

Calculations Based on Frame Difference

Any group of frames capable of having lenses edged from one pattern will, regardless of eyesize, all have the same frame difference (that is $A - B$). The frame difference number should be marked on the pattern. This marking is for the convenience of the operator during the multifocal lens layout process.

It will be recalled that in order to calculate seg drop or raise that the B dimension of the frame must be known. If the B dimension of the frame size to be used is unknown, it must be either measured using the frame itself (if available) or calculated using the pattern as a basis. This is done by subtracting the frame difference stamped on the pattern from the eyesize.

Example:

A "lenses only" order must be completed for a frame having an eyesize of 48. The frame is not available at the laboratory. Bifocal height has been specified as 18 mm and the frame difference measurement on the pattern is stamped ▢ 4.5. (This means that the pattern is made for the boxing system and, according to that system, the difference of $A - B$ is 4.5 mm.) How much seg drop or raise is required?

Solution:

To calculate seg drop, the B dimension of the lens must be known. The B dimension is calculated as follows:

$$B = \text{eyesize} - \text{frame difference},$$

which in this case will be

$$B = 48 - 4.5$$
$$= 43.5 \text{ mm}.$$

Therefore,

$$\text{seg drop} = \text{seg height} - \frac{B}{2}$$
$$= 18 - \frac{43.5}{2}$$
$$= -3.75 \text{ mm}.$$

(As previously explained, had the frame difference not been marked on the pattern, it could have been figured by measuring both A and B pattern dimensions using a ruler, measuring gauge, or Box-o-Graph.)

Terminology

No matter how carefully a lens is marked, unless the pattern is accurately made, the MRP of the finished lens will not be correctly placed. Layout calculations

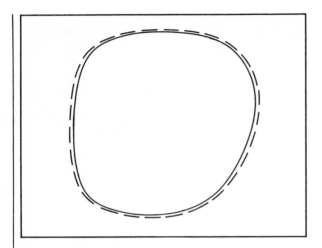

Figure 6–4. *In the figure shown, as the horizontal eye (A) increases by 2 mm; the lens increases in size by 1 mm in every direction.*

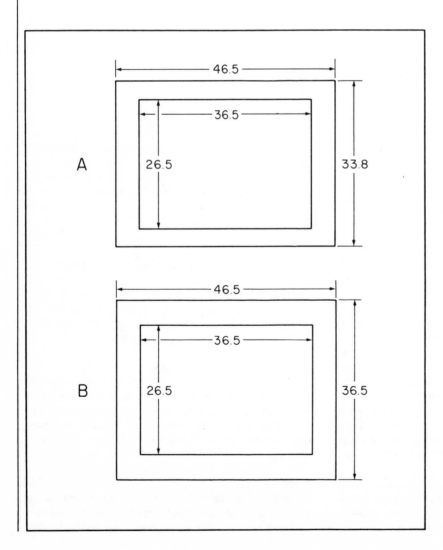

Figure 6–5. *A. These squares have exactly the same shape. B. Here the outer square, created from the inner "pattern" is not the same shape, even though the "frame difference" remains as 10 mm. To be the same shape, both dimensions must increase by equal portions.*

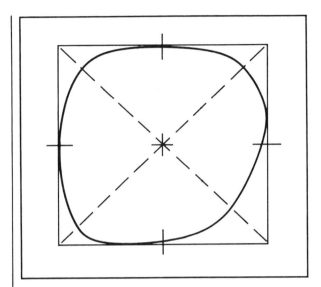

Figure 6–6. *The geometric (boxing) center of a pattern or lens is always at the center of the enclosing box, regardless of where pattern holes are drilled or MRP's are placed.*

for decentration are based on the assumption that the pattern's center of rotation will be at its geometric or boxing center.[2]

When a lens that required decentration is being positioned on a protractor or centering device, the MRP is decentered away from the origin on the protractor or centering screen. The origin of the protractor or screen denotes the future position of the block. This block is attached to the lens at the point that should become the boxing (geometric) center[3] of the lens after it has been edged. Because of the mechanics of the edging system, when the lens is placed in the edger, the center of the block becomes the center of rotation for the lens as it is ground. It only stands to reason, then, that if the middle mounting hole is not at the proper position on the pattern, the lens cannot be positioned in the frame as expected. (As previously discussed, the geometrical center of a pattern (or lens) is the center of the rectangle that completely surrounds the pattern, with each side touching it, as Figure 6–6 illustrates.) Even though the central mounting hole for the pattern should be located directly on the geomet-

rical center, this unfortunately does not happen in every case.

The *mechanical center* of a pattern is that point around which the pattern rotates. (Other names for the mechanical center are the *cutting center* or *edging center*.) It is readily identifiable since it is quite logically found in the middle of the central mounting hole. If the pattern is made for the boxing system, boxing and mechanical centers are coincident.

When the pattern is intentionally constructed so that the center hole does not correspond to the geometrical center of the pattern, it is usually done for the purpose of raising the location of the MRP's, or because the pattern was made for a system other than the boxing system.

For Raising MRP's

Moving the mechanical center of the pattern upward might be considered advantageous in the case of an especially deep frame where the wearer will undoubtedly be looking through an area of the lens opening well above the geometrical center. Because the deviation in location was done ostensibly on optical grounds, the pattern has been referred to by some as being *optically centered;* this pattern is shown in Figure 6–7B. The standard method of pattern construction where mechanical and geometrical centers are coincident with one another is re-

---

[2]Layout calculations for British Standards are based on the assumption that the pattern will rotate around the datum center.

[3]Using British Standards, the datum center.

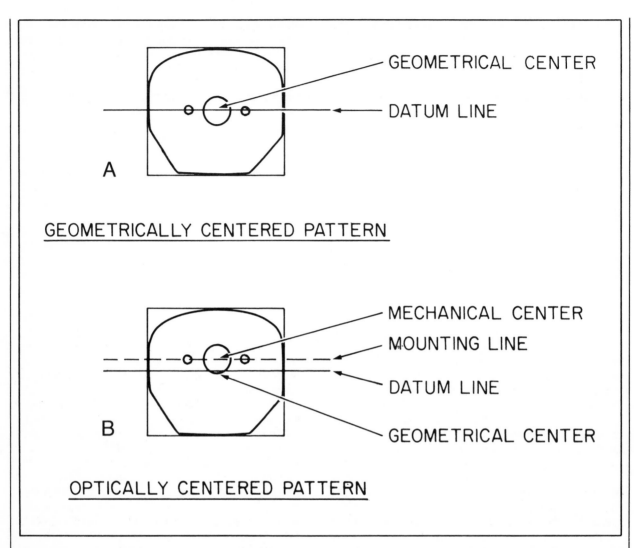

GEOMETRICAL CENTER

DATUM LINE

A

GEOMETRICALLY CENTERED PATTERN

MECHANICAL CENTER

MOUNTING LINE

DATUM LINE

GEOMETRICAL CENTER

B

OPTICALLY CENTERED PATTERN

Figure 6–7. *In this figure,* A *is the conventional construction. The geometrical center is also the mechanical center.*

ferred to as a *geometrically centered pattern,* which is illustrated in Figure 6–7(A). This terminology somehow makes the nonstandard "optically centered pattern" sound as if it is of superior design. This is not the case, since the astute dispenser can overcome potential problems by specifying the vertical location of the major reference points.

Additional Terminology
There are additional terms used to refer to patterns. In conformity with terminology used for ophthalmic lenses, patterns can also be said to have a horizon-

tal *datum line* passing through the boxing or geometrical center.

The horizontal line that passes through the mechanical center of the pattern is referred to as the *mounting line.*[4] When the mechanical center and boxing center coincide, the datum and mounting lines are one and the same. Yet this coincidence is not always the case, as in Figure 6–7B.

---

[4]The location of the pattern mounting line will not necessarily correspond to the frame mounting line, which is arbitrarily defined according to frame construction.

The question now arises as to how the previously marked cutting line of the lens corresponds to the datum and mounting lines. Recall that the cutting line is denoted by the horizontal portion of the cross placed on the uncut lens during marking. It becomes the reference line for blocking and subsequent edging, and is placed to ensure that cylinder axis and major reference point will fall at the desired location. This cutting line becomes the midline for the location of the block, and because the center of the block corresponds to the center of the pattern during edging, the cutting line will always be in the same horizontal plane as the mounting line. Thus, with the lens block placed on the cutting line, cutting and mounting lines will always correspond. Yet it can be seen that when the mechanical center of the pattern is raised, the cutting line of the lens and the datum line no longer correspond. To prevent frustration and lens spoilage, remember this point.

THE CONSEQUENCES OF NONCOINCIDENT MOUNTING AND DATUM LINES

When the mechanical center of a pattern is above its geometrical or boxing center, the MRP of the edged lens will be above its boxing center. (For example, if the pattern's mechanical center is 3 mm above its boxing center, then the MRP of the edged lens will be 3 mm above the boxing center of the edged lens.) If both right and left lenses are of approximately the same power, and both will be edged using the same pattern, a slight vertical elevation will be of no great consequence. Both MRP's will be elevated to the same level, ensuring that there will be no induced vertical prism.

However, consider what may happen at a later point in time if only one lens is to be replaced. If the practitioner who replaces the lens does not have the original pattern, a new one will be made according to standard centering methods. During the fabrication process the MRP height of the nonreplaced lens should be measured. In this manner any potential problem will be avoided, as the MRP of the new lens will be raised to the appropriate matching height. If this is not done and the technician relies solely upon the information given on the order, there will be a discrepancy in the vertical heights of the two lenses. This induces a vertical prismatic effect, making the prescription unacceptable.

When an "optically centered pattern" is used to edge multifocals, noncompensation can be disastrous! For instance, a pattern has a mounting line that is 3 mm higher than the datum line. For bifocals whose desired height is specified as 18 mm, the technician makes all calculations for seg drop on the assumption that this drop is occurring from the centrally placed datum line. Yet in actuality the blocked lens is centered 3 mm *above* the datum line. Consequently instead of having bifocals placed at 18 mm, the top of the bifocal line is at 21 mm!

How to Compensate for Optically Centered Patterns

Compensation for either MRP positioning or multifocal height must be made at the time of lens centration and marking. Once the lens is marked and blocked, no more compensation is possible.

To compensate, the technician must know the distance between pattern boxing and mechanical centers. This can be ascertained by first finding the pattern's *B* dimension, then measuring the vertical distance from the lowest part of the pattern (bottom of the enclosing rectangle) to the mounting line. This measure, less half the *B* dimension, gives the difference between geometrical and mechanical centers.

For multifocal height compensation, the seg top line must be lowered during centration (layout) by the same number of millimeters as the pattern's mounting line is above the datum line. In other words, because of the way the pattern is made, the whole lens will be positioned higher in the frame than it would otherwise be. To compensate for this, lower it during layout.

Example:

During layout the operator checks the pattern and finds it to be optically centered with the mechanical center 3 mm above the boxing center. Pertinent prescription data are as follows:

PD = 66/62
Seg height = 20 mm
Seg style = Flat Top 25
Frame dimensions: A = 52 mm
                                  B = 42 mm
                              DBL = 18 mm

What is the correct amount of seg raise or drop and how would the correctly positioned lens appear before marking?

Solution:

First calculate the seg raise or drop in the conventional manner and then make compensation for the pattern.

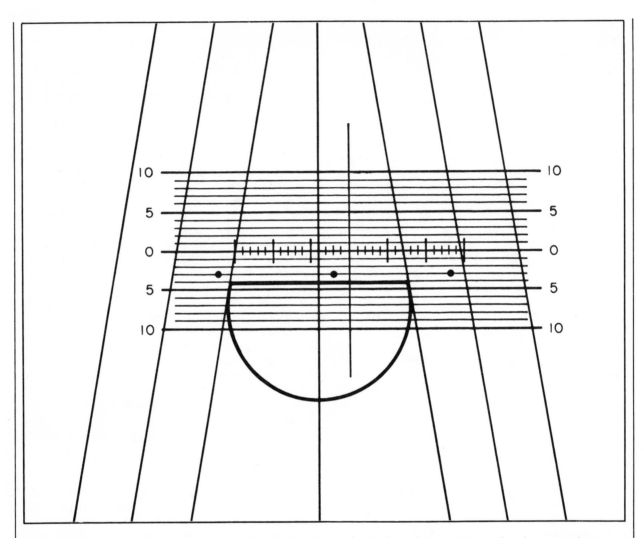

Figure 6–8. *For patterns with a vertically displaced mechanical center, compensation in centration must occur. In the example shown, a seg drop of −1 mm is calculated, but the pattern's mechanical center is 3 mm above its boxing center. Therefore a −4 mm drop is required to achieve the expected segment height.*

$$\text{seg raise or drop} = \text{seg height} - \frac{B}{2}$$

$$= 20 - \frac{42}{2}$$

$$= 20 - 21$$

seg drop = −1 (a minus direction denotes seg drop)

Without compensation the seg would be dropped 1 mm. However, because of the pattern the seg will be raised an additional 3 mm. Therefore the seg must be placed 3 mm lower during layout (−3 additional).

$$\text{seg drop} = -1 -3$$
$$= -4$$

Thus the seg is positioned 4 mm below the horizontal reference line and is ready for marking, as shown in Figure 6–8.

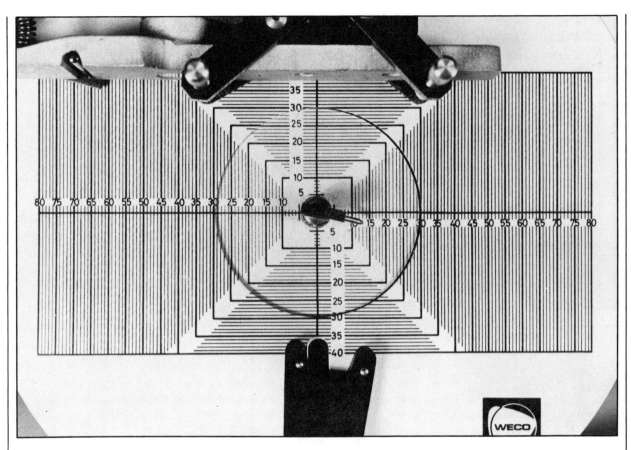

Figure 6–9. *When a technician centers a frame on a pattern maker, the grid assists in alignment.*

PATTERN MAKING

Because of the vast number of available frame styles, it is impossible to have a complete library of patterns so that the correct pattern is available for every frame presented for lens fabrication. Ordering a pattern for every single frame that passes through the laboratory is totally impractical. The delays caused would not be acceptable to the wearer, not to mention the volume of paperwork that would be generated. For this reason a system for making patterns is a necessity.

Systems for pattern making vary in methodology and cost, from a system that consists of a marking pen and pair of shears, up to models having automatic tracing systems. In spite of the variety of available products, there are certain commonalities for all systems.

Frame Setup for Pattern Making

In order to make a pattern the frame must be on hand or, at the very minimum, a labeled tracing from that frame. To make a pattern directly from a frame, all pattern makers require that the frame be properly centered for tracing. This is done so that the mechanical center of the pattern will end up corresponding to the boxing center of the lens shape.

The centering grid on a pattern maker may vary in its construction, but basically it consists of measured distances left, right, up and down from an origin. This central origin represents the position that the mechanical (rotational) center of the pattern will oc-

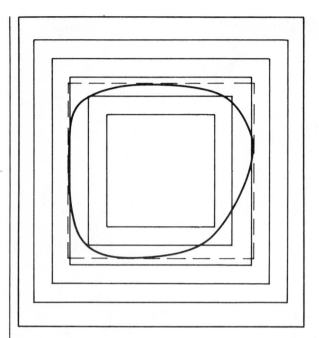

Figure 6–10. *When the technician centers a frame's lens opening for pattern making according to the boxing system, the left extremity must be equal to the right, while the upper and lower extremities must be equal.*

cupy, as Figure 6–9 shows. The lens opening of the frame must then be centered so that the geometric center of its shape is precisely at the middle of the grid origin. This is done, as in Figure 6–10, by making the outermost points to the left and right occupy the same distance from the origin. The uppermost and lowermost points must also be equidistant from the origin.[5]

In actually carrying out this procedure, the frame must be initially oriented with its frame front face down on a centering grid. To ensure that the datum line of the pattern will correspond to the frame datum line and not be tilted, the top of the frame is pressed against a horizontal bar (see Figure 6–11). This horizontal bar will slide up and down, but will not tilt. Tilting the frame causes an off-axis pattern, making it impossible to cut a cylinder lens at the right axis. When centering is achieved, the frame is clamped securely into place and is ready for tracing.

---

[5]To make a pattern for the datum system, the top and bottom reference lines are the highest and lowest tangents to the lens shape, exactly as in the boxing system. However, the left and right reference points are different. Because the pattern's mechanical center must fall at the datum center, the frame must be moved so that the distances from the grid origin to the left and right points striking the eyewire *on the datum line* are equal.

Tracing is most often accomplished by rotating the mounted frame on the pattern maker while a stylus rests inside the frame groove. The stylus is mechanically linked to a cutting mechanism that uses a pantographic system to cut the pattern from a pattern blank. The pattern blank is marked with an *N*, indicating the nasal side. This blank should be placed in the pattern maker so that it indeed corresponds to the nasal side of the frame when cut.

Most "homemade" patterns are cut precisely for the size of the frame. This avoids shape distortion caused by large differences in pattern and finished lens sizes, as was previously described. Maintaining a 1-to-1 eyesize/pattern size ratio may understandably require the use of larger pattern blanks for certain frames. (Pattern blanks are shown in Figure 6–12.) Once the pattern is cut, it may require some smoothing of the edges, depending upon the sophistication of the cutting mechanism. When smoothing is necessary, it may be accomplished with a medium-fine file. File only as much as necessary to remove roughness so the basic shape or size is not changed.

Cut-out Patterns

A system of pattern making that allows the frame shape to be traced directly onto the pattern blank is shown in Figure 6–13.

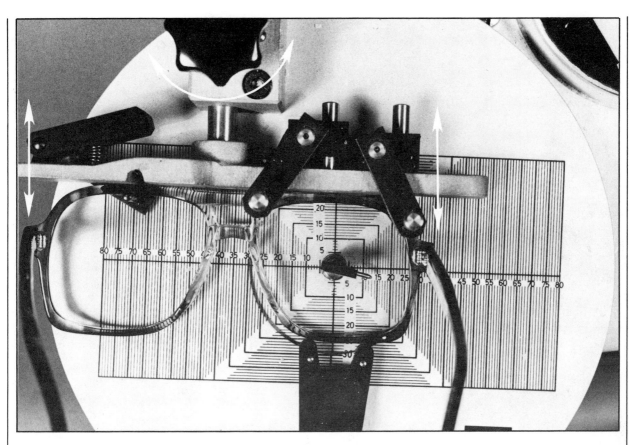

Figure 6–11. *The horizontal bar on a pattern maker gives stability to the frame during the tracing process while simultaneously keeping it level. If tilted, a correct axis is not possible. In the figure shown, the horizontal bar must be raised slightly to allow equal measures both above and below the grid origin.*

The frame is placed on a squaring block containing the pattern to be used. Printed on the pattern is a gridlike scale system to allow for centering. Once the frame is properly centered, the shape is traced around the inside of the eyewire (as in Figure 6–14). Then small, sturdy cutting shears are used to cut around the marked shape (see Figure 6–15). A file or the side of a hand edger wheel is used to smooth off rough edges, as Figure 6–16 shows. A pattern made in this manner cannot be assumed to have the same size as the frame's eyesize, unless compensation is made.

Making a Pattern from a Lens Tracing

Upon occasion a special order will be received that lists no frame name, but only a tracing of the lens that is presently being worn in the frame. Such a request is difficult to fill properly, and indeed cannot be adequately filled unless certain specifications are given. These are:

1. The size of the lens. (Do not assume that the tracing is the same size as the lens. When a lens is traced, the tracing is naturally larger than the lens, or if the frame eyewire were traced, it is considerably smaller.)
2. The distance between lenses (DBL) to allow calculation for decentration.
3. The 180-degree line. (If the lens is traced in an even slightly rotated position, the cylinder axis will be incorrect.)

One possibility for filling such a request is to find a pattern that most closely approximates the shape and

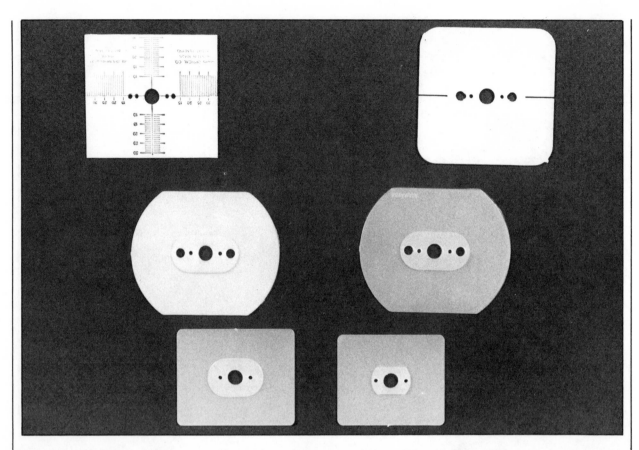

Figure 6–12. *Pattern blanks come in a variety of shapes and sizes. When cutting patterns on a 1-to-1 ratio, the blank when centered must be large enough to completely cover the frame's lens opening.*

will not cut any corners from the required shape. The lens is edged, then reshaped by hand until correct, holding the lens up to the tracing for comparison.

Another method is to carefully mark the datum line on the tracing, then draw a vertical line through the geometrical center. A pattern blank capable of being cut with shears may also be marked in the same manner, as in Figure 6–17. The tracing is cut out and placed on the pattern blank so that horizontal and vertical markings align (see Figure 6–18), then traced about with a marking pen (as in Figure 6–19). The marked shape is then cut from the blank in the same manner as was seen in Figure 6–15. Such a pattern should be checked for center displacement using the method that will be described shortly, so as to ensure accuracy of the PD and seg height.

Edgers That Make Patterns
Some edgers are adaptable, as they allow the practitioner to make a pattern by grinding the pattern blank on the edger wheel as if it were a lens. Keep in mind, though, that such a system requires exactly the same amount of time and accuracy in correctly positioning the frame as is required in operating a standard pattern marker.

Using Lenses as Patterns
An old or paired lens may be used as a pattern on some edgers having an adapting kit. When this is done, the pattern lens must be precisely clamped on-center and at the correct 180-degree meridian. In addition, the pressure must be set at its lightest so as not to chip the pattern lens. To help prevent

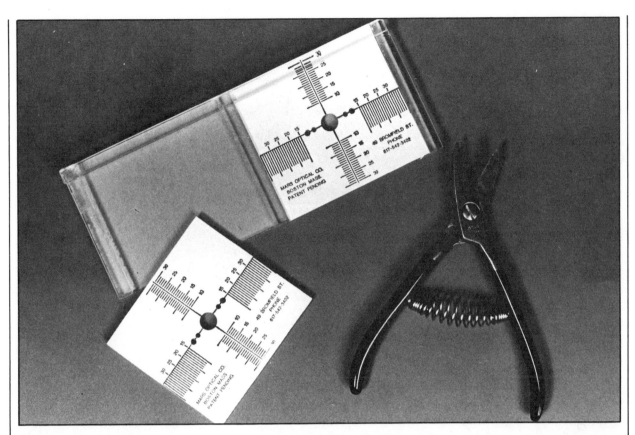

Figure 6–13. *Using principles identical to those of the more expensive pattern making instruments, kits are available for making patterns by hand. (Mars Pattern Kit supplied courtesy of Mars Optical Co.)*

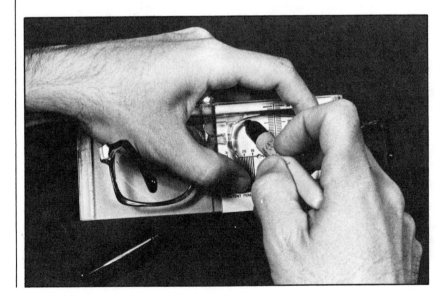

Figure 6–14. *The pattern is first positioned by holding it securely against the upper horizontal bar and sliding the pattern vertically in its holder until the correct vertical alignment is achieved. Sliding the frame left or right gives a centered horizontal alignment. The shape is traced using the pen provided. Take care to avoid marking the frame with the pen.*

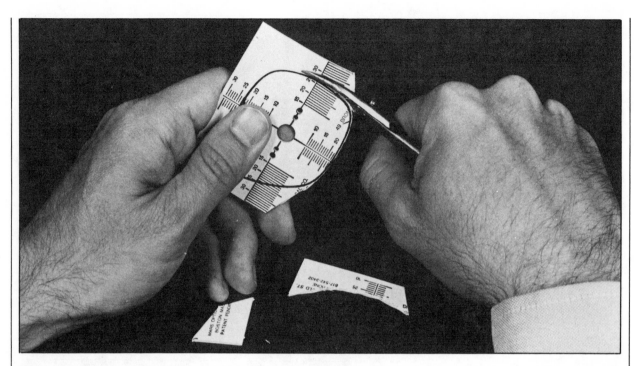

Figure 6–15. *Curved cutting shears help to cut around corners.*

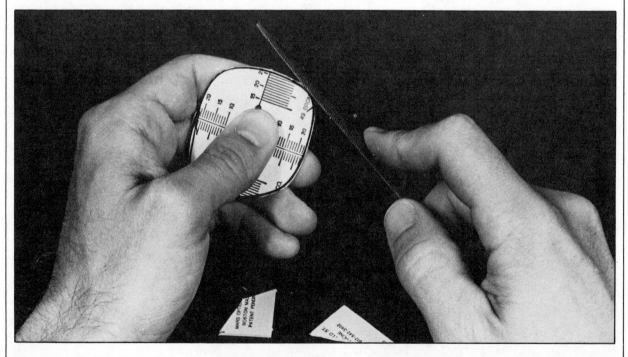

Figure 6–16. *Smoothing pattern roughness with a file gives better size and shape.*

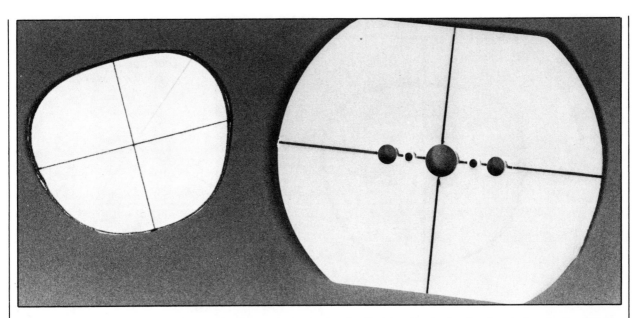

Figure 6–17. *A pattern can be made from a lens tracing by first boxing in the tracing to locate the boxing center. (A horizontal should have been indicated in some manner on the tracing to assure axis accuracy.) If a premarked pattern blank is unavailable, a standard blank can be marked.*

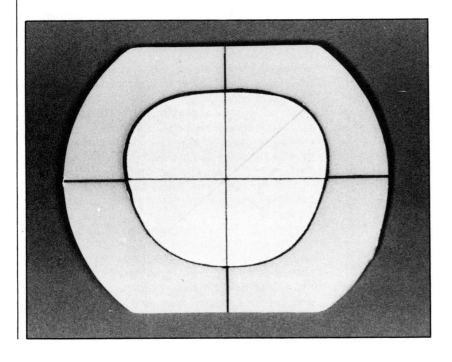

Figure 6–18. *The cut-out tracing substitutes for a frame. It is placed on the pattern blank so that the boxing center corresponds to the mechanical center of the blank.*

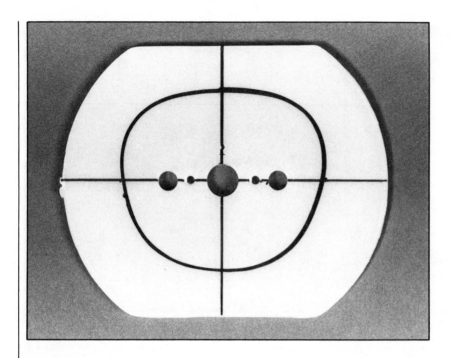

chipping, some practitioners smear petroleum jelly on the edger's clapper plate upon which the lens turns in order to reduce friction.

Checking Pattern Shape

Some practitioners consider it advisable to check the newly cut pattern's size and shape. As Figure 6–20 shows, this may be done by physically inserting the pattern in the frame as if it were a lens. This is done without heating the frame. Areas of slight shape distortion may be corrected by filing or by hand grinding against the side of a ceramic hand edging wheel (as shown in Figure 6–21). The face of a diamond hand edger also may be used.

If the pattern fits tightly into the frame it can be assumed that the pattern is .5 mm smaller than required. If the fit is acceptable, but not especially tight, the pattern is a full millimeter smaller. Appropriate compensation can then be made when the edger is set for lens size.

Compensation for Pattern Central Hole Displacement

Despite careful setup for cutting patterns, errors can occur that cause a displacement of the pattern's central hole (mechanical center). Unfortunately, the amount of lateral displacement that occurs in the pattern will cause double the amount of error in the resulting PD. This occurs because of the fact that the lenses will be displaced in opposite directions! However, if the error is discovered before the lenses are marked, an appropriate compensation may be made, which is carried out in the same manner as in compensating for the optically centered pattern.

A Simple Pattern Measuring System

In order to make any kind of compensation for displacement, first determine if a displacement has occurred, and if so, to what extent. The simplest of such systems can be made from a piece of centimeter graph paper. A central x,y coordinate cross is drawn and circles carefully added by drawing through the holes of an existing pattern. These circles must not be displaced and should be checked to ensure that they are absolutely centered. Numbers are added for ease of reference, in the manner shown in Figure 6–22. The pattern may now be placed on the completed sheet so that the drawn circles may be seen through the holes. The outermost point on the pattern in each of the four directions should be noted. For the pattern to pass as acceptable, top and bottom numbers must be identical. The numbers in the horizontal meridian to the far left and right must also match.

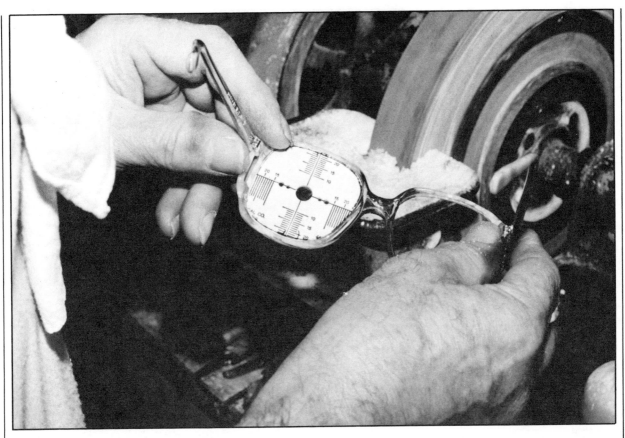

Figure 6–20. *To help in better shape duplication, handmade patterns may be slipped into the frame. Inconsistencies in shape between frame and pattern are more readily apparent and can be filed or ground into better conformity.*

As may be remembered from an earlier section in this chapter, a homemade graph paper system is not the only available method for checking of pattern accuracy. A system using identical methods is available on a Box-o-Graph, as was seen in Figure 6–3.

Other systems have also been devised by individual laboratories. One such device enables the pattern to be mounted, then turned every 90 degrees so that each side may be measured with a horizontal bar connected to a digital readout. Each pattern made locally can then be checked for accuracy and any required compensation immediately calculated.

Determining Direction and Amount of Error

Once an error has been discovered, the amount of error and its direction must be determined. The most straightforward manner to determine a lateral error, for example, is to slide the pattern left or right until both horizontal measures are the same. The amount of displacement of the pattern's central hole gives a direct reading of the error. (The primary disadvantage to this system is the difficulty in determining accurately just how far the pattern center has moved.) Displacement is noted as being toward the nasal or temporal side of the pattern and not as left or right. This system can be illustrated by the following example.

Example:
A pattern is checked for accuracy and is found to be vertically centered, but horizontally off. How can the error be corrected?

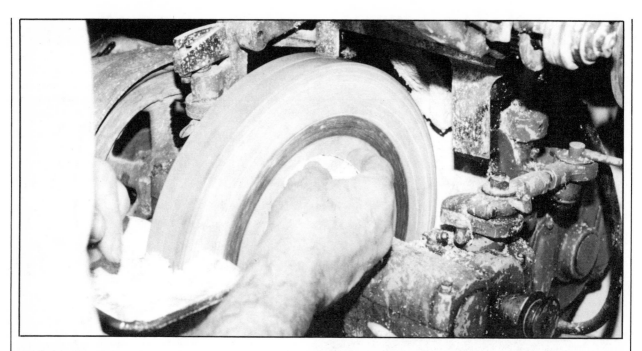

Figure 6–21. *Smoothing or reshaping the edge of a handmade pattern on the side of a hand edger is a fast alternative to filing.*

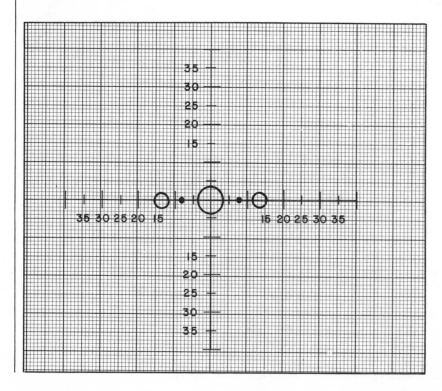

Figure 6–22. *A grid to check pattern size and central hole placement can be made from ordinary millimeter graph paper.*

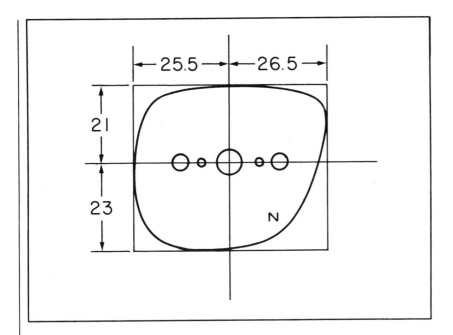

Figure 6–23. *Were this pattern to be used for a multifocal prescription, the distance and near PD's would both be 2 mm too large. The segment height would also be a millimeter higher than anticipated.*

Solution:

The pattern is shifted until both left and right sides are equal. In this position the central hole is 1 mm too far temporally, as Figure 6–23 illustrates. If the lens were marked and blocked normally it would be edged with the MRP exactly where the central pattern hole is, i.e., 1 mm too far outward. This also means that the PD would be 2 mm larger than ordered. Therefore, to compensate, each lens must be decentered an extra millimeter inward, above and beyond the otherwise calculated amount.

It can be readily seen that compensation must take place in the opposite direction from the direction of pattern center displacement. (See Table 6–1.)

Table 6–1. Pattern Center Displacement Compensation

If the pattern center is displaced	The lens must be decentered
Temporally	Nasally
Nasally	Temporally
Upward	Downward
Downward	Upward

A more accurate method for determining correct compensation is to leave the pattern centered, but to note the distance of opposing sides from the mechanical center (central hole center) and calculate the compensation. Beginning in the vertical dimension it can be seen that the distance above the mounting line intersecting the mechanical center plus the distance below will give the *B* dimension. If the pattern is correct, the distance to the top minus the distance to the bottom equals zero. If they are not equal, the difference between the two measures divided by 2 gives the required compensation. Expressed as a formula this would be written as

$$\frac{top - bottom}{2} = \text{vertical compensation required.}$$

If the results are positive the lens must be raised; if negative, lowered.

The same system applies to lateral compensation.

$$\frac{temporal - nasal}{2} = \text{lateral compensation.}$$

Thus, if the result is a positive number the mechanical center is displaced too far nasalward, requiring that the lens be decentered outward. However, if a negative number results, the mechanical center is too far temporalward, requiring the lens to be decentered inward.

Example:

The pattern shown in Figure 6–23 is in error both vertically and laterally. Were this pattern to be used, what compensations would be necessary to ensure the accuracy of seg height and PD?

Solution:

Horizontal and vertical components are considered separately. To determine the vertical displacement of the mechanical center, note that the pattern top is 21 mm high while the bottom is 23. Therefore

$$\frac{21 - 23}{2} = -1.$$

This means that the lens MRP or seg height must be lowered 1 mm more than otherwise calculated.

For lateral compensation, note the temporal measurement is 25.5 mm and the nasal 26.5 mm. Therefore

$$\frac{25.5 - 26.5}{2} = -0.5 \text{ mm.}$$

This means that the MRP must be decentered in by .5 millimeter. This is in addition to the amount normally required.

Horizontal Alignment for Datum Centered Patterns

To determine whether a pattern is made according to the datum system, measure the *C* dimension of the pattern. If the mechanical center is located at the midpoint of the *C,* the pattern is a datum system pattern. Unless both *A* and *C* dimensions are equal, boxing calculated decentration will produce an incorrect PD. There are two means by which the pattern can nevertheless be used. The first is to treat that pattern as if the mechanical center had been "misplaced" and then appropriately compensate by using the method outlined previously.

The second means is more direct: Calculate decentration in the manner commonly employed if British Standards are used. The frame is measured along the datum line, from the inside temporal edge of one eyewire to the inside nasal edge of the other. (See Figure A1–2 in Appendix 1.) This measure is actually the same as the datum center distance and is equal to the datum length (same as boxing *C*) plus the datum DBL. The PD is subtracted from this measure and divided by two to obtain the datum decentration per lens.

$$\frac{(\text{datum length} + \text{datum DBL}) - \text{PD}}{2}$$
$$= \text{datum decentration per lens.}$$

For a more complete explanation of the two systems, refer to Appendix 1.

PATTERNLESS SYSTEMS

A *patternless system* for edging lenses is one that stores all lens shape information in a central computer, then recalls the shape when a code number is input. The central computer is hooked up to the lens edger so that the grinding mechanism may be computer driven.

Despite the advantage of not having to always keep patterns on hand, patterns are required initially. Information is fed into the system by a tracing of the pattern's rotational movement.

PATTERN ON THE EDGER

When a pattern is placed on the edger, it must be positioned so that the lens being cut will be edged for the individual wearer's eye. It must then be reversed for the paired lens. Usually this may be quickly visualized. If, for example, the convex side of the lens as it would be in the edger faces left, then a right lens requires that the nasal side of the pattern be nearest the operator.

PROFICIENCY TEST QUESTIONS

1. A pattern has an *A* dimension of 46 and a pattern difference of 5. If the *A* dimension of the lens to be cut is 50, what will the *B* dimension of the lens be?
   a. 45
   b. 55
   c. 46
   d. 54
   e. 41

2. A pattern is marked with a frame difference of 7 mm. If the lens eyesize is 50 mm and the seg height is to be 19 mm, how large is the seg drop?
   a. −2.5 mm
   b. −6 mm
   c. −9.5 mm
   d. −1 mm
   e. none of the above is correct.

3. If a pattern has a frame difference of 10, and a 50-mm eyesize frame has a *B* dimension of 40, what *B* dimension does a 55-mm eyesize have?
   a. 44 mm
   b. 45 mm
   c. 46 mm
   d. 40 mm
   e. none of the above is correct.

4. A pattern has a pattern difference of 7. How much seg drop is indicated for a frame with an *A* dimension of 52 and a seg height of 17 mm?
   a. −12.5 mm
   b. −9 mm
   c. −7.5 mm
   d. −5.5 mm
   e. none of the above is correct.

5. If a pattern is made for use with the boxing system, where will it have its central hole?
   a. Boxing center
   b. Datum center
   c. Optical center
   d. Major reference point

6. What is the point on a pattern around which it *always* rotates?
   a. Boxing center
   b. Datum center
   c. Mechanical center
   d. Optical center

e. Major reference point

7. Which three terms are always synonymous?
   a. Datum center
   b. Cutting center
   c. Mechanical center
   d. Boxing center
   e. Edging center

8. T or F Optically centered patterns invariably produce superior results from an optical standpoint.

9. What is the name given to the horizontal line that *always* passes through the mechanical center of the pattern?
   a. Datum line
   b. Mounting line
   c. B line

10. For the following Rx, an optically centered pattern having its mechanical center 3 mm above the geometrical center is used. How much decentration per lens is in order?

    +4.75D sph
    +4.50D sph
    height of OC's = 25 mm
    A = 49
    B = 47
    ED = 54
    DBL = 18
    PD = 63

11. A frame has the following dimensions:

    A = 46
    B = 42
    C = 46
    DBL = 18

    The pattern to be used has the mechanical center 2.5 mm above the boxing center. If the correct seg height for the prescription is 18 mm, what drop below the horizontal reference line is correct?
    a. −3 mm
    b. −2.5 mm
    c. −20.5 mm
    d. −5.5 mm
    e. None of the above is correct.

12. When someone makes a pattern to be used with the datum system, what must be set first?
    a. The uppermost and lowermost points must be made vertically equidistant from the grid origin.

117

b. The left and right sides of the lens opening must be made equidistant from the grid origin.

c. It is unimportant which is done first.

13. If a lens is to be made from a tracing that was done from an old lens, which of the following need not be specially marked or described?
    a. Eyesize
    b. 180-degree line
    c. DBL
    d. Cylinder axis position in old lens

14. If an old lens were spotted at its boxing center, placed with this spot over the pattern hole, and traced onto a pattern blank, which parameter would be most likely to be in error if the pattern were cut out and used?
    a. PD
    b. Seg height
    c. Cylinder axis
    d. Sphere power

15. A homemade pattern is placed on a Box-o-Graph to check it for accuracy. From the mechanical center, the outermost tangents in each direction are as follows:

    top 23 mm
    bottom 23 mm
    nasal 26 mm
    temporal 24 mm

    What decentration compensation must be made during layout?
    a. Decenter each lens an additional 1 mm in.
    b. Decenter each lens 1 mm *less* in than would be otherwise indicated.
    c. Decenter each lens an additional 2 mm in.
    d. Decenter each lens 2 mm *less* in than would otherwise be indicated.

16. If a pattern center is displaced nasally, how must the lens be decentered to compensate for the error?
    a. Nasally
    b. Temporally
    c. The decentration depends upon lens power.

17. A pattern made on a pattern maker has the central hole displaced 1 mm too high and 1 mm too far nasally. For a single vision lens, how much vertical and horizontal decentration is required to obtain a properly centered lens when the lens is placed in a frame having the following dimensions?

    A = 46
    B = 43
    C = 45
    ED = 48
    DBL = 18
    wearer's PD = 60

    a. 2 in, 1 up
    b. 3 in, 1 up
    c. 3 in, 1 down
    d. 1 in, 1 down
    e. None of the above is correct.

18. When using a datum centered pattern, decentration per lens equals which of the following?
    a. $\dfrac{A + \text{boxing DBL} - \text{PD}}{2}$
    b. $\dfrac{A + \text{datum DBL} - \text{PD}}{2}$
    c. $\dfrac{C + \text{datum DBL} - \text{PD}}{2}$
    d. $\dfrac{A + \text{MBL} - \text{PD}}{2}$

Chapter 7

Edging

The process of lens edging has not always been one of placing an entire lens blank in an automatic diamond wheel edger and cutting the lens to finished form in one operation. In the past, much more of the process was done by hand.

CUTTING AND CHIPPING

The cutting and chipping process used so regularly in the past consisted of outlining the desired lens shape on the glass lens with an appropriate marking instrument. The shape was then cut into the lens surface using a glass cutter (as shown in Figures 7–1, 7–2, and 7–3). The glass cutter did not cut through the glass, but simply scored the surface so that the outermost unwanted portions of the lens would break away clean along the scored line.

Then a more refined system was developed that made use of the lens pattern, as Figure 7–4 shows; this method allowed the lens to be scored in the exact outline of the desired shape. In both free-hand or guided scoring, the lens was cut several millimeters larger than required to allow room for some inaccuracy in breaking away of the lens and for an even lens edge finish.

After lens cutting, the outermost areas of glass were removed using chipping pliers that were, and still are, available in a variety of designs (see Figure 7–5). The outer lens areas may be removed by loosely grasping the lens near the scored section, as Figure 7–6A shows, and breaking it away with a twist, as in Figure 7–6B.

Lenses may also be chipped to size without being scored. Chipping pliers are used to "nibble" away the glass a little at a time from the edge, while slightly squeezing the plier, combined with twisting the hand via the forearm in a rotational movement away from the individual. The other hand holds the lens near the edge being chipped, as in Figure 7–7. After chipping to shape, the lens can be hand edged to size using a ceramic wheel. All scoring and chipping procedures are, of course, only applicable with glass lenses.

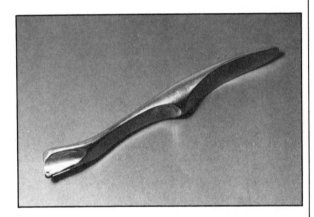

Figure 7–1. A "cutting spoon" has a small cutting wheel that cuts and rolls across a surface to create a scored line.

AUTOMATIC EDGING WITH CERAMIC WHEELS

Automatic diamond wheel edgers had as their forerunner the automatic rimless edger with a ceramic wheel. This equipment put a flat edge on the lenses, which was sufficient for the majority of prescription work being done at the time. If any other edge configuration was used it had to be done by hand.

The ceramic wheel itself is composed of grit and a bonding agent that is cast to shape, fired in a kiln, then machined to proper specifications.[1]

When the abrasive material wears, losing its cutting ability, the bonding agent either dissolves or falls apart, allowing the worn grit to fall away, exposing fresh, sharp material. This principle still applies with higher-speed, diamond bond wheels. Ceramic wheels give an excellent, smooth finish and are still used, though not exclusively, for hand edging. Ceramic wheels have a long life because, with the exception of the central hub, they are composed entirely of abrasive grit and bonding material.

[1]Hans Hirschhorn, "Modern Edging Methods—Part I," *The Optical Index,* Vol. 55, No. 4, April 1980, p. 93.

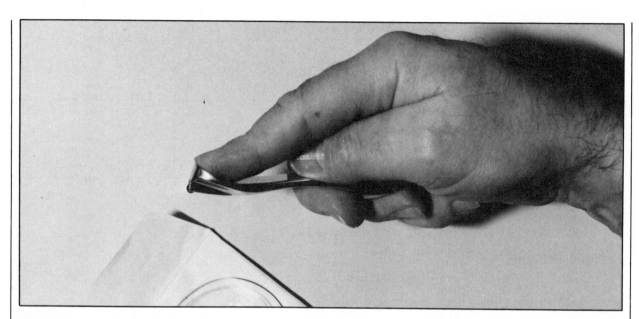

Figure 7–2. *Holding the cutting spoon for optimum control.*

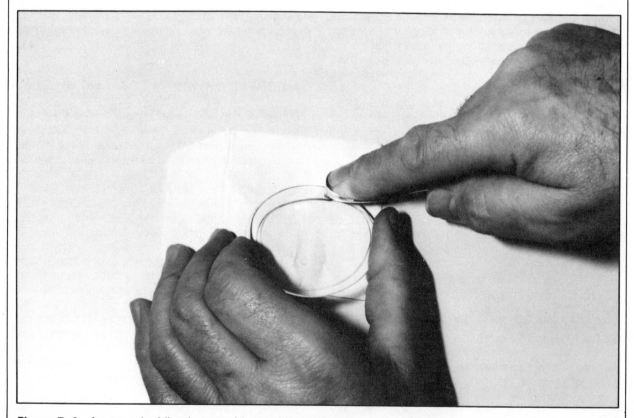

Figure 7–3. *A premarked line is scored by tracing around the shape a single time.*

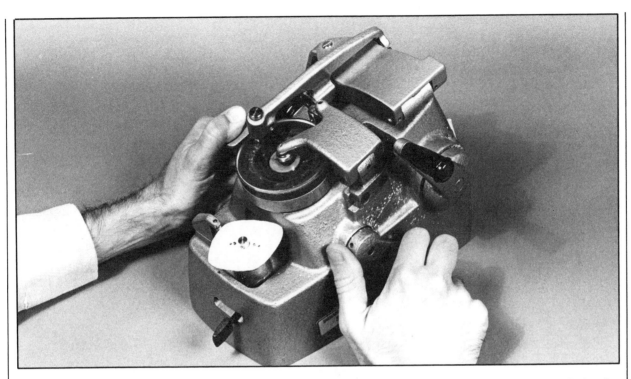

Figure 7–4. *The same function as the cutting spoon can be performed on a lens cutter with the help of a pattern.*

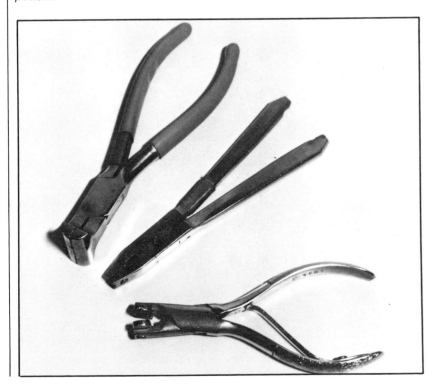

Figure 7–5. *Chipping pliers come in a variety of designs, allowing for the preference of the individual and the thickness of the lens being chipped or broken away.*

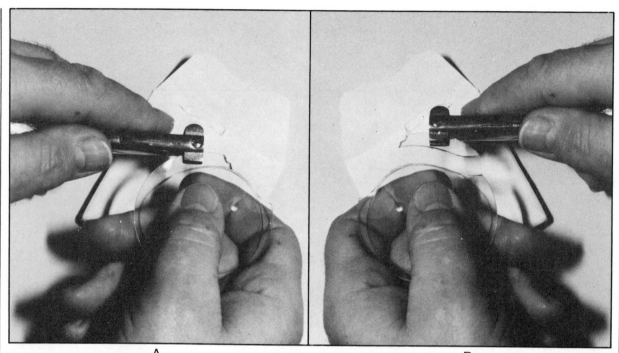

A   B

Figure 7–6. A *The lens is grasped near the scored section for support as sections are snapped off.* B *Scored lenses that are not excessively thick break off in fairly large pieces even if very little force is exerted.*

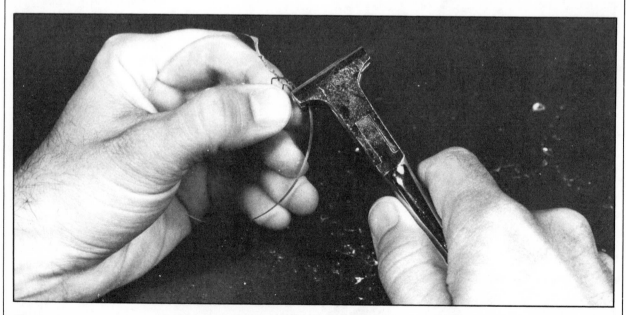

Figure 7–7. *Lenses may be chipped without scoring by nibbling away at the edge with a turning motion of the pliers.*

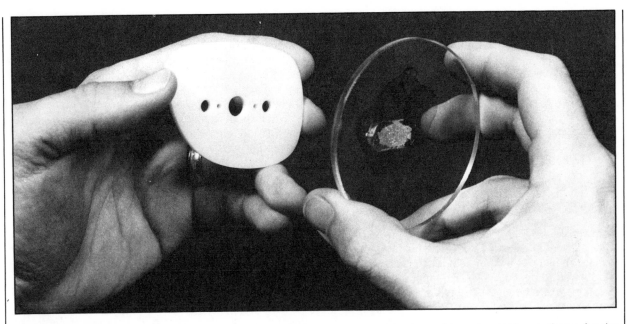

Figure 7–8. *When a lens is placed into the edger, the pattern must be turned to cut a right eye shape for the right lens. Fortunately most lens blocks are made to prohibit the lens from being placed in the edger upside-down.*

THE EDGING PROCESS

The basic principles in lens edging have remained approximately the same since automatic ceramic edgers were first developed. Of course vast improvements in edger wheel construction, machine cycling patterns, and bevel placement and style have occurred over time.

The edging process generally begins when the operator places the pattern on the edger so that it is properly oriented to cut either the left or right lens. (By convention, most operators begin with the right lens.) Assuming the front surface of the lens is facing left, then the pattern will, in most cases, be right side up with the nasal half in the direction of the operator (see Figure 7–8). The lens must then also be oriented right side up. Fortunately most blocking systems are now constructed so that they will not fit the edger chuck if oriented upside-down.

For the left lens, the pattern must be removed and turned around so that the nasal side is away from the operator. Then the edger must be set so that it will cut the lens to the required size.

Edger Settings
It stands to reason that if all lens patterns were exactly the same size as the required finished lens,

then no size setting would be required. The edger could duplicate the pattern exactly in a 1-to-1 relationship. However, this would mean that instead of having one pattern for each frame shape, a separate pattern would be required for every available size!

This raises the question of pattern size. When patterns were first used with rimless edgers, far fewer shapes were available. So that the operator would know how to set the machine, it was necessary for all patterns to have one standard size. The "standard size" was set by the manufacturer such that American Optical patterns, for instance, were 37 mm in their *A* dimension, Shuron patterns were 36.5 mm, and some European types were standardized at 40 mm.

What this meant was, if an instrument was calibrated for a 37-mm pattern, when a 42-mm eyesize lens was required, the instrument dial could be set for 42 mm, and the lens would cut out to have an *A* dimension of exactly 42 mm. This assumes, of course, that the requisite 37-mm pattern was used. Eventually, within the United States, a standard pattern size of 36.5 mm evolved.

Any of the previously mentioned small standard pattern sizes was appropriate when most eyewear was being fit in very conservative sizes. With the advent of major frame style changes, lenses began to be edged for sizes significantly larger than the pattern, giving rise to problems of "pattern distortion." Because an equal amount of glass was being added to the original shape in every direction, the integrity of the original shape was being lost. The only feasible solution was to issue a pattern for larger style frames that was closer to the actual lens size being cut.

Now if the pattern is larger than the standard size, compensation in the edger setting must be made. Without compensation the lens will be edged larger than the frame eyesize. If the lens is 2 mm larger than the standard, the lens will be 2 mm larger than the frame eyesize.

Example 1:

A pattern is supplied for a certain frame. This pattern measures 46.5 in its *A* dimension. Suppose the lens is to be edged for a 50-mm eyesize. If the edger is calibrated for a pattern size standard of 36.5 mm, what size lens will be edged if the edger sizing dial is set for 50 mm?

Solution:

For this edger, a 36.5-mm pattern is expected to produce the lens size at which the dial is set. If a 50-mm lens is desired, the dial is set at 50 mm. However, since the pattern is 10 mm too large, the lens produced will also be 10 mm too large. Setting the edger at 50 mm in conjunction with this pattern will produce a lens having a 60-mm eyesize.

Example 2:

In order to produce a lens of the correct eyesize for Example 1, at what setting would the edger sizing dial have to be?

Solution:

Since this 46.5-mm pattern, being 10 mm larger than the standard, produces lenses 10 mm too big, then 10 mm must be subtracted from the required eyesize.

$$50 \text{ mm} - 10 \text{ mm} = 40 \text{ mm}.$$

To arrive at a 50-mm lens, the edger must be set for 40 mm.

Set Numbers

Whenever a compensation must be made for a pattern that deviates from a given standard size, that numerical compensation is referred to as the *set number*. Because patterns are now almost always larger than the standard, this difference must be subtracted from the eyesize. For this reason, set numbers are seen as negative numbers.

Patterns that accompany a manufacturer's frame in most cases have a set number stamped directly on the pattern. Knowing the eyesize and pattern set number should allow an edger setting to be made directly without measuring the pattern. It is advisable, though, to check each new pattern for accuracy when first received.

Example:

A lens is to be edged for a frame having an *A* dimension of 53 mm. The pattern has the set number −5 stamped on it. What is the proper edger setting? If measured, what would the expected *A* dimension of the pattern be?

Solution:

"Set −5" means that 5 mm must be deducted from the desired lens size. Therefore, the edger setting is 53 − 5 = 48 mm. If the edger is set for 48 mm using this pattern, a 53-mm lens will be ground. "Set −5" also means that the pattern is 5 mm larger than the standard size, which in the U.S. would be 36.5 mm. This pattern can be expected to have an *A* dimension of 41.5 mm.

Generally, edger dials are marked in one of three ways. The first is a direct eyesize reading as in Figure 7–9. The edger is set exactly as previously described, with pattern set numbers being subtracted from the eyesize to obtain the setting. When such an edger is calibrated for a standard size pattern whose *A* dimension is 36.5 mm, setting the edger at 36.5 mm will always produce a lens of exactly the same size as the pattern. In other words, if a pattern is made directly from a frame and duplicates the frame size, then a 36.5-mm setting will give the correct lens size.

Example 1:

A frame has a 55-mm eyesize. A pattern is made on a 1-to-1 ratio and when finished also measures 55 mm. What is the set number for the pattern? What must the edger setting be?

Solution:

Since pattern set number = standard size − actual pattern size, then in this instance

$$\text{pattern size} = 36.5 - 55$$
$$= -18.5 \text{ mm}.$$

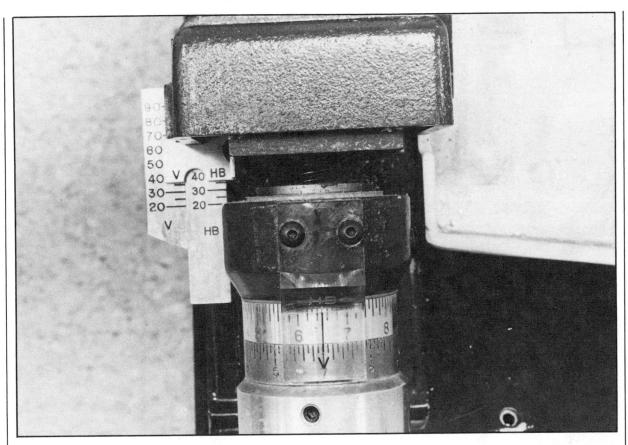

Figure 7–9. *This type of edger dial allows eyesize to be set directly—after having compensated for the pattern set number, of course. There are two separate scales. One is for the V-bevel wheel, the other for the hidden bevel.*

The pattern set number has been determined to be −18.5.

Now since

edger setting = eyesize + set number,

then for our example

edger setting = 55 − 18.5
= 36.5 mm.

To introduce the second edger dial configuration, let us begin by considering a second example.

Example 2:

Suppose that after having made this 55-mm pattern, the operator wishes later to use it for a 57-mm eyesize frame. How far from the 36.5-mm setting must the edger dial be moved and in which direction in order to achieve the correct lens size for the 57 mm frame?

Solution:

To make a lens 2 mm bigger than the previous one, set the edger 2 mm greater than it was before, or at 38.5 mm. Calculating in the traditional manner gives identical results:

edger setting = 57 − 18.5
= 38.5 mm.

A Second Dial Configuration

From the preceding information it can be seen that there is a certain dial setting on every edger at which

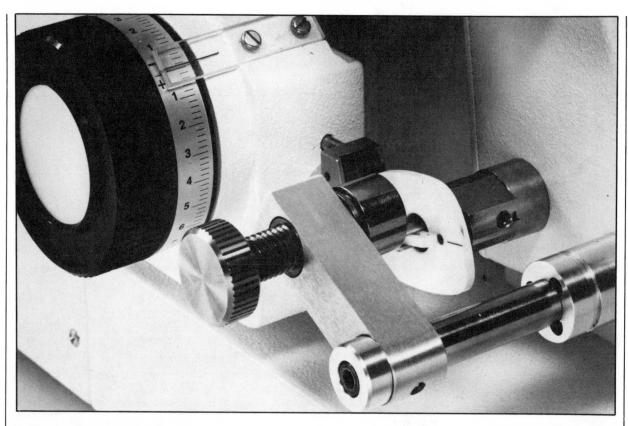

Figure 7–10. *If a pattern is used having the same size as the lens to be ground, a plus-minus scale would require a zero setting. If the pattern is not the same size as the lens, then the size difference is added or subtracted by means of the dial. (Photo courtesy of Essilor.)*

lenses will be produced at exactly the same size as the pattern being used. For those edgers just described that have a direct millimeter scale reading, the setting for edging 1-to-1 corresponds to the "standard" pattern size. In the previous examples the standard setting was 36.5. The second system of edger dial calibration eliminates the direct eyesize readings and instead places a "zero" at that point where a 1-to-1 pattern/lens ratio prevails. The dial is still marked off in millimeters, but it is numbered above and below the zero. (See Figure 7–10.)

The operator dials in the difference in millimeters between the lens size and the desired pattern size. With this type of system,

$$\text{edger setting} = \text{lens size} - \text{pattern size.}$$

Taking the previously given example: In this second system of edger setting when a 55 mm pattern is used and a 57 mm edged lens is desired

$$\begin{aligned} \text{edger setting} &= 57 \text{ mm} - 55 \text{ mm} \\ &= +2 \text{ mm,} \end{aligned}$$

meaning that the dial is turned to a plus two reading.

There are advantages to both systems. The strict eyesize dial works best when premanufactured patterns with printed set numbers are used. But when homemade patterns are used, many practitioners prefer the second system of a zero position with markings to indicate how much larger or smaller the lens should be than the pattern.

A Combination System

The third system is really a combination of the previous two. Both types of scales are printed on the dial. If the standard size chosen for the pattern is 36.5 mm, the zero mark will of necessity be printed

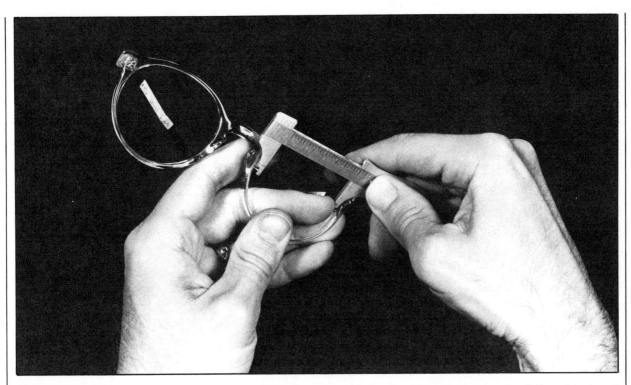

Figure 7–11. *In the boxing system, the vernier caliper can only be used to measure eyesize if the widest part of the shape is confined to one horizontal plane; as, for example, when* A *and* C *dimensions are equal. (With the datum system, the vernier may always be used, as the eyesize is the width along the datum line.)*

adjacent to that size number.

It should be noted that when an edger is equipped with more than two grinding wheels there may be more than one complete set of scales on the edger dial, as Figure 7–9 illustrates. Each scale may be independently recalibrated for grinding wheel wear since groove depth on each wheel may vary, influencing the final lens size.

DEVIATIONS FROM CALCULATED EDGER SETTINGS

During the course of time the experienced lab technician will find that certain frames run somewhat larger or smaller than actually marked. Therefore, it is not unusual to find that if the technician relies totally on the marked frame size to set the edger, the lens may not fit the frame.

To assure a correct fit, the eyesize can be measured. In measuring, remember that when using the boxing system the *A* dimension is the distance between two parallel vertical lines enclosing the lens or lens opening in the frame, and not necessarily the width of the lens across the middle (*C*) as used in the datum system. (See Appendix A, Figure A1–4.)

When the technician measures a frame for a boxing system *A* dimension, if the frame is equal to the *C* dimension, the widest portion of the lens opening is right in the middle. Therefore, the frame can be measured directly using an appropriate set of calipers or a slide gauge, as Figure 7–11 shows. In this manner no estimate for depth of frame groove is needed, since the measuring device fits directly into the groove. The *C* dimension can always be measured directly. When it is not possible to obtain the widest dimension on a horizontal plane, a millimeter

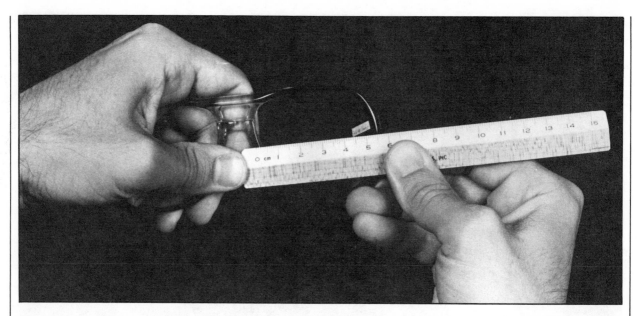

Figure 7–12. *When measuring the eyesize according to the boxing system, the ruler is held horizontally with the zero as far left as the most lefthand edge of the lens groove. The reading corresponds to the farthest righthand lens groove location.*

rule may be used, as shown in Figure 7–12. The same degree of accuracy cannot be expected using this method, as the locations of the far left and right points are only visually estimated.

For frames made from certain materials, the lenses often are edged somewhat larger to assure a secure fit. The nature of the material dictates how much larger the lenses are edged; the amounts given as guidelines are shown in Table 7–1.

Table 7–1. Size Compensation When Edging for Frames of Various Materials

Material used	Size after edging
Acetate	Marked size or .5 mm larger than measured size
Propionate	Marked size or .5 mm larger than measured size
Nylon	0.2 mm larger than the measured size
Optyl	0.6 to 1.0 mm oversize
Metal	On size

LENS CHUCKING

After a final determination of correct edger setting is made, the lens block is slipped into the edger chuck (See Figure 7–13) and clamped in place. This process is referred to as *lens chucking* and may be done manually or with the aid of compressed air.

Manual Chucking

When the process is done manually, the lens is clamped by any of a variety of methods, such as lowering a handle or turning a handwheel. Figure 7–14 shows how this brings a holding pad up against the positioned lens surface. The lens should be clamped firmly, but not with excessive pressure, and the handle should be locked in place. Too little pressure can cause lens slippage on the block, while too much pressure contributes to lens breakage during edging.

In most cases the material used for the holding pad is felt or a felt-like substance that is compressible, but has resilience. Because of the nature of the pad, the lens may be squeezed in place regardless of variations in curvature that naturally occur with different lens powers.

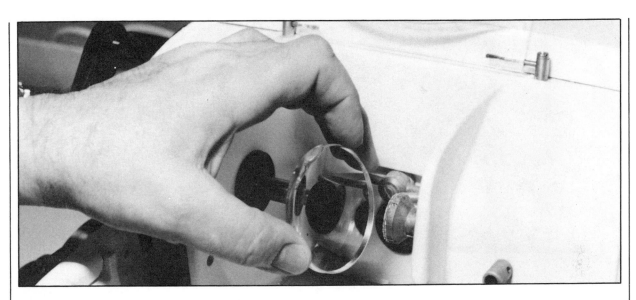

Figure 7–13. Chucking a lens for edging.

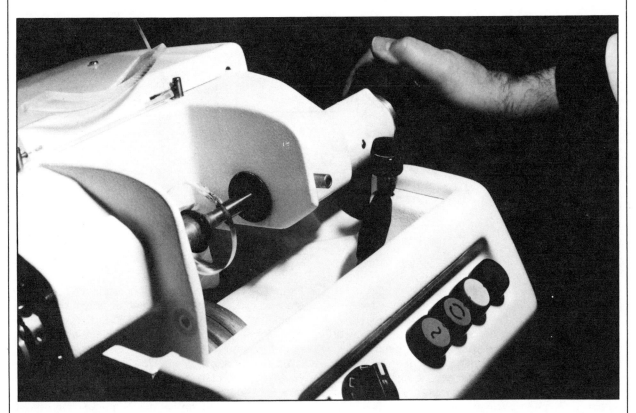

Figure 7–14. The felt pad is brought against the lens until the lens is secure, squeezing water from the pad. Excessive tightness is not required. Lenses may be chucked manually or pneumatically.

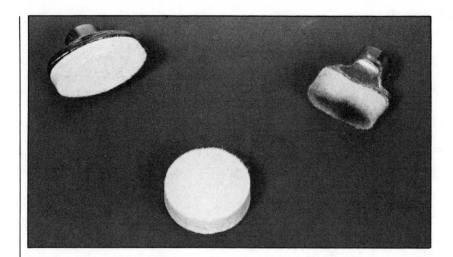

Figure 7–15. A variety of felt pad shapes are available, depending upon need. The large, round shape holds the lens well, but is inappropriate for half-eye shapes.

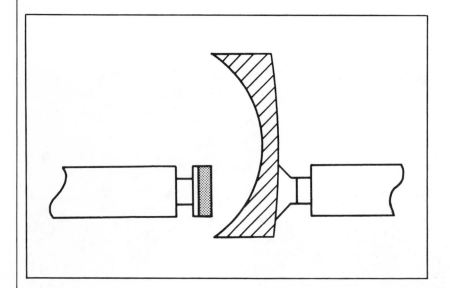

Figure 7–16. A high-powered lens with much decentration or a lens having a large amount of prism may not be held as securely using a conventional chucking system.

When the lens to be edged will be large in its finished form, a larger holding pad may be used. For most lenses the standard felt pad works well, but if the finished lens will be small, as in the case of lenses for half-eye frames, the large metal-backed pad will strike the wheel during edging, doing severe damage to the wheel. In this case a smaller oval or football shape is required. (See Figure 7–15.) In cases of strong prism or much decentration with high-powered lenses, the firmness of the hold decreases as a wedge effect occurs in clamping, as

Figure 7–16 shows. This problem has been addressed by a number of manufacturers, who have developed a swivel cone, shown in Figure 7–17, and other forms of articulating lens holders whereby an even pressure to the contact area is restored.

When an unusual situation arises in which the bevel must be placed at or near to the back surface of a thick lens, the construction of the edger wheel may not allow enough flat grinding area on the front surface. Some edgers overcome the problem by allowing the right and left halves of the chucking

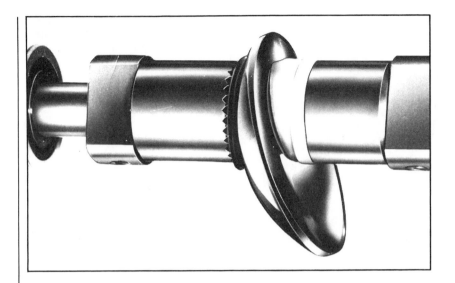

Figure 7–17. *One system devised for securely holding greatly decentered or prism lenses is a patented swivel cone nose. (Photo courtesy of Essilor.)*

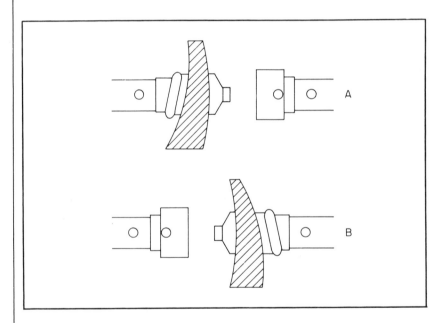

A

B

Figure 7–18. *To grind a thick lens with the bevel toward the back may require more diamond wheel width on the forward side of the lens groove than available. One solution is to use a clamping inversion system that allows the lens to be reversed in the edger. (Naturally, then the pattern must be turned around as well.) (Redrawn and used with permission of Universal-Briot.)*

clamps to be reversed, in what is termed a clamping inversion system. Thus the lens is blocked on the back, allowing the wide shelf of the edger wheel to be used to full advantage. (See Figure 7–18.)

Air Chucking

Although manual lens chucking is not difficult, when a large number of lenses are being run through the edger daily, *air chucking*, or *pneumatic chucking*,

may be advisable. An air line is run from a compressor to the specially adapted edger so that when a lever is tripped, the felt pad is pressed against the lens and held in place by the force of the compressed air. Pressure requirements vary, depending on lens type and its construction. Glass lenses may allow 80 pounds per square inch, while most plastic lenses are chucked at 50 to 60 psi. Plastic multifocals with wide segment ledges—such as flattop 35's or

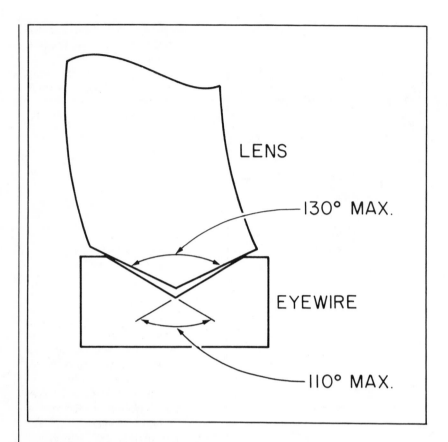

Figure 7–19. *The lens bevel angle must always be greater than the groove angle in the eyewire.*

segs with a near add of +3.00D and over—require still lower pressures. High pressures cause these lenses to crack along the ledge. It is obvious that all operators must keep their fingers clear of the clamping area since the full force of pressure occurs instantaneously.

Not only does air chucking reduce operator fatigue, but it also cuts edging time by a few seconds per lens. Although this may not be a factor in low-volume labs, if the edger is used over the course of a full day a measurable amount of time can be saved.

BEVEL SELECTION

When a lens is cut to size for placement in a spectacle frame, the edge must be shaped in such a way that it will stay securely in place. For lenses held in place by means of a groove in the frame eyewire, the American National Standards Institute[2] states

[2]*Requirements for Dress Ophthalmic Frames* (ANSI Z80. 5–1979), p. 8, American National Standards Institute, 1450 Broadway, New York, NY 10018.

that a frame eyewire groove angle should not be greater than 110 degrees, nor should a lens bevel angle be greater than 130 degrees. These minimum and maximum bevel angles are summarized in Figure 7–19. The bevel angle must always be greater than the groove angle. In making the bevel angle larger, the lens has less tendency to chip around its periphery through strain on the bevel apex.

In spite of constraints placed on permissible bevel angles, much latitude remains about the permissible overall shape of the lens edge.

Placement of Apex for Hand-Bevelled Lenses

In the past, when lenses were hand-bevelled, the main requirement for achieving a good cosmetic effect was the placement of the bevel apex. Figure 7–20 illustrates that for low-powered lenses having relatively thin edges, the apex was best positioned at the center of the lens edge. However, when lens edges became thicker, as with high-minus power, the center bevel positioning was not as cosmetically suitable. Positioning the bevel apex right in the center of the lens having a thick edge makes the lens

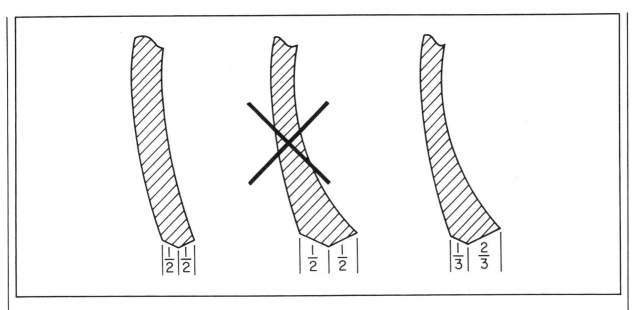

Figure 7–20. *For thin lenses, the bevel apex is approximately placed in the middle of the edge. As the lens becomes thicker, it should be moved toward the front. A ⅓, ⅔ ratio is correct.*

"spill out" the front of the frame. Not only did the wearer know the lenses are thick, everybody else did too! Therefore, in order to correct this problem, the apex of the bevel was pushed forward such that it was one-third of the edge thickness from the front, as the righthand lens in Figure 7–20 shows. When this was done, the major portion of the lens was behind the frontal plane of the spectacles and less of the lens bevel was seen from the front. Although reflections from the larger bevelled surface on the posterior lens edge still was seen as a concentric ring effect, the overall appearance was better.

Placement of Apex by Automatic Edger Wheels

The quality of edge design was vastly improved with the development of a grooved automatic edger wheel. This wheel allowed a bevel to be placed on a thick lens edge at any position while the remainder of the bevel was edged flat, as in Figure 7–21.

American Optical Company referred to the resulting bevel as a *Hide-a-Bevel.* When the lens with this style bevel is inserted into a spectacle frame, the finished prescription appears considerably better cosmetically, because the bevel will often completely disappear into the frame groove. Because of forward placement, the front of the lens does not protrude, and the concentric ring effect, though still present, is reduced by the more favorable edge angle. Such an edge is only feasible with an automatic edger.

The first automatic edgers had only one wheel, requiring that the lens first be reduced in size by the previously described chipping process. The wheel itself was ceramic, giving an excellent, smooth edge finish, but requiring a longer cycle to complete the process. Although some edgers still offer ceramic wheels for finishing off the lens edge, most are now equipped with a wheel using a diamond abrasive, which cuts much faster.

Current Bevelling Systems

Roughing Wheels

To replace the troublesome and risky process of chipping a lens down to a slightly larger pre-edging size, automatic edgers now have a roughing cycle.

The complete blank received from the surfacing lab or lens stock is placed in the edger. As the cycle begins, the lens blank is brought into contact with a coarse diamond wheel called a *roughing wheel,* which cuts it down rapidly. (This wheel is sometimes referred to as a *hogging wheel.*) When the roughing cycle is complete, the lens will have the correct shape as dictated by the pattern, but will be slightly large.

The lens may then pass to the second phase of edging, in which a finer *finishing wheel* puts the

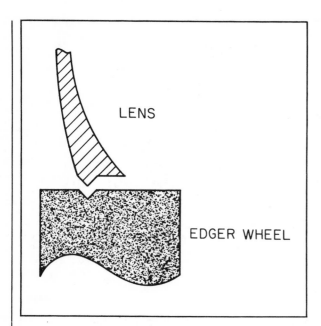

LENS

EDGER WHEEL

Figure 7–21. *Much cosmetic advantage was gained with the introduction of the so-called hidden bevel.*

correct edge on the lens while cutting it to its final size. There are separate size adjustments within the edger for the roughing wheel that must be checked periodically. If the roughing wheel sizing is set to cut the lens *too* small, there will still be coarse chip marks on the lens edge after the finishing wheel completes its work. But if the roughing wheel cuts the lens a great deal *larger* than the finished size, the finishing wheel must take off the remaining material, reducing its life span and increasing edging time. The difference (measured in millimeters) between the size of lens produced by the roughing wheel and the finished lens size is known as the *wheel differential* (or *grinding allowance*) and is important for efficient edger operation (see also Chapter 10 for a discussion on maintenance).

It is possible to edge glass and plastic lenses on the same wheels. If the wheel is suitable for glass, it will also work for conventional plastic, as long as the great majority of lenses being used are glass. If too many plastic lenses are edged at one time on the conventional roughing wheel without interspersing a good number of glass lenses, plastic material fills up the space between diamond particles, causing the wheel to "load." This reduces wheel efficiency and can also produce severe edge chipping (flaking) of glass lenses.

Fortunately there are roughing wheels produced that are especially designed for plastic lenses. These are considerably coarser than those designed for glass, with a greater distance between larger diamond grit particles. Although wheels designed for glass may be used intermittently for conventional plastic lenses, wheels designed for plastic should *never* be used for glass. Therefore, when a large percent of the lab's lens production is plastic lenses, the lab must be equipped with either two separate edgers or an edger that has two roughing wheels, one for glass and one for plastic.

Finishing Wheels
Once a lens is rough edged to shape, it must be bevelled on a finishing wheel. There are a large variety of finishing wheel designs available. Which wheel is best for a particular lab will depend upon several factors.

1. *Flat.* The simplest design in bevels is not really a bevel at all, but a flat edge. The flat edge is appropriate for rimless style eyewear. Seldom is a flat edge produced on a special flat wheel; they are usually ground on the flat portion of a grooved wheel used for another style of bevel as well. If the edger does not have a computer controlled program that places and keeps the lens on the flat portion automatically, it may be necessary to prevent the lens from slipping into the groove manually. This can be done, as Figure 7–22 illustrates, by moving a stop mechanism far enough over to cover the groove of the wheel. As the lens is automatically lowered onto the wheel,

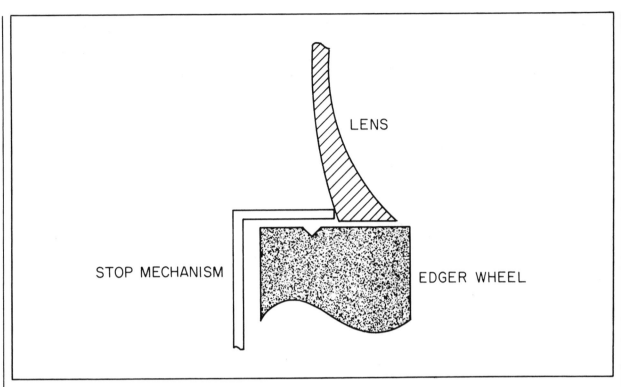

Figure 7–22. *A lens may be edged flat on the non-grooved portion of an otherwise flat wheel. Some method of preventing the lens from gravitating to the groove must be employed, as in the figure shown.*

the operator may be required to manually move the descending carriage head on the edger toward the flat portion of the wheel and help hold it there during edging.

In the case of a manual operation for rimless lenses, it will be necessary to compensate for the lack of a bevel in setting the eyesize. The eyesize should be set larger by an amount equal to twice the wheel groove depth. This usually totals about 2 mm. Therefore, if a 48-mm lens size is desired, the edger must be set as if the desired result were 50 mm.

Another method used is to change the set number on the pattern so that the computation is automatically done with the initial edger setting. For example, a rimless pattern is marked "set-15." Normally for a 54-mm eyesize, a 39-mm setting is selected, then increased by twice the groove depth to approximately 41 mm. If, however, the pattern were remarked to a "set-13," the operator could simply subtract

$$54 - 13 = 41$$

to obtain the correct setting. When electing this option, take care to check every rimless pattern before adding it to the pattern file to avoid costly mistakes.

2. *V-Bevel.* The V-bevel wheel is the most elementary design and duplicates results that could be accomplished by hand. The wheel is shaped like a V and, as a general rule, standard V-bevel wheels are used with a free-floating carriage or head system. That is to say, the lens is allowed to position itself in the groove and will "float," or gravitate to the middle of the groove itself. Because of the free-floating situation, a 50-50 bevel will result with the groove apex in the middle of the lens.

A system has been devised in an attempt to use the standard V-bevel wheel configuration and still position the apex of the lens bevel more toward the front of the lens. This is done by using two different grits of diamond on the same wheel, as

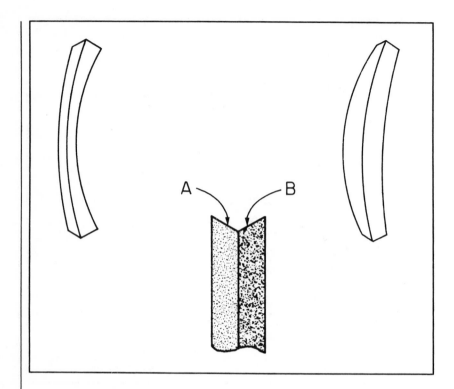

Figure 7–23. *Some V-bevels contain two different grits. The grit on surface* A *would be a finer grit, which cuts the front edge, while* B, *a coarser grit, cuts the back.*

Figure 7–23 shows. The side of the V-bevel that edges the front part of the lens edge contains a finer diamond grit and consequently edges more slowly. The rear surface side, being coarser, cuts into the edge faster, removing more material and causing the apex of the bevel to be positioned toward the front. Often the wheel is actually two halves, fastening together left and right to make one complete wheel.

3. *Special V (Plus/Minus V).* A special design variation uses the V-bevel free-float concept, yet produces a cosmetically better edge than the standard V. (See Figure 7–24.) Instead of having a lens with a relatively steep-angled edge, the edge flattens out a bit both on the front and back. With the help of a two-grit system or a mechanical stop mechanism preventing the lens from moving too far in one direction, the result may be a more controlled bevel location. This type of bevel is quite adequate for powers of up to +6.00 or −8.00D. (It should be remembered that power limitations are only a guideline. Thickness also increases as a function of lens size.) Lenses having a power of not over +6.00 or −8.00D may be edged with a special V-bevel. Beyond these

powers, another style wheel used in conjunction with a guided bevel system of edging produces results which some regard as more suitable.

4. *Double V's.* A configuration that combines two bevel grooves on one wheel and can be used in a free-float situation for either plus or minus lenses is known as the *double V.* (See Figure 7–25.) The minus lens side has a somewhat more shallow groove and produces a lens with a flat portion behind the forward-displaced bevel. Plus lenses are edged in the second groove. A thin lens gives a more conventional 50/50 V-bevel, while a thicker lens may be edged so less of the front bevel is exposed to view. For lenses of considerable thickness, a guided bevel system produces more favorable results.

5. *Mini-bevels.* A bevel system capable of producing a flat edge either in front of or behind the bevel of the lens may be referred to as a *Hide-a-Bevel* or *mini-bevel,* shown in Figure 7–26.[3] Actually, a

---

[3]Although many term this type of bevel a *hidden bevel,* the expression "hidden bevel" has become a more general term which may refer to the type of edges produced by special V's, double V's or mini-bevels.

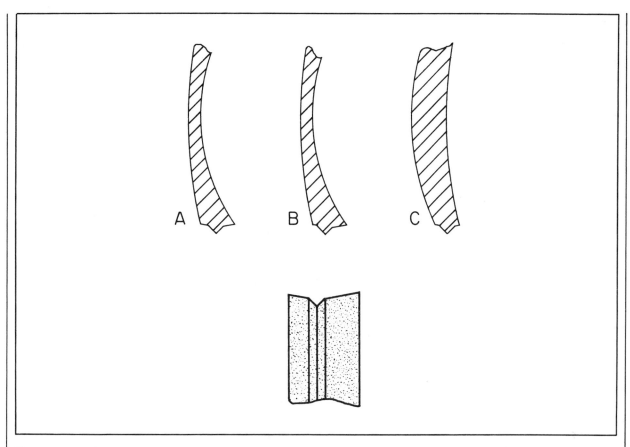

Figure 7–24. *The special V wheel may produce either* A *or* B *on high-minus lenses, depending upon factors such as wheel grit and placement controls. Lens* C *is a high-plus lens.*

mini-bevel is generally accepted as being smaller than the original Hide-a-Bevel design. The smaller bevel is especially well suited for metal-rimmed frames having shallow grooves.

To obtain the best results with a mini-bevel, the bevel must be guided.

Free-Float Bevel Systems

One method of guiding the bevel is to allow a "free-float" situation for the lens on the edger wheel, but restrict how far across the wheel groove the lens is permitted to float. This is done by means of a stop mechanism, often made from a nylon material to prevent lens scratching and sometimes referred to as a "nylon finger." When a finished lens edge will be no wider than the groove in the edger wheel, the nylon finger is not used so as to allow an unrestricted free float of the lens in the groove, producing an equal sided 50-50 bevel. When the finished minus lens is wider than the wheel groove width, however, the nylon finger is moved in close to the groove. The front surface of the lens touches this stop mechanism and, at least for lenses having low base curves, the bevel is produced at an even distance from the front surface of the lens, as in Figure 7–27.

Another system for positioning the bevel is by means of a small guide wheel that tracks along the front surface of the lens as the lens rotates in the edger. Although the possibility of marring the front of the lens is small with a more conventional style stop mechanism, the guide wheel further reduces this chance.

Non-Float Bevel Systems

Although most systems allow the edger head to float freely on the wheel, there are methods that restrict the horizontal movement of the lens as it turns in the edger. When an operator attempts to control bevel

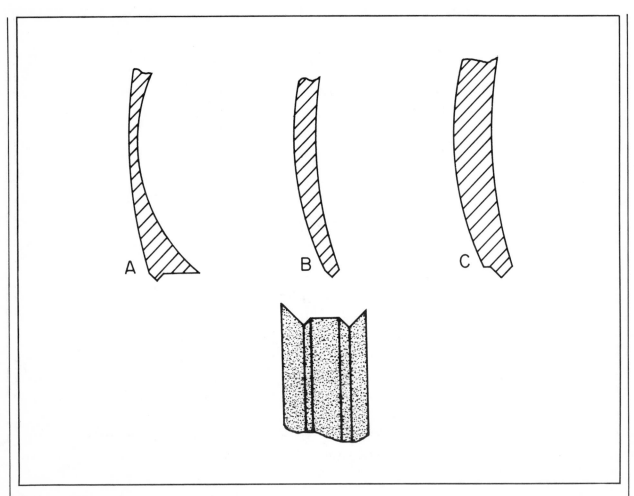

Figure 7–25. *The double-V wheel produces bevels such as that shown on lens A for minus lenses. Plus lenses can be edged as seen in lenses B and C.*

placement in this manner, the problem is complicated by the fact that spectacle lenses normally have a curved front surface. If the front surface were always flat, the lens could merely be locked in position so that only vertical movement would be permitted as the pattern and lens rotated on the wheel. Yet because the lens is curved, if the lens does not move left and right as it turns, its edge will run completely out of the groove. And to further complicate the issue, all lenses do not have the same front curvature, making necessary horizontal edger movement a variable, even for points the same radius away from the edging center! (See Figure 7–28.)

This problem may be overcome by controlling horizontal movement using a panhard rod principle. To understand the principle, think of a pole in an empty pond. One end of a rod is attached halfway up the pole. The other end of the rod has a float on it that rests on the bottom of the pool, as illustrated in Figure 7–29. Now as water is added to the pool, the float causes the free end of the rod to rise. As it begins to rise, the free end describes an arc. A horizontal movement is caused by a vertical rise in the water level.

With a lens edger, the rotating pattern used causes the blocked lens and chucking assembly to move up and down as it turns.

By attaching one end of a rod to a stationary part of the edger and the other end to the lens assembly, as the lens moves up and down it will also be forced

138

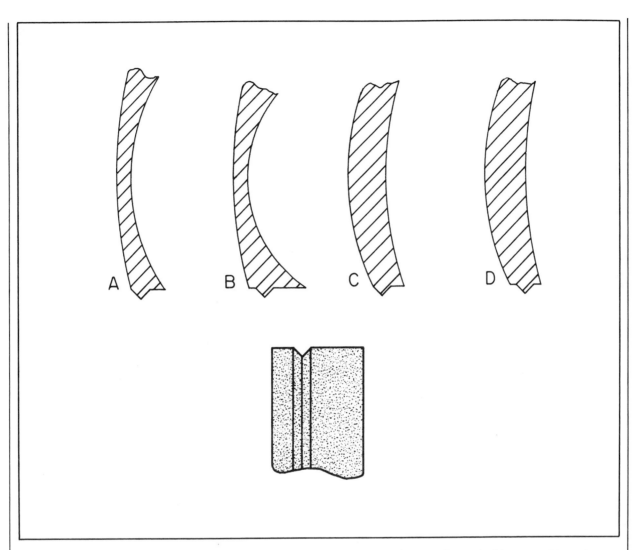

Figure 7–26. *Mini-bevels should not be automatically placed at the front surface of all lenses, although most minus lenses look best when ground this way, as in A. High-minus lenses are often better edged with the bevel slightly back from the front surface, as seen in B. This keeps the back edge from touching the wearer's face, and with plastic frames may better hide thickness. Moderately thick-edged plus lenses, as shown in C, are edged in a manner similar to that of moderately powered minus lenses. Thick-edged plus lenses often do well with the bevel more toward the midline, as in D. However, when edges are excessively thick on plus lenses, the thickness may be due to having selected too large a lens blank for the eyesize (see Chapter 1).*

to move back and forth horizontally in a controlled manner, as Figure 7–30 shows. The more the lens is raised by the pattern (this is equivalent to a rise in water level), the farther the lens will be displaced horizontally (the float moves farther from the pole).

In order for the bevel to end up on the lens at the right place, two factors are important. First, the end of the rod (panhard rod) must be attached to the "pole" at the correct height. The height of attachment primarily controls how far the lens will be pushed or pulled horizontally as its level rises and falls. Moving the height of attachment up causes a more pro-

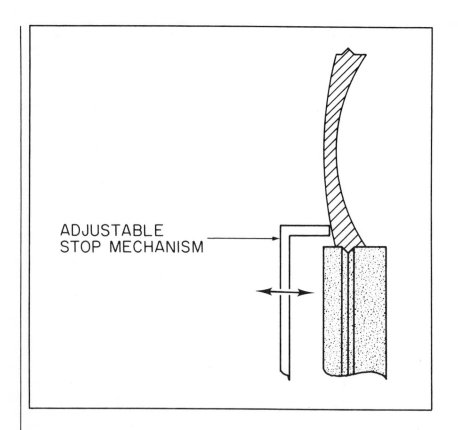

ADJUSTABLE
STOP MECHANISM

Figure 7–27. *If an edger uses a free-float system, an adjustable stop mechanism may be used to regulate the distance that the lens bevel will be ground from the front surface.*

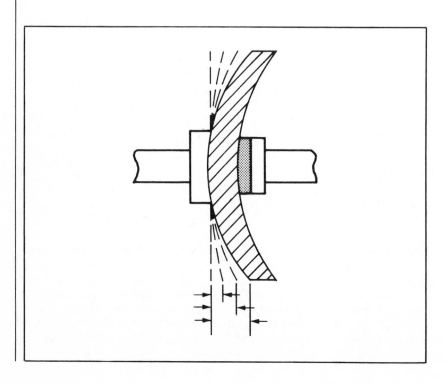

Figure 7–28. *Lens base curves vary. The higher the curve is and the larger the lens, the farther back from the chucked central portion will the edge be placed. Were the lens to be locked in a stationary horizontal location and only allowed to move up and down during edging, the bevel would move completely off the edge on long corners.*

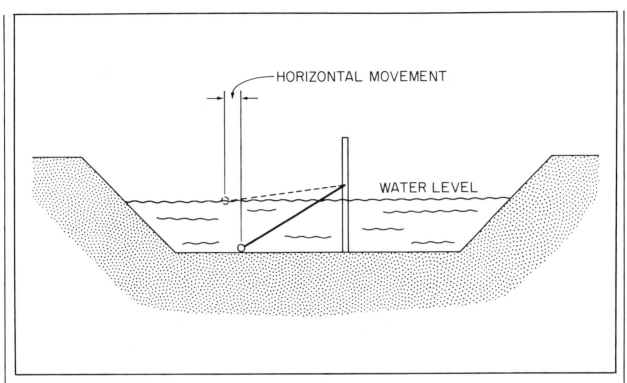

HORIZONTAL MOVEMENT

WATER LEVEL

Figure 7–29. *The panhard rod principle works in much the same manner as a float on a stick.*

nounced horizontal movement. This is needed for lenses with high base curves.

Second, the panhard rod must be of the correct length. This ensures that the edge of the lens will be over the edger wheel groove. Shortening the rod length will cause the bevel to move toward the front of the lens, while lengthening it will place the bevel toward the rear surface.

It can be seen that any guided bevel system requires two settings. The first allows for lens steepness (base curve) so that the bevel does not travel off the lens edge because of "long corners." Once the operator correctly allows for lens steepness, the bevel should always be at a given distance from the front of the lens. The second setting allows this given distance to be altered according to optical or cosmetic needs.

With some sturdy metal frames it may be advantageous to make the bevel fit the frame, rather than the lens, as shown in Figures 7-31 A and B. To serve these needs, only a non-floating guided bevel system

is needed.

A Guided Bevel System for Mass Production

When a great number of lenses of the same shape and base curve must be produced, as in the case of sun or safety glasses, one system for accurately positioning the location of the bevel is to use a *curved pattern.* The pattern must be a duplicate of the lens to be edged and must have exactly the same size as the lens. It must also have the same curvature, be for the same eye (right or left), and be grooved so as to fit the frame perfectly. When using this pattern, a special clapper plate is used, having a groove into which the bevelled pattern fits. This restricts the pattern and therefore also the edger head from floating freely on the wheel. Thus, using the pattern, an otherwise free-floating edging system may be transformed into a guided bevel system that controls both horizontal and vertical lens movement on the edger wheel.

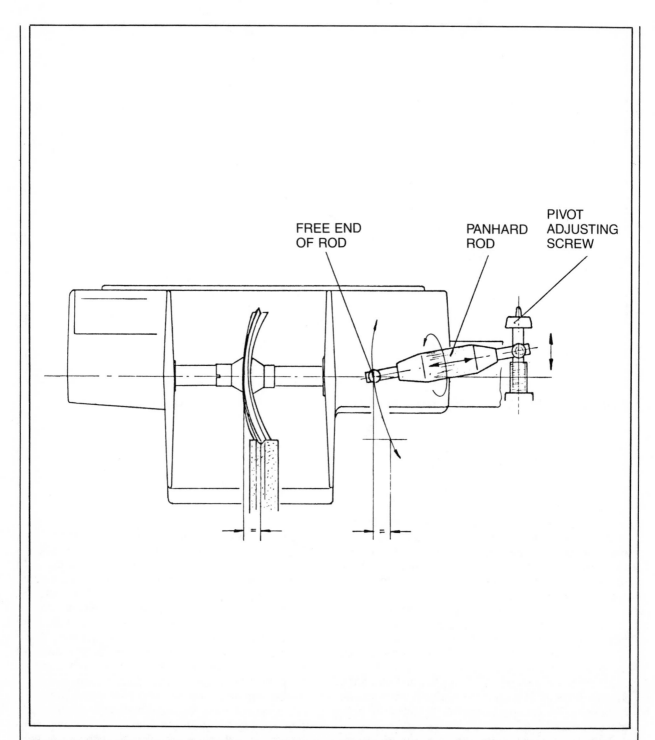

FREE END
OF ROD

PANHARD
ROD

PIVOT
ADJUSTING
SCREW

Figure 7–30. *The panhard rod may be lengthened or shortened to move the bevel to the back or front of the lens. By adjusting the stationary point of attachment of the panhard rod up or down by means of the pivot adjusting screw, the path of the free end of the rod changes. This allows for correct bevel placement compensation for lens base curve differences. (Drawing courtesy of WECO.)*

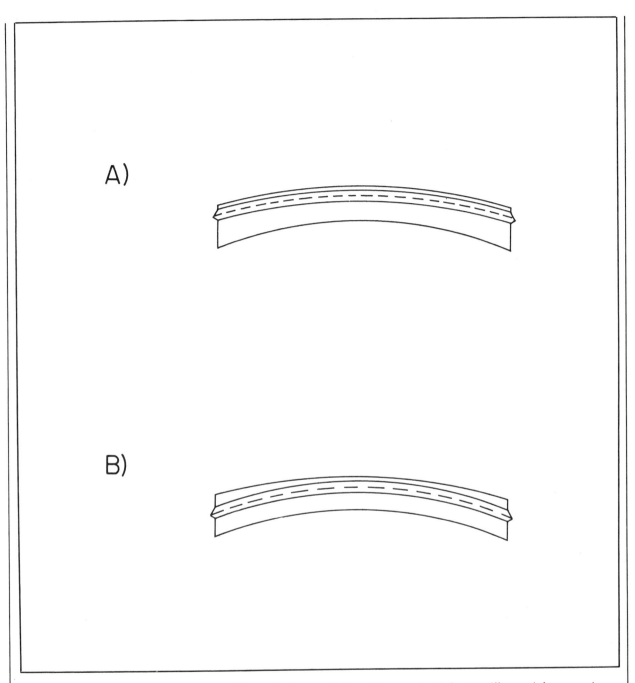

Figure 7–31. *These lenses are seen from the top and have been edged for a stiff metal frame using a guided bevel system of edging. The frame to be used was manufactured to accept a lens with an average front curve (usually +6.00D). The upper rims of the frame front are pressed to fit this average curve and are not easily bent to a new conformation. Because the front curve of the lens is flatter than the curve of the frame, the bevel on lens A will not fit properly. However, if the lens is edged using a guided bevel system, the bevel can be made to fit the frame, rather than simply follow the front curve of the lens. The bevel shown in B will conform to the curve of the frame.*

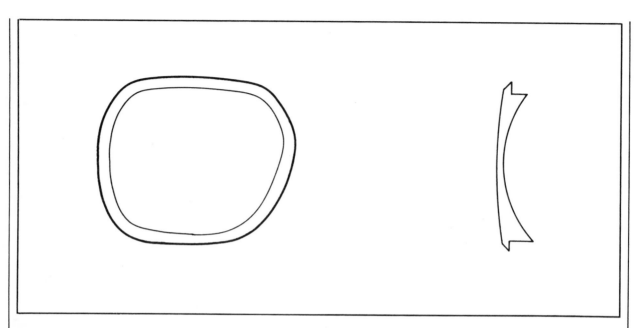

Figure 7–32. *The first type of facet looks much like a hidden bevel were the ledge to be ground deeply into the lens.*

The Facet

The *facet* is an edge configuration used with high-minus lenses to reduce edge thickness and weight, and can take two forms. One consists of grinding a squared-off portion away from the back of the lens, as is shown in Figure 7–32. When this facet is used, a reduction in usable optics by more than 5 or 6 mm is not necessary, nor even desirable cosmetically, as even with only this small reduction, a considerable amount of edge thickness can be eliminated.

It is also useful in removing lens edge thickness that otherwise restricts the fitting of an adjustable nosepad frame.

The facet shown in Figure 7-32 is usually ground on the lens after it first has been edged to a hidden bevel configuration. Thereafter the "ledge" of the hidden bevel is further removed using the edge of the stone.

A second type of facet (advanced primarily by Tura) is used with rimless eyewear and resembles the bevelled edge appearance on custom ground mirrors. A relatively steep bevel is ground onto the front edge of the lens, then highly polished. Instead of making the lenses look awkward because of thickness, such lenses look almost as if the edge was designed thicker to accommodate the bevelled glass effect. An important aspect of the design is the sharp corners of the lens shape. These lenses must be a plastic material. The bevelling can be done completely by hand with patience and skill, or in conjunction with an edger wheel designed especially for the purpose. In either case the edges must afterwards be polished as is described in Chapter 9.

Frame/Bevel Relationships

Up to this point, consideration in choosing a bevel style has been limited to discussing edger wheel types, as is summarized in Table 7–2. Another major consideration not to be overlooked depends upon the frame for which the lens is being edged. With some frames, the required bevel style will be immediately obvious. (See Table 7–3.) A rimless mounting, for example, requires that the lens have a flat edge.

Table 7–2. Edger Wheel Configurations

Wheel type	Lens recommendations	Mounting circumstances	Comments
Flat	Any power permissible; high minus unattractive	Rimless; Nylon Supra	Usually a part of another wheel
V-bevel (free float)	Low power lenses; plano sunlenses; plano safety lenses	Normal grooved frames	Thick edges yield poor results
Special V (free-float) (Plus/Minus V)	All lenses where nonguided bevel placement suffices; generally from +6.00D to −8.00D of lens power	Normal grooved frames	Extremely versatile
Double V's (free float)	For low and mid-power lenses up to ±5.0D	Normal grooved frames	Attractive results similar to guided bevel
Mini-bevel (guided or free float)	For high-powered lenses	For normal grooved frames or shallow grooved metal frames	Can result in skillful looking job when properly guided
Facet, type 1 (guided)	Thick-edged lenses	Normal grooved frames	When minimizing weight reduction and edge thickness is important; usually a part of another wheel; is a cosmetic compromise at best
Facet, Tura	High-minus lenses	Rimless mountings designed especially for this facet	Limited to plastic lenses

Table 7–3. Appropriate Lens Bevels for Basic Frame Types

Frame type	Lens power	Lens bevel recommendations
Rimless	High-minus	Flat (rimless not recommended) Facet, Tura (for specially designed rimless mountings)
	High-plus	Flat (excellent choice for rimless)
	Low-plus and minus	Flat (fine for rimless)
Metal eyewire	High-minus	Mini-bevel, bevel toward the front
	High-plus With large decentration and/or large frame difference	Mini-bevel
	With small frame difference and an ED which approaches the frame *A* dimensions	V-bevel
	Low-plus and minus	V-bevel, special V or double V's
Plastic	High-minus	Mini-bevel; bevel toward front, but not necessarily at the front
	High-plus a. With large decentration and/or large frame difference	Mini-bevel; bevel slightly front of center
	b. With small frame difference and an ED that approaches *A*	V-bevel
	Low-plus and minus	V-bevel, special V or double V's (bevel placement depends greatly upon how wide the frame's rim is and where in the rim the groove is placed)

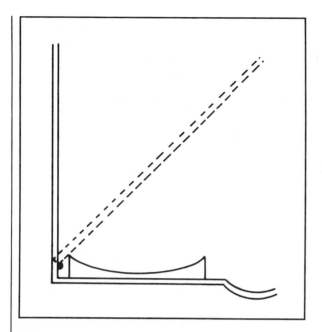

Figure 7–33. *If no consideration is given to edge thickness during the frame selection process, it may not even be possible to close the temples!*

Metal or Combination Frames

For metal frames or combination frames with metal chassis, standard V-bevels, or variations on V's work well.

When the minus power of a lens increases, a mini-bevel with the bevel apex toward the front is well suited. It should be remembered, though, that after a certain amount of edge thickness is reached, nosepad positioning will be interfered with and it may no longer be possible to close the temples completely. In this situation, lens edges are easily chipped if a temple is forced against them, as Figure 7–33 illustrates.

There are alternatives that can be chosen to reduce this problem. These include using a facet or going to a myodisc configuration. Since the difficulty often stems back to a poorly chosen frame, an alternative selection could be made, or the next smaller eyesize in the same frame considered. If the use of a standard V-bevel is ruled out, the tempered area of the lens can be modified through hand edging. (See Table 7–4.)

An option that avoids lens modification altogether may be carried out on the frame by bending the endpiece outward. In compensation, the temple is bent inward near its point of attachment. Unfortunately, this is a cosmetically undesirable situation.

For plastic frames, the high-minus lens uses a hidden bevel. For extremely high-minus full-field lenses, it may not be desirable to place the bevel at the extreme front edge of the lens, but rather a slight amount back to avoid too much lens protruding from the back of the frame. Many plastic frames are especially designed to accommodate high-minus lenses. The frame groove position should be observed before edging the lens to take full advantage of the camouflage effect designed into the frame.

Table 7–4. Alternatives in Handling Obstructively Thick Edges

1. Use a facet.
2. Go to a myodisc construction
   a. by surfacing.
   b. by hand edging and polishing.
3. Use a smaller eyesize.
4. Modify specific portions of the edge by hand.
5. Bend the frame endpiece outward, with a compensating sharp bend in the temple near the butt portion.
6. Move the bevel farther back from the front of the lens.

High-plus lenses should be given the same consideration for plastic frames as was described previously for metal.

Bevel Placement for Anisometropic Corrections

A prescription in which the right and left eyes differ significantly from one another in power corrects a condition known as *anisometropia.* Because prescription lenses either magnify, as with plus lenses, or minify, as with minus lenses, an Rx with differing powers right and left will cause different amounts of magnification. In order to reduce magnification differences so that one eye's perception of objects is not greatly larger than the other eye's,[4] magnification can be altered by changing the vertex distance (distance from lens to eye).[5]

Moving a plus lens farther from the eye increases its magnifying properties while the opposite effect

occurs with minus lenses (see Table 7–5). By placing the lens bevel toward the front or back of the lens, a change in vertex distance will be effected, thereby also bringing about a change in magnification. Table 7–6 summarizes how this may be used to advantage.

Table 7–5. Magnification Effects of Spectacle Lenses

Lens type	Action	Effect
Plus	Moving the lens *farther* from the eye	Increases magnification
	Moving the lens *closer* to the eye	Decreases magnification
Minus	Moving the lens *farther* from the eye	Increases minification (i.e., decreases magnification)
	Moving the lens *closer* to the eye	Decreases minification (i.e., increases magnification)

[4]Anisometropia can either be due to axial length differences in the eye, or differences in the powers of the eyes' refracting surfaces. If the anisometropia is due solely to refractive ametropia, then no attempt need be made to compensate for magnification differences. (Instances of refractive ametropia appear to be in the minority.) Correction is usually attempted by the matching of base curves and, to a degree, lens thicknesses.

[5]Magnification can also be altered by a change in the front curve of a lens or by a change in lens thickness.

Table 7–6. Unequal Right Eye/Left Eye Power Combinations Bevel Placement for Reducing Magnification Differences

Power combinations	Lens power	Bevel placement
High-plus with lower-plus	High-plus → Lower-plus →	Bevel toward front of lens edge Bevel toward rear of lens edge
High-minus with lower-minus	High-minus → Lower-minus →	Bevel toward front of lens edge Bevel toward rear of lens edge
Plus one eye, minus other eye	Plus Minus	Bevel as far to front of lens edge as possible for both lenses

ADJUSTING PRESSURE OF THE LENS AGAINST THE WHEEL

The pressure exerted by the edger as it presses the lens against the wheel can be varied. Heavy pressure should be used when glass lenses with especially thick edges are being ground. In fact, in most any instance when a mini-bevel or hidden bevel is a must, somewhat heavier pressure is advisable.

To edge lenses without mechanically guiding the bevel location, a somewhat heavier pressure is advisable. Edging without enough pressure in a free-float situation will not cause the lens to gravitate as forcefully to the groove.

In general, less pressure is required for plastic lenses than for glass. The exception is the polycarbonate lens, which should be run at the greatest pressure that will not cause it to slip off the block. This procedure reduces the amount of *flash (swarf),* which is a shredded-wheat-like accumulation of plastic on the lens edge.

It is recommended that high-index lenses be run on low pressure. Since high-index glass yields rapidly to wheel abrasion, edging cycle time is not usually reduced.

Because pressure from the edger head is eventually exerted on the pattern against the clapper plate, when using a thin pattern, pressure should be reduced. The smallest pressure possible will be used if an actual lens is serving as a pattern. (This is only possible on edgers specifically designed to allow this procedure.)

Beyond these general guidelines, the best counterbalance pressures will be found through experience with the machine. (Comparative pressures are shown in Figure 7–34.) Too much pressure will cause a drag on the motor and excessive wheel wear and can sometimes be detected by the presence of a hump on the lens edge not indicated by pattern shape. Too little pressure slows the edging process, cutting into production time.

THE EDGING CYCLE

Before edging the first of a number of lenses, allow the machine to run through one complete cycle empty. This serves to wet the felt chucking clamps, which helps to reduce lens slippage. The wheel should be observed during this empty cycle to verify that it is being flooded with an adequate supply of coolant. Flooding the wheel with coolant before edging begins ensures less drag from a dry wheel, extending wheel life.

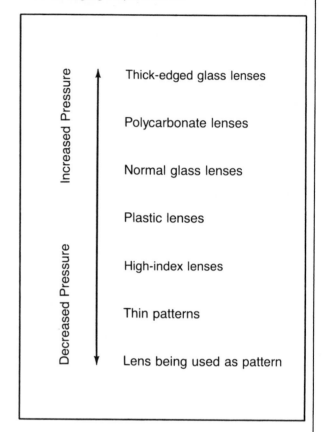

Figure 7–34. *Edger counterweight pressure as related to edging requirements.*

The Roughing Cycle
The roughing cycle takes the lens down rapidly to within 2 to 2.5 mm of finished lens size. The function of this wide, flat wheel is to remove lens material rapidly so that the finer, slower-cutting finishing wheel can operate more efficiently.

Wheel Wear
The most basic of edger types lowers the lens onto the roughing wheel repeatedly in one spot. In time, though, the wheel will develop a shallow groove in that area. As long as wheel differential is readjusted to allow for this depth change, no major problems will develop. The primary disadvantage, however, is that eventually the abrasive surface at the center of the groove will wear through. This requires replace-

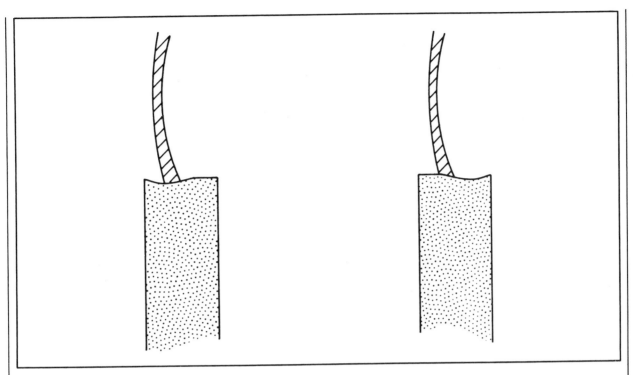

Figure 7–35. *When a roughing wheel begins to wear from continuous use (lefthand illustration), wheel life may be prolonged by turning the wheel so that the wear becomes more even. After turning, the wheel should be dressed before using. (See Chapter 11, "Diamond Wheels.")*

ment of a wheel even though much good abrasive area remains. Because the most severely worn area is usually somewhat off-center, removing the wheel and turning it around periodically will permit more evenness of wear and a longer life, as Figure 7–35 illustrates. Before use, however, the wheel must be redressed with an abrasive stick.

A few wheel manufacturers offer a wheel that comes in two halves. By interchanging the halves right for left, as in Figure 7–36, the worn central area will now be at the outer edge while the thicker edge portion cuts in the middle of the wheel.

The next step in evenness of wheel wear is to use an edger that has the capacity to drop the lens onto the wheel in two or more different positions. This can be done manually by preference of the operator, or automatically, depending upon the sophistication of the edger. The term used by some for such an automatic option is *levelator*. It can be overridden so that an especially thick lens will not be positioned half off the wheel.

Another solution to uneven wheel wear is to make the lens move laterally back-and-forth across the wheel as the lens is ground.

Rotation During Edging

Most edgers have a lens rotating system that is activated when the pattern presses against a clapper plate. The lens is lowered onto the wheel and does not move until sufficient lens stock is edged away, allowing the pattern to touch the clapper plate. At this point the lens rotates. Upon a slight rotational movement, the unedged portion of the lens lifts the pattern off the plate, halting rotation until enough lens stock is removed to allow the pattern to drop back again. The process repeats itself until at least slightly over one full revolution is completed.

A second system utilizes *intermittent rotation*. In this system the lens rotates continuously, regardless of whether or not the pattern is in contact with the plate. To avoid having the lens turn endlessly as it awaits the complete edging of an especially stubborn

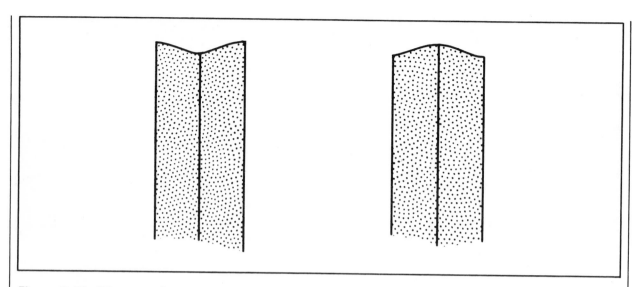

Figure 7–36. *When a split-style roughing wheel wears, the right and left halves may be reversed to allow full utilization of all the abrasive surface material.*

area, the edger reverses rotation as soon as the pattern touches the plate. In this manner the machine grinds back and forth over an area where a large amount of lens stock must be removed until the task is complete, then moves on to the next area. After an uninterrupted revolution has been completed without the pattern leaving the plate, the roughing cycle finishes.

Cycling Pause
Normally the rough-edged lens goes directly to the finishing cycle without interruption. Some edgers allow for a pause between cycles so that a specific bevel finishing setting can be made.

It should be noted that any edger may be stopped manually after roughing by simply cutting the power. However, unless it has a reset capability, the cycle will have to be allowed to complete itself, with or without the lens, before another lens can be edged.

The Finishing Cycle
A lens normally enters the finishing cycle directly from the roughing cycle. The final bevel style ground will depend upon the edger wheel in use.

If there is doubt as to whether the lens blank will be large enough, it is useful to run a test lens. For example, suppose that a certain style bifocal is specified for segment location so that the likelihood of creating an air space between frame rim and lens

edge exists. Although the lens blank may be the largest available, it still may border on being too small. Rather than risk ruining the lens, it is advisable to use a previously rejected blank of the same design, and edge it to the specified size and shape first. If the lens does not cut out, possible arrangements for using a smaller eyesize or an altered seg position can be considered.

Trial Rotation
For lenses where bevel placement is critical, a test lens of similar power can also be run. A better option, though, is one that allows a trial rotation of the lens in the edger, without actual bevelling taking place. For edgers so equipped, the system works as follows.

First, the edger is set for cycling pause so that when the lens completes the roughing cycle it stops before going onto the finishing wheel. A change is made to a non-float, guided bevel mode. If a trial rotation option is available, the machine can be set so that the lens rotates at a position close to, but not in contact with, the wheel. By observing the lens turning in close proximity to the finishing groove while occasionally halting its rotation, the operator can make necessary adjustments ahead of time to assure optimum bevel placement.

To be absolutely sure of the future bevel location, the edger can be set 2 mm larger than the final size

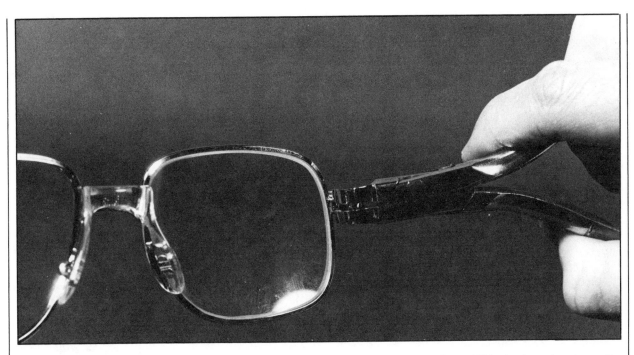

Figure 7–37. *A lens may be checked for size accuracy using a pair of pliers. With the lens in place, the barrels are simply squeezed together, eliminating continuous insertion and removal of the eyewire screw.*

and then run. The edger will lightly trace out the proposed location of the bevel. If this location is satisfactory, appropriate modifications for either base curve or forward bevel placement may be made.

Emergency Stops

As with any type of equipment, occasionally it becomes necessary to stop the operation in mid-cycle. Just how this is done varies with the manufacturer and could be handled by such things as a red "panic button," or a "reset" button on the machine that lifts the lens and resets the machine to start. If the machine has no such feature, the operator may do any one or more of the following, depending upon the nature of the problem.

1. Lift the lens off the wheel by manually raising the edger head.
2. Turn the machine off.
3. Turn the size setting to a high reading so that the lens no longer touches the grinding wheel.

It is almost inevitable that the need for an emergency stop will occur sometime. The time to know how to react is before the first lens is ever edged. When a need arises to act quickly, it is too late to look things up in an instruction manual.

Checking Size Accuracy

Once a lens has been edged, the block should not be removed until it is certain that the lens will fit into the frame exactly. This is especially true for metal frames, where very small size increments determine the difference between ill- and well-fitting lenses.

To check lens size accuracy for a metal frame, place the lens in the eyewire with the block still on. Then, using a thin-nosed pair of pliers, squeeze the two sections of the eyewire together, as in Figure 7–37. This will draw the eyewire around the lens. If the upper and lower halves of the barrel fail to come together, the lens is still too large. The eyewire should close fully, leaving no gaps between the lens and the eyewire, yet without putting undue stress on a lens.

Undue stress from a metal eyewire will cause a plastic lens to warp and a glass lens to exhibit stress when viewed with the aid of a colmascope.[6] Figure 7–38 shows how the strain appears with a colmascope.

---

[6]A colmascope consists of a light source behind two crossed polaroids. When a lens is placed between two polaroids, internal lens stress becomes visually apparent.

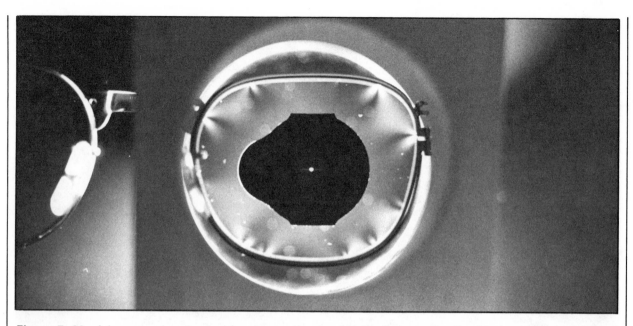

Figure 7–38. *A lens may be checked for stress using back-lighted, crossed polaroids (a colmascope). Here the adhesive pad block is still on the lens so that it may be re-edged easily. The bright marks around the periphery of the lens will show up with a rainbow effect and indicate entirely too much strain. Were such a lens to be dispensed, it would easily chip or flake at the edge at one or more of these strain points, especially if dropped or knocked against an object.*

While the block remains on the lens, an operator may make slight steps in size reduction by running the lens through the finishing cycle again. However, once the lens is removed, it is extremely difficult to reblock the lens accurately enough to allow an even removal of only a few tenths of a millimeter.

Because plastic frames stretch upon lens insertion, some variation in lens size is possible without serious consequences. Such lens size variation is not possible when using a metal frame, since the frame will not expand or contract. It is best to have the frame in the lab when the lenses are edged, but if this is not the case, a more accurate indication of size than a rule or box-o-graph can be obtained using a circumference gauge. By knowing the circumference necessary for each eyesize of a given metal frame, precision in duplication is possible. Therefore, for metal frames which are uniformly manufactured to precisely repeatable sizes, an exact fit can be obtained without the frame being in the laboratory.

VARIATIONS IN LENS MATERIALS

Although the edging process remains approximately the same in spite of differences in lens materials, there are some aspects that require special attention. These will be discussed separately on the basis of the lens material used.

Crown Glass

Crown glass has been considered to be the standard material for ophthalmic lenses. Unless otherwise specified, it is generally assumed that lens fabrication equipment being ordered is for glass. Crown glass for ophthalmic use has an index of 1.523. Glass lenses are also referred to as *mineral lenses*.

Photochromic Glass

Photochromic glass, which darkens as light intensity increases, is treated almost the same as crown glass during the edging process. Because of its composition, the photochromic lens generates more heat when being edged and is harder on edger wheels. As a result, some wheels have been designed for use in situations where a high percentage of photochromic lenses are used. These wheels work for standard glass lenses as well, so there is no need to segregate work into photochromic and non-photochromic.

When edging a large proportion of photochromic lenses, the coolant must be of good quality and of sufficient concentration to produce the desired effect. Failure to maintain a clean, efficient coolant flow will cause unnecessarily rough lens edges and a reduced abrasive wheel life.

Photochromic glass must be chemically treated in a bath whose composition varies from that used for crown glass lenses. This is discussed in more detail in the section concerned with safety specifications.

Photochromic glass has an index of 1.523, making surface curves for photochromic lenses identical to crown glass surface curves of equal refractive power.

High-Index Lenses

Some clear glass lenses are made from materials that result in a higher refractive index than the standard crown glass lens. Common refractive indices for these so-called high-index lenses are 1.60, 1.70 and 1.80.

Because of basic property differences in the material, high-index lenses should be edged with less pressure than standard crown lenses. Although not required (nor especially convenient), edging high-index lenses with a ceramic wheel instead of the standard diamond impregnated wheel will result in a reduced number of microcracks at the lens edge.

It is advisable to avoid large temperature shocks with high-index glass, as when a warm lens is rinsed with cold water. A standard crown lens can generally withstand a 70°C difference in temperature, whereas a 50°C maximum difference is average for high-index.[7]

It is recommended that high-index lenses not be notched or drilled, since these processes reduce impact resistance.

Lenses Made from Plastic

Edging of plastic CR-39[8] lenses can be done on the same equipment and with the same edger wheels as are used for glass *if* relatively few of the lenses are plastic. When the percentage of plastic lenses increases, the plastic begins to glaze the wheel. *Glaze* means that the spaces between abrasive diamond cutting edges become clogged with plastic, preventing good, clean cutting.

A glazed wheel results in increased cutting time for lenses being edged. It also causes the edges of the glass lenses to chip to a depth of 4–5 mm into the lens surface, ruining the lens. This will not occur when only a few plastic lenses are interspersed with glass because the wheel is cleaned by the glass before plastic can build up to a glaze.

The solution to the problem of glazing can be handled in one of two ways. The first is to simply add another edger having a roughing wheel specifically designed for plastic. This type of wheel is considerably coarser than those used for glass. The second solution is an edger with three cutting wheels. Most three-wheel edgers are designed with one roughing wheel and two finishing wheels. With two finishing wheels greater versatility in bevel style is achieved.

It is possible, however, to specify one finishing and two roughing wheels. One roughing wheel may then be used for glass, and the second for plastic. All lenses may use the same finishing wheel, as the same kind of wheel is often used for both plastic and glass. Take extreme care to be certain that glass lenses are not inadvertently allowed to edge on the wheel designed for plastic, as wheel damage can occur.

The three-wheel edger design for both plastic and glass would be best for a small office lab where not all lenses are edged in-house. It can also be useful where limited floor space is available. As soon as volume begins to indicate the need, separate edgers for glass and plastic should be obtained. This is especially true when one remembers that it is possible to operate two edgers simultaneously, increasing efficiency. (If polycarbonate lenses are to be edged, keep in mind that a CR-39 lens can be cut on an edger that has been adapted to handle polycarbonate.)

When plastic lenses are edged, ground plastic material in the coolant causes foaming. If nothing is done to retard foaming, the bubbly froth begins overflowing the tank and spilling onto the floor like a fountain full of laundry detergent! Defoaming agents may be added directly to the coolant to suppress foaming, or a defoaming spray may be used on the surface whenever foaming begins, as Figure 7–39 indicates.

Plastic lenses may also be edged on edgers designed to cut the lens to size with a small router blade, rather than through traditional grinding meth-

---

[7]"High-Lite, S-1005 High Index, Low Density," Schott Optical Glass, Inc., Duryea, Pennsylvania, 1979.

[8]Columbia Resin 39, a trademark of Pittsburgh Plate Glass Co.

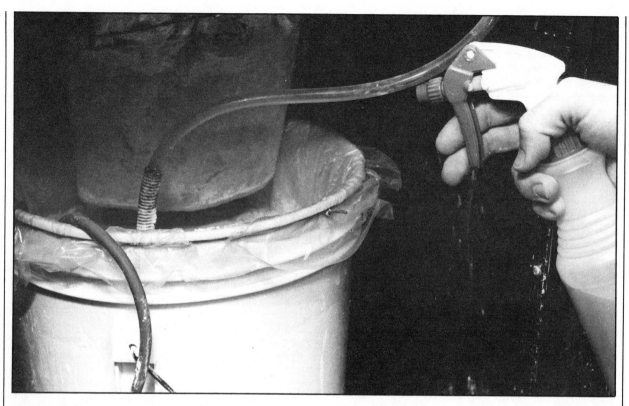

Figure 7–39. *Plastic lenses can cause coolant foaming during edging. A defoaming agent can be added to the coolant and foam can be reduced by spraying with a defoaming liquid.*

ods. This will be discussed in more detail in the next section, which deals with polycarbonate lenses.

Polycarbonate Lenses

Polycarbonate lenses are highly impact resistant and have been used for some time as protective lenses in industrial situations. They are also available for prescription use.

Although of a higher refractive index (1.586) than even crown glass, polycarbonate is a softer material and easily scratched unless coated. A protective coating is standard.

Care should be taken to ensure that all surfaces or points which come into contact with the lens are free from rough edges or burrs. Lensometer marking points should not be overlooked.

Lenses should be free of dirt and oils in order to avoid surface deblocking or slipping. For this reason, it is best to grip the lenses by their edges.

The use of *protective* surface adhesive tapes is not recommended, as the lens coating can be pulled off when the tape is removed.

The method of choice for blocking polycarbonate is an adhesive pad system.

Special Methods for Edging Polycarbonate

Because of the nature of the lens material, attempts to edge these lenses on wheels designed for glass or CR-39 material are totally useless. The wheel quickly loads with material and the lens rides on the spinning wheel without being cut. In order to solve the problem, three separate methods were developed.

Milling Cutters

The *first method* employs a toothed *milling cutter*. The teeth of the cutter are shaped to produce a bevel on the lens edge. The lens is brought to the appropriate shape as the cutter blades chop off parts of the lens, as opposed to the grinding action of most wheels. Using a milling cutter wheel is especially practical for the industrial production of plano safety lenses where the edger is fed by an

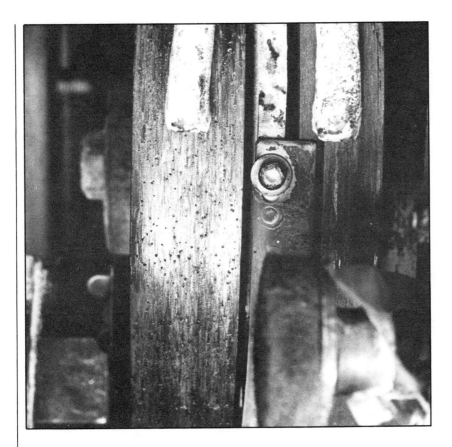

Figure 7–40. *Diamond particles are more widely spaced on wheels used in the edging of polycarbonate lenses.*

automatic loader. However, stringent safety precautions must be taken if milling cutter wheels are to be used for manually operated prescription edgers. The edger must be equipped with a safety brake that stops the wheel when the cover is lifted.

Milling cutters must rotate fast enough so the cutter wheel neither gives a ragged edge nor induces stress in the lens. If there are too few "bites" or chops per minute, stress develops in the lens. This stress will later result either in a cracked lens or in surface crazing. The minimum number of bites per minute required for a stress-free lens is 32,000.[9] Bites per minute may be found by multiplying the RPM (revolutions per minute) of the motor times the number of teeth on the milling cutter.

When a lens has been edged with a milling cutter, fine, evenly-spaced cutting marks are visible along

the bevel. For non-industrial use, it may be necessary to hand polish the edge for a better cosmetic result.

Diamond Wheels

As mentioned before, attempts made to edge polycarbonate lenses on conventional wheels meet with failure. CR-39 is a *thermosetting* material, meaning that once it has been molded to the correct shape, it cannot be remolded. Polycarbonate, however, is *thermoplastic.* When an edging technique is used that generates a significant amount of heat, the polycarbonate material softens and quickly loads up on the edger wheel. Therefore it became necessary to develop a special type of *diamond wheel.*

Figure 7–40 shows one style roughing wheel used; an electroplated wheel with a single layer of large, blocky, coarsely-spaced diamond crystals.

Even the finishing wheel must be specially designed, using a metal-bonding technique and smaller diamond crystals.

The edging process can be performed either wet,

---

[9]Ronald C. Wiand, "New Methods for Edging Polycarbonate Lenses," a paper given at the Optical Laboratories Association annual meeting, Atlanta, Georgia, Nov. 20-22, 1980.

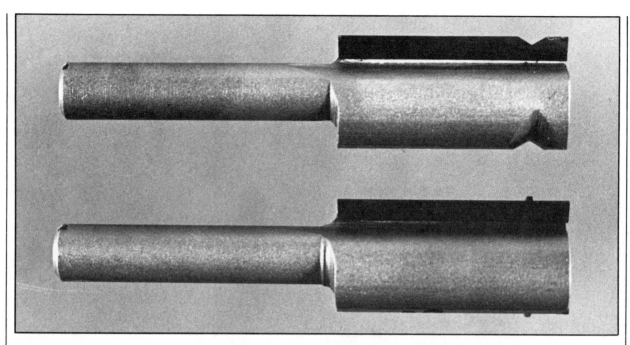

Figure 7–41. *Polycarbonate and CR-39 plastic lenses can be edged using a router blade and no coolant. The upper blade is used to produce a hidden bevel, the lower blade for grooving a lens to accept a nylon cord as with nylon supra style frames. (Photo courtesy of National Optronics, Incorporated.)*

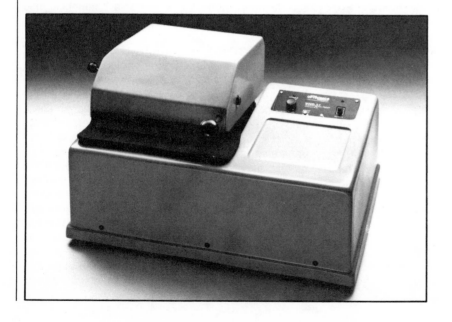

Figure 7–42. *One example of a router style plastic lens bevel edger. (Courtesy of National Optronics, Incorporated.)*

using coolants, or dry. However, a combination of both processes yields a more stress-free lens. In this combination process, the lens is rough edged with no coolant. During the finishing cycle the coolant pump is activated and the edging process completed.

Even though these wheels are specifically developed for polycarbonate, they may also be used for CR-39 lenses.

Router Blades

A *third type* of edger that utilizes a completely different system can also be used for either CR-39 or polycarbonate. Such edgers cut the lens to size using a small, rapidly rotating *router blade.* (See Figure 7–41.) It is not possible to adapt a conventional edger to router-blade edging. These are intended for plastic lenses only and cannot, under any circumstances, be used for glass. (See Figure 7–42.)

When a lens is edged with a router blade, there is no coolant required, as small chips of lens are removed with a slicing action. Because there is no coolant, chips are drawn out of the edging chamber with a vacuum pump. Speed of edging is increased considerably, reducing the actual cutting cycle to anywhere from 13 to 35 seconds.

Even when using a router blade, some system for controlling bevel location is still required. Although bevel placement systems can vary, one such system utilizes a guide wheel that rolls on the front surface periphery of the lens during rotation.

Special router blades are available that, instead of bevelling the edge, will groove it for use with frames having a nylon cord lens retention system.

When the router-blade system is used for the softer polycarbonate lens, an extremely high number of cuts per minute are required, as was the case when using a milling cutter. In contrast, the harder CR-39 material is edged at a slower cutting speed. (Hardness of material must not be equated with impact resistance, as the softer polycarbonate lens is by far the more resistant to breakage.)

How Edgers for Polycarbonate Differ From Conventional Edgers

There are certain points at which diamond wheel edgers adapted for polycarbonate differ from conventional edgers. For example, a fine mesh screen or nylon stocking is needed between the drain and above the coolant to filter out chips created during dry edging. The drain part itself is larger to facilitate waste chip outflow.

As might be imagined, the adaptation of a conventional edger for polycarbonate is feasible. It is even possible to install a toggle switch between edger and coolant pump that allows the advantage of coolant flow during the finishing cycle only. Before deciding to adapt an existing edger, however, the relative benefits gained in cost savings should be carefully weighed.

Stress in Polycarbonate Lenses Due to Edging

If the speed of the milling cutter, diamond wheel, or router blade is too slow, stress develops in a lens. Edging-induced lens stress can also result from dull cutting surfaces on the wheel or blade. Although stressed, lenses may still edge rapidly and look acceptable from a cosmetic viewpoint. In other words, if the lens is subjected to stress created by attempts to cut off overly large chips of lens (a slow cutter) or normal-sized chips with a blunt instrument (dull cutter), stress is absorbed by the lens. As Table 7–7 lists, over a period of time, lens stress is released in the form of cracking or surface crazing.

Table 7–7. When Stress in Polycarbonate is Too High after Edging

Problem	Solution
Cutter blades too dull or diamond wheel becoming dulled	Resharpen or replace blades. Send diamond wheel in for rework
Head pressure too high	Bring head pressure back
RPM of motor too slow	Increase motor speed or increase number of teeth in milling cutter
Too few teeth in milling cutter wheel for RPM of motor	Increase motor speed or increase number of teeth in milling cutter
Lenses being edged dry (This may not become a problem unless several other combined factors cause stress to reach a borderline level)	Consider using a coolant on the final cutting cycle

General Electric, the developer of polycarbonate, has determined that a polycarbonate lens should not be subjected to any stress during the manufacturing process that exceeds 1,000 pounds per square inch (PSI). General Electric also has developed tests that can be performed on the lens to indicate if this level of stress has been exceeded.

One such test indicates whether the lens has been subjected to a level of stress of 500 PSI or greater. This is done by brushing the edge of the

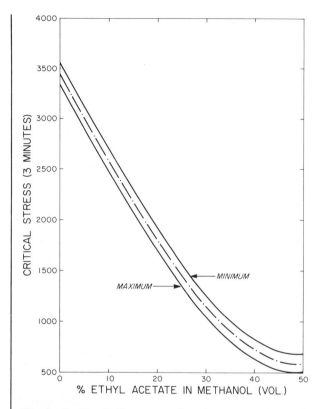

Figure 7–43. *As the proportional measurements of a mixture containing ethyl acetate and methanol are varied, the detectable stress in polycarbonate material will also vary.*

lens with carbon tetrachloride. If hairline cracks or crazing appear, a stress of 500 PSI has been exceeded. (Carbon tetrachloride is a toxic material and should only be used in a well-ventilated area.)

A second test is done using a mixture of ethyl acetate and methanol. Use extreme care, as this chemical mixture is quite flammable and toxic. The stress sensitivity of the solution increases with the addition of ethyl acetate. Pure methanol will detect stress over 3,400 PSI. Therefore, combining the two in varying proportions allows a go/no-go type test for any desired level. (See Figure 7–43.) The normally used combination is 1 to 1, which detects stress that could range from 500 to 700 PSI. Maximum allowable stress could be checked by using 35% ethyl acetate and 65% methanol by volume. The test itself is carried out by emersing the lens in the solution for three minutes, then examining the edge for hairline cracks or crazing. Such a solution should be used for one lens only. Both carbon tetrachloride and ethyl acetate/methanol tests should be done on a lens intended solely for testing purposes.

Completing the Process

Like other lenses, polycarbonate lenses should be safety bevelled. There are variations in this process that are discussed in the section on hand edging.

It is important that the lens be edged and mounted stress-free to avoid future cracking or surface crazing. Although improper edging techniques can be the greatest source of stress in a polycarbonate lens, mounting the lenses too tightly will also yield significant stress.

Cleaning of polycarbonate lenses may not employ harsh chemicals. A mild detergent should prove sufficient.

Laminated Lenses

When lenses are composed of two or more materials laminated together, the lens must be edged on a wheel that is compatible with both materials.

For example, Corlon[10] lenses are made with the front half of crown or photochromic glass laminated together with a back half composed of optical quality polyurethane material. The lenses are edged on a standard glass edger. However, in the case of the Corlon lens, the coolant tank should be equipped with a filter to trap small slivers of polyurethane material and prevent their recirculation.

---

[10]Corlon is manufactured by Corning Glass Works.

PROFICIENCY TEST QUESTIONS

1. There are definite relationships between pattern size and edger setting. Assuming a standard pattern size of 36.5 mm, fill in the missing information for each of the lens size/pattern size combinations listed below.

Eyesize	Pattern Size	Set Number	Edger Setting
50	36.5	a	b
48	c	−10	d
45	e	f	37
g	44.5	h	44
50	36.5	i	j
k	l	−5	57
50	51.5	m	n
52	50	o	p

2. If a pattern is marked, "set-5," what is the pattern's *A* dimension? (Assume a U.S. standard.)
   a. 37.5
   b. 41
   c. 45
   d. 41.5
   e. Cannot be determined from information given

3. A pattern measures 56 mm. If the frame to be used is a 58 □ 20, what edger setting will result in a correctly edged lens?
   a. Set at 36.5 mm
   b. Set at 38.5 mm
   c. Set at 54 mm
   d. Set at 56 mm
   e. Set at 58 mm

4. A pattern has a *B* dimension of 47 and a pattern difference of 4. What is the pattern set number?
   a. −14.5
   b. −4
   c. −6.5
   d. −40.5
   e. None of the above is correct.

5. A pattern has a size of 36.5 mm, and is marked □ 6. If the edger is correctly calibrated and set for 52 mm, what will the *B* dimension of the edged lens measure?
   a. 42.5 mm
   b. 30.5 mm
   c. 46 mm

d. 58 mm
   e. None of the above is correct.

6. An edger has a setting dial with a zero, plus-minus scale. A pattern has an *A* dimension of 53. The frame has an *A* dimension of 49. What would the edger setting be?
   a. −2 mm
   b. −12.5 mm
   c. −16.5 mm
   d. −4 mm
   e. None of the above is correct.

7. An edger has a setting dial with a zero, plus-minus scale. The pattern is marked "set-10." The frame has an *A* dimension of 52. To what is the edger dial set? (Assume the pattern to be marked for U.S. Standards.)
   a. −10
   b. +5.5
   c. 62
   d. −15.6
   e. None of the above is correct.

8. The edging cycle is interrupted after roughing. The pattern set number is "set-10" and the edger has been set on 40 mm. The lens measures 52.5 mm across the *A* dimension. Assuming the lens will be the correct size when completely edged, what is the wheel differential of the edger?

9. For cutting a rimless lens on an edger not programmed for flat edging, the stop mechanism is set to prevent the lens from entering the groove. The edger setting must be compensated by which of the following?
   a. Adding the groove depth to the calculated edger setting
   b. Subtracting the groove depth from the calculated edger setting
   c. Adding twice the groove depth to the calculated edger setting
   d. Subtracting twice the groove depth from the calculated edger setting.

10. Some V-bevels are made to cause the lens bevel apex to be more toward the front of the lens. This is done by what procedure?
   a. Making the groove steeper.
   b. Making the groove deeper.
   c. Using a coarser grade diamond grit on the front side of the groove than on the back

d. Using a finer grade diamond grit on the front side of the groove than on the back
e. None of the above will cause the desired effect.

11. A lens is to be edged for the following frame:

    A = 48, B = 38, DBL = 20, ED = 48

    The wearer's PD is 64.
    If the lens is a minus lens, where will it be thicker?
    a. At the top or bottom
    b. Nasally
    c. Temporally

12. If the lens above were a plus lens, which edge would be thickest?
    a. The top or bottom edge
    b. The nasal edge
    c. The temporal edge

13. Choose the statement about a regular facet (non-Tura style) that is false.
    a. When the facet is used, edge thickness is reduced.
    b. Lens field of view will be increased slightly due to a reduction in the concentric ring effect.
    c. A reduction of usable optics by more than 5 or 6 mm is not necessary.
    d. The facet follows the basic shape of the lens.
    e. The facet is produced by using the edge of the stone (edger wheel).

14. T or F   According to ANSI standards the frame groove angle must be greater than the lens bevel angle.

15. A high-plus lens with a large amount of decentration and/or a large frame difference is best edged using a:
    a. facet
    b. V-bevel
    c. mini-bevel
    d. myodisc configuration

16. In the edging process for progressive add lenses when a fitting cross system is used for facial measurement, what is the reference point for edging?
    a. MRP
    b. Fitting cross

17. What does the counterbalance adjustment on the edger do?
    a. Controls where the lens first comes in contact with the edger finishing wheel
    b. Controls where the lens comes to rest on the edger finishing wheel after it has initially made contact
    c. Controls the placement of the bevel on the lens edge
    d. Controls when the lens is lifted from the roughing to the finishing wheel
    e. Controls the amount of weight the float carriage exerts on the lens in contact with the edger wheels

18. How much larger should a roughed lens be than when finished?
    a. 1.5 to 2.0 mm
    b. 2.0 to 2.5 mm
    c. 2.5 to 3.0 mm
    d. 3.0 to 3.5 mm
    e. 3.5 to 4.0 mm

19. For edging lenses on a free-float system, the lens will track in the edger wheel groove more accurately with what level of pressure?
    a. Lighter head pressure
    b. Heavier head pressure
    c. Tracking is unaffected by head pressure.

20. On a polycarbonate lens, what reduces edge swarf?
    a. Decreasing head pressure
    b. Increasing head pressure

21. Which factors increase stress in a polycarbonate lens?
    a. A slower cutter blade
    b. Too many teeth on the milling cutter
    c. A dull cutting mechanism
    d. Low edging pressure

22. Which of the following lenses is thermosetting?
    a. CR-39
    b. Polycarbonate

23. Match the refractive indices to the correct lens material.
    crown glass _____   a. 1.425
    polycarbonate _____   b. 1.498
    CR-39 _____   c. 1.523
    high-lite glass _____   d. 1.530
                                 e. 1.586

f. 1.621
g. 1.70

24. For a prescription of

R: −4.00 −2.00 × 180
L: −7.00 −2.00 × 180

if an attempt were made to equalize magnification by changing vertex distances, which of the following would happen?
a. Right bevel would be moved toward the front of the lens and the left bevel somewhat more toward the middle of the lens edge.
b. Left bevel would be moved toward the front of the lens and the right bevel somewhat more toward the middle of the lens edge.
c. Both bevels would be moved toward the front of the lens.
d. Both bevels would be moved to a more central location.

25. T or F   A hump on the edge of a lens that is not a part of the pattern shape indicates not enough head pressure during edging.

26. Place the lens types in order, from those requiring the least edger head pressure to those requiring the most:
a. 1,2,3,4   1. plastic lenses
b. 4,3,2,1   2. glass lenses
c. 3,1,2,4   3. polycarbonate lenses
d. 4,1,2,3   4. high index lenses
e. 1,4,2,3

27. Moving a plus lens farther from the eye does which of the following?
a. Increases its magnification
b. Decreases its magnification
c. Does not affect magnification

28. T or F   The groove for a nylon cord lens retention system can be produced on some edgers.

29. Which response is true of a thermoplastic material?
a. It cannot be remolded once it has been originally molded, even when heated.
b. It can be remolded once it has been molded, if heated sufficiently.
c. It becomes harder if heated.

Chapter 8
Deblocking

The method used to deblock a lens depends, of course, upon what blocking method was used. Some are self-evident, such as breaking the seal of a suction blocked lens by lifting the edge of the suction cup.

DEBLOCKING METAL ALLOY BLOCKED LENSES

One of the fastest methods of deblocking an alloy blocked lens is by *shock* or *impact deblocking*. A short hollow fiber tube with a diameter slightly larger than the block itself is used. The lens is placed face down on the tube with the block inside. Figure 8–1 shows how the lens is held in place with one finger, while the shock deblocker is slapped against a flat surface. Sudden impact causes the block to drop off. (This method is not recommended for plastic lenses.) Because some alloy blocks are so small and lightweight, this method may not always prove satisfactory.

Metal blocks may also be removed using a large-jawed plier. The jaws are oriented so that they span the longest axis of the block, as in Figure 8–2.

Deblocking is *not* accomplished by pulling the block off, but rather by squeezing. As pressure is applied to the longer axis, slight flexing of the metal occurs, breaking the seal between lens and alloy. The pliers themselves never touch the lens. This method works best on glass lenses, as the lens does not flex with the metal as a plastic lens could.

The third method uses a hot water bath to melt the alloy off the lens. It is not necessary to have a special deblocking unit in order to use this method, especially if hot water deblocking is used primarily as a backup method for especially stubborn cases, or when special caution is required. Some technicians have used a hot pot such as might be used to heat water for tea at an office. The lens is placed in a teflon strainer. The strainer allows the lens to be immersed in the water. When the alloy liquifies, it runs through the strainer, leaving a deblocked lens that can be retrieved easily. Some practitioners have used a spring clip clothespin instead of or in conjunction with the strainer. The clothespin is clipped to one edge of the lens and immersed.

To retrieve the liquid alloy, the entire contents of the pot are poured into another container. (The bulk

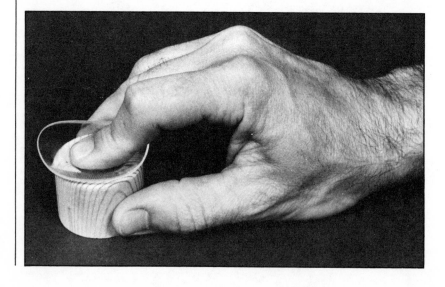

Figure 8–1. Shock deblocking of metal alloy blocked lenses can be achieved using a wood cylinder with a central hole large enough to accept the width of the block.

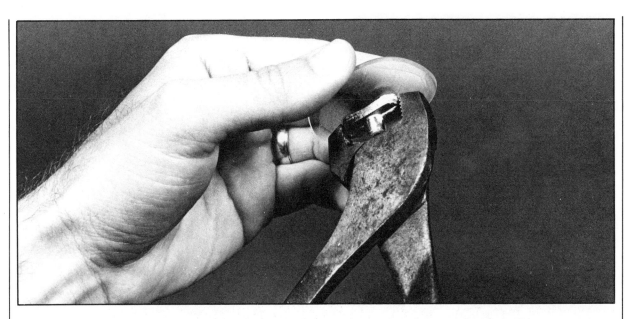

Figure 8–2. *When pliers are used to deblock an alloy blocked lens, squeeze the long axis of the block to deblock—do not pull.*

of the hot water may be poured back into the pot if desired, as the alloy remains on the bottom of the container.) For convenience it is best to use a somewhat flexible container. When the alloy has cooled and hardened, it can then be easily removed by flexing the container as one might a plastic ice tray.

Metal blocks are most easily removed from plastic lenses. Because a plastic lens flexes when pressure is applied, a block can be made to drop off by applying a twisting motion to the lens, as Figure 8–3 shows. Because the alloy will not flex to the same extent, the bond between alloy and lens breaks, releasing the block.

Remelting the Alloy

Before returning the alloy blocks to the blocking unit for remelting, it is best to rinse them to remove lens spray and coolant contaminants. This reduces problems with stopped up blocker feed lines and general alloy contamination.

Alloy blocks should be remelted a few at a time if the metal blocker is being used so as not to alter the alloy temperature too greatly. This is not of great concern if lenses are not to be blocked immediately.

When more than one type of alloy is being used in the lab, take care that cross-contamination does not occur, as unexpected changes in melting temperature can result.

DEBLOCKING ADHESIVE PAD BLOCKED LENSES

Blocks applied to the lens with an adhesive pad system are removed by a twisting motion. The method used to accomplish this requires a tool (see Figure 8–4) that firmly holds the block while the lens is twisted. The usual holding tool is shaped to accept the block exactly like the edger chuck does.

As a precautionary measure, it is advisable to hold the lens with a lab towel while twisting; Figure 8–5 shows the correct position. If the lens is held in the palm of the hand without a towel the technician can get small surface cuts, since sharp edges have not been removed by hand edging.

Just a reminder: A lens should not be deblocked until there is no doubt that it will fit into the frame readily. It is much easier to take a lens down in size on an automatic edger than to hand edge it to size.

Table 8–1 summarizes the deblocking methods discussed in this chapter.

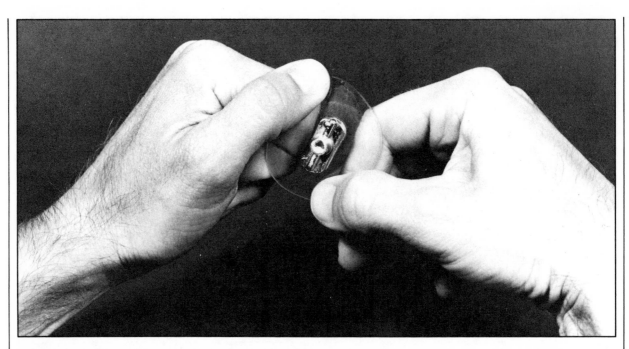

Figure 8–3. *If a plastic lens is twisted slightly, adhesion is broken and the alloy block will drop off.*

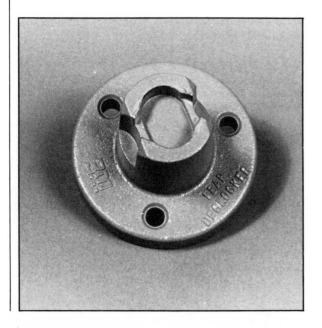

Figure 8–4. *An adhesive pad deblocker is simply a holding mechanism for the block. Deblocking occurs when the lens is twisted off the block.*

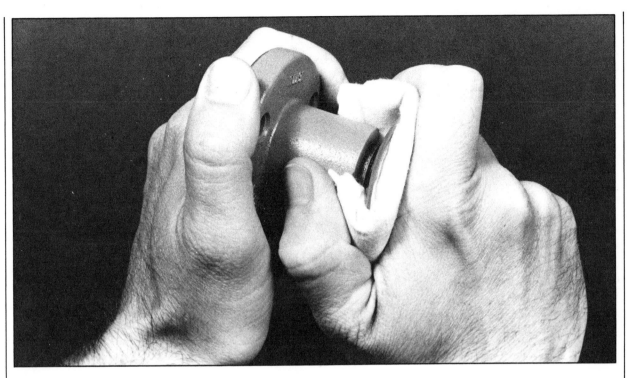

Figure 8–5. *Although many practitioners deblock lenses without the use of a lab towel, small cuts can be avoided by padding the edges of the lenses.*

Table 8–1. Deblocking Methods

Blocking Method Employed	Block Removal Techniques
Pressure blocking	"Deblocking" accomplished by removing lens from edger
Suction blocking	Break seal by lifting edge of suction cup with fingernail Twist off

Metal alloy blocking	For glass lenses
	    Impact or shock
	    Plier pressure
	    Hot water
	
	For plastic lenses
	    Torque lens
	    Hot water

Adhesive pad blocking	Twist off

PROFICIENCY TEST QUESTIONS

1. Which method is inappropriate for deblocking metal alloy blocked lenses?
   a. Shock
   b. Twist off
   c. Plier pressure
   d. Hot water
   e. All of the above are appropriate.

2. T or F   Deblocking of metal alloy blocked lenses is accomplished by grasping the block across the short dimension and pulling it off.

3. What type of container is best to use when allowing retrieved molten alloy to cool?
   a. Cast iron pan
   b. Aluminum pan
   c. Corning or Pyrex style dish
   d. Plastic container

4. How may an adhesive pad blocked lens be deblocked?
   a. Impact or shock
   b. A twist-off motion
   c. Torquing the lens
   d. Peeling the pad off with the fingernail
   e. Using hot water

5. T or F   Regardless of blocking method, the safest way to deblock a plastic lens is with hot water.

6. T or F   A lens should not be deblocked until there is no doubt that it will fit into the frame readily.

Chapter 9
Hand Edging

PURPOSES

Hand edging is most commonly used to (1) smooth edge surfaces and (2) remove sharp edges from a lens after it has been machine edged. The first process is referred to as *edge smoothing* and the second as *safety* or *pin bevelling.* Hand edging may also be used to reduce a lens in size somewhat or to reshape the lens.

TYPES OF HAND EDGERS

In simplest terms, a *hand edger* is an abrasive wheel mounted so that the operator is allowed free access to manually grind lens edges.

The most traditional style of hand edger is a large diameter wheel with a 1½-inch wide edge, as shown in Figure 9–1. The wheel is ceramic and may be retrued often to remove surface irregularities. Since the wheel is ceramic down to the hub, it has an extremely long life.

Deviations from this basic hand edger design have occurred with the advent of diamond faced wheels. The cost of constructing a wheel with a diamond abrasive that must cover such a large surface area encouraged the development of alternate designs.

Some manufacturers have maintained the basic design, but reduced the wheel diameter and/or the edge width. Reducing edge width understandably restricts the horizontal working area available.

A more commonly occurring design for diamond

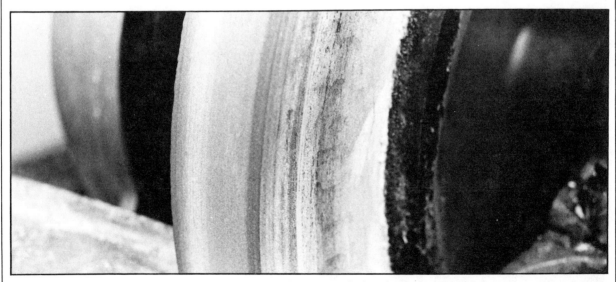

Figure 9–1. Although it requires occasional retruing, a ceramic hand edging wheel has an exceptionally long life because of its depth.

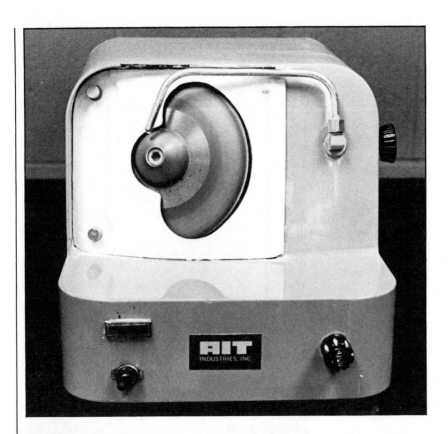

Figure 9–2. *A face-type hand edger reduces the amount of diamond required by placing the abrasive on the side of the wheel.*

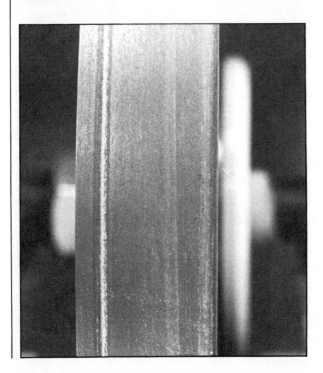

Figure 9–3. *A grooved wheel is not for the purpose of smoothing both bevel surfaces of normal lenses simultaneously. It allows lenses with hidden bevel edge shapes to be reduced in size without destroying the edge configuration.*

hand edgers is the one in Figure 9–2, which uses the face of a rotating wheel for grinding, rather than using the edge. In this manner, a larger working area is obtained from fewer square units of diamond impregnated surface. A disadvantage of the face-type edger is that such a design does not allow use of the corner of the wheel for hard-to-reach sections of the bevel. In compensation, a central curved hub is provided.

Occasionally, the flat area on an automatic edger wheel is used to hand edge a lens. This will only prove satisfactory if the edger design allows free access to the wheel and if lenses are edged periodically and in limited numbers.

One option worth considering when selecting a hand edger is the kind of V-grooved wheel shown in Figure 9–3. This groove allows an edged, hidden-bevel lens to be reduced in size. Unless this option is available, a size reduction or shape modification by hand is possible only if the hidden bevel is changed to a standard V.

AVAILABLE WHEEL TYPES

Wheels having varying amounts of abrasiveness may be chosen for hand edging, depending upon the primary use of the wheel. As mentioned before, there are two main purposes for hand edging. The first is reduction of lens size or lens shape alteration. The second is the removal of microchips and the smoothing of sharp edges. The wheel type selected depends upon which functions are carried out more frequently.

Ceramic Wheels
The ceramic wheel can give an excellent finish and is the wheel many practitioners prefer. It gives especially good results with glass lenses. Although a ceramic wheel is available in more than one grit size, the most commonly used is a fine grit that generally has a brown or green color. If a ceramic stone is selected for plastic lenses, a coarser grit is preferable and the wheel color is generally blue. The blue stone will cut a glass lens slightly faster than brown or green stones.

Diamond Wheels
A great amount of versatility is available using different types of diamond wheels. As would be expected, those wheels having an extra-fine grit are excellent for pin bevelling, while a rough grit is used for rapid removal of lens edge substance.

Hand edger wheels have a tendency to "load" with plastic in the same manner as do automatic edger wheels. Therefore, diamond hand edger wheels made especially for plastic are available. *Wheels designed for plastic are to be used with plastic lenses only. Wheels designed for glass will accept both glass and plastic.*

Here is an example of a common selection of hand edger wheel grits:

    Plastic: Rough
    Plastic: Fine
    Glass/Plastic: Rough
    Glass/Plastic: Medium-rough
    Glass/Plastic: Fine
    Glass/Plastic: Extra-fine

Grit types and their purposes are listed in Table 9–1. If only one wheel must be chosen for all purposes, the fine-grit wheel will prove to be the most versatile. It allows smooth pin bevelling, yet can still be used to take size down. A super-fine wheel is for pin bevelling and edge smoothing only. In contrast, rough wheels are excellent for rapid shape reduction or alteration, but cannot be expected to adequately perform smoothing tasks.

For maximum efficiency, use two wheels of different grits in close proximity to one another.

Table 9–1. Hand Edger Wheel Grit Types and Their Purposes

Type	Primary purpose(s)
Rough	Removing edge stock rapidly
Medium	Removing edge stock
Fine	Pin bevelling and edge smoothing; also removes edge stock moderately well
Extra-fine	Pin bevelling and edge smoothing

PREPARING THE WHEEL

Before hand edging, the wheel must be wet. Some hand edgers have a coolant recycling system with a pump and coolant tank below the unit. Others use tap water that does not recirculate, but simply drains out. In either case, a steady drip on the wheel is required. Because of the smoothness of most wheels, the thumb may be drawn across the face of the spinning wheel to ensure that the entire surface

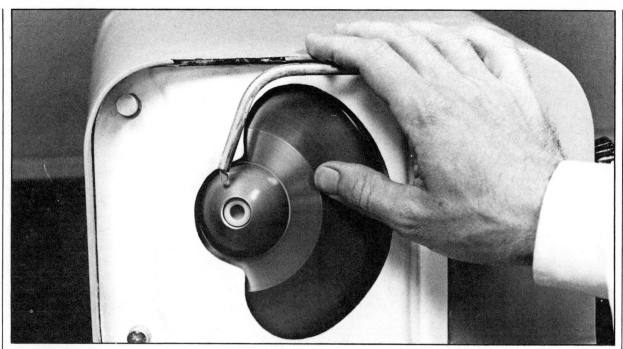

Figure 9–4. *Drawing the thumb across the hand wheel assures even wetting before grinding begins.*

is wetted; this method is illustrated in Figure 9–4.

Some wheels use a sponge to prevent splashing and to spread the water evenly over the surface. The sponge should be wetted and positioned before turning the unit on. It must also be removed whenever the unit is turned off. If this is not done, ceramic wheels will absorb water from the sponge and swell, creating a lump on the wheel.

HOW HAND EDGING IS DONE

The most basic procedure in hand edging consists of edge smoothing and pin bevelling. At the same time the smoothing process is being carried out, the technician checks the quality of bevel for both angle and apex position. As was previously illustrated in Figure 7–20, the apex of the bevel should be centrally placed for thin lenses, but placed a third of the way from the front for thicker-edged lenses.

The first step in hand edging consists of rotating the rear surface of the bevel on the face of the hand stone. Technique is all-important, beginning with how the lens is held.

Holding the Lens

The left hand[1] is rested on the hand rest and the lens is grasped between thumb and forefinger with both hands. The right thumb and forefinger will act as a pivotal point while the left thumb and forefinger will guide the lens.

Assuming that the apical angle on the bevel is as needed, the lens is held with the back surface of the lens bevel flat against the cutting plane of the wheel. Figure 9–5 shows this in cross section from the side; thus seen it makes an angle with the cutting plane of the wheel of approximately 41 degrees.

Were the lens to be viewed from the front, the angle that the lens makes with the horizontal plane could vary considerably, depending upon the personal preference of the operator. However, an angle of approximately 60 degrees will allow the operator a good view of the lens without leaning sideways, while still taking advantage of the upward pull of the wheel. The lens is held on its 180-degree cutting line, as shown in Figure 9–6.

---

[1]The sequence will be explained from the righthanded point of view. Those who are lefthanded should substitute left for right and right for left. Pictures visualized in mirror image will give the lefthanded perspective. (Holding the book in front of a large mirror will show correct left hand positioning.)

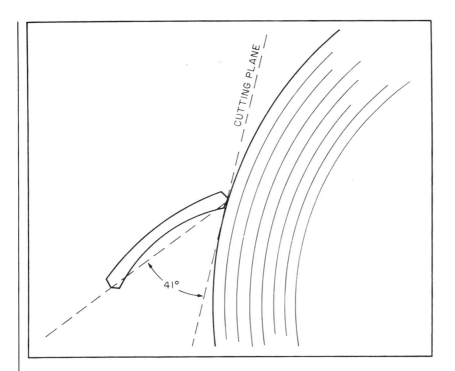

Figure 9–5. *During edge smoothing, the back bevel surface is smoothed first. This helps to position the apex. The lens is held somewhere near a 41-degree angle with the cutting plane. It is angled downward considerably more than it will be when the front bevel surface is smoothed.*

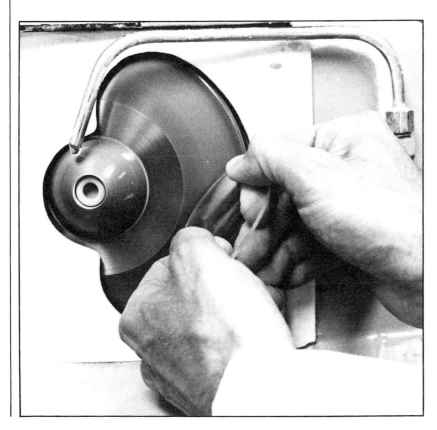

Figure 9–6. *By tilting the lens to approximately 60 degrees, and rotating it clockwise, the upward pull of the wheel can be used to advantage. (Lefthanders tilt to the mirror image and rotate the lens counterclockwise.)*

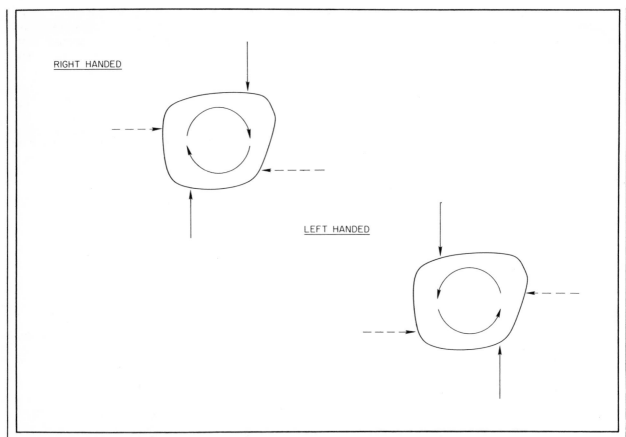

Figure 9–7. *It is best to start edging a lens from a point just past a lens corner.*

Lens rotation will be clockwise[2] so that it turns with the wheel. As Figure 9–7 demonstrates, the best place to begin is just past a lens corner.

The lens is held tightly between right thumb and forefinger. This point on the lens becomes the pivotal point. Figure 9–8 shows how the left thumb and forefinger (primarily the thumb) guide the lens across the surface of the wheel. As the lens turns 180 degrees, the left forefinger is removed from the lens and the thumb guides it on around, as illustrated in Figure 9–9.

Pressure and Rotational Speed

The finer the wheel grit, the more pressure may be

applied. However, there are several variables that affect how much pressure is appropriate.

As could be expected, if the lens edge is especially thick, then more pressure may be applied. Note, though, that this is true primarily for the back side of the bevel, since it contains the bulk of the surface area.

Pressure on the lens against the wheel must be slackened as the corners are smoothed. As lens/wheel contact area reduces, if the overall force being applied is not reduced, pressure per square inch will increase dramatically.

An alternative to reducing pressure against the lens as corners are rounded is to increase the speed of rotation. Since less time is spent in contact with the wheel, cutting is reduced.

In actual practice, both speed of rotation and force

[2]Lefthanders rotate counterclockwise with the lens at 120 degrees instead of 60 degrees.

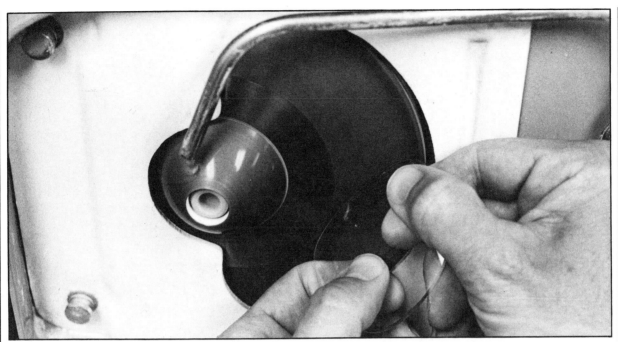

Figure 9–8. *To begin, hold the lens with thumb and forefingers as shown. The right thumb and forefinger serve as a pivotal point. The left thumb and forefinger guide the lens onto the wheel, controlling speed.*

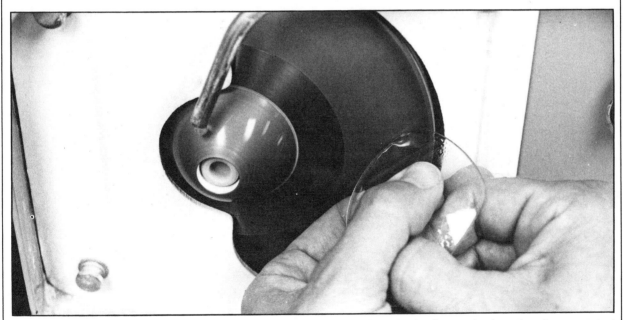

Figure 9–9. *The lens is not removed from the wheel surface often. In the figure, the lens has been rotated a full 180 degrees. The right hand still functions as a pivotal point, the left as a guide. By now moving the left finger out from under the lens, further uninterrupted rotation may be accomplished using the thumb of the left hand.*

against the wheel are simultaneously varied. (See Table 9–2.)

Listening to the Wheel

A great deal can be learned about the edge quality of the finished lens by listening to the sound of the wheel during hand edging.

The wheel should make a constant, unbroken sound. There are several reasons why the wheel might emit a wavy, irregular tone, all of which relate to faulty technique.

If the angle of lens *tilt* is being altered, a wavy sound occurs. This will result in a wavy bevel apex and incomplete, irregular removal of the "frosted" appearance of the bevel face.

Variations in the intensity of the sound indicate that *pressure* on the lens is uneven. An uneven, wavy bevel will result and a possible alteration in the basic shape of the lens could occur. Applying too much pressure on corners will cause corner gaps between lens and frame that will be evident after mounting.

Short, choppy sounds indicate that the lens is being lifted from the wheel too often. The best technique is to use a smooth, long motion.

A smooth sound interrupted by periodic wavy sounds indicates an attempt to regrip the lens without lifting it from the wheel. Each time the grip is changed, the lens must be lifted. It is impossible to maintain a correct wheel/lens relationship while simultaneously shifting the grip on the lens.

The following list summarizes the basic rules of hand edging.

1. A constant angle between the wheel face and lens must be maintained.
2. Never reposition a grip on the lens while the lens is against the wheel.
3. Travel as far around the bevel as possible before lifting the lens from the wheel.
4. Listen to the sound of the lens on the wheel.

How to Practice Edge Smoothing

Practice proper smoothing by choosing a lens large enough to allow an easy grip. A low-minus lens has an optimum edge configuration. A lens that has not previously been hand smoothed will still have a slightly frosted look to the bevel.

After each major "pass" around the lens, wipe the lens edge dry and check the frosted area. If all the white is being removed near just the apex, for example, the lens is being held consistently at the wrong angle. However, if the frost that remains is erratically positioned and is sometimes near the apex, and other times is near the lens surface, the hands must be rested more firmly on the hand rest and attention given to maintaining a consistent angle of tilt.

Until satisfactory results are obtained consistently while edge smoothing, an operator should not expect to perform lens size reductions or shape modifications with much success.

Sequence of Hand Edging Steps

As mentioned, the sequencing of steps in hand edging and pin bevelling begins with the back surface of the bevel. In most instances, if the bevel apex has not been optimally placed by the automatic edger, the apex needs to be moved toward the front. For this reason smoothing begins with the rear surface. If extra pressure is applied during the smoothing process, the bevel moves forward. When the

---

Table 9–2. Factors Affecting Cutting Speed in Hand Edging

Cutting speed will increase . . .	Cutting speed will decrease . . .
if pressure against the wheel is increased.	if pressure against the wheel is decreased.
if speed of rotation is decreased.	if speed of rotation is increased.
if a rougher grit wheel is used.	if a finer grit wheel is used.
at a corner of the lens shape.	along a straight side of the lens shape.
as lens edge thickness decreases.	as lens edge thickness increases.

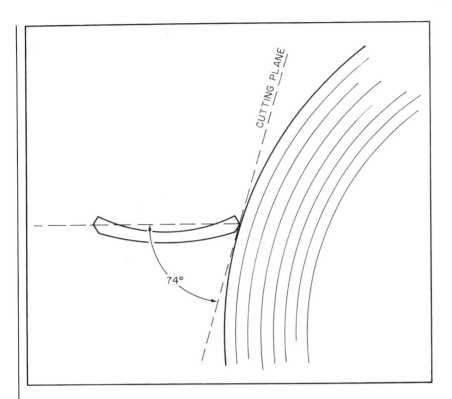

CUTTING PLANE

74°

Figure 9–10. *A common mistake in hand edging is to make the lens bevel too sharp. The near horizontal position of the lens shown in the figure is correct, but invariably seems wrong to the novice.*

bevel apex has been properly placed, the front surface of the bevel is smoothed. Because of bevel configuration, however, the angle between the cutting plane of the wheel and the lens is considerably greater than it was for the front surface. As Figure 9–10 shows, the angle is approximately 74 degrees, but can appear to be almost at right angles to the wheel, depending upon where the wheel is contacted. Front bevel smoothing is done lightly, so as not to alter bevel positioning.

Table 9–3 lists the proper steps for hand edging.

Table 9–3. Order for Hand Edging

	Approximate angle to wheel cutting plane
1. Rear face of bevel (and rimless rear pin bevel)	41°
2. Front face of bevel (and rimless front pin bevel)	74°
3. Front pin bevel	37°
4. Rear pin bevel	37°
5. Apex pin bevel	Held vertically at right angles

Pin Bevelling

Following smoothing, the lens undergoes pin bevelling. This is first at the intersection of front lens and bevel surfaces, followed by the rear lens and bevel intersection, and concluded with the apex of the bevel.

There are two primary reasons for pin bevelling. The first is a safety precaution. If the intersection is allowed to remain as a sharp corner, the risk of chipping or flaking at the interface between the two surfaces is considerably higher. Hence the alternate term, *safety bevel*. The second reason is to remove *microchips* or "stars" left as the abrasive wheel grinds away lens material. Microchips are seen by holding the lens up to a light source and turning it slightly. Star-like reflections on the edge indicate their presence.

The basic procedure for pin bevelling is the same as for edge smoothing. For front and rear surfaces the lens is held in the same manner, except that the angle the lens forms with the cutting plane is only half what it was for the smoothing process. Figure 9–11 compares angles for grinding types of bevels. Very little pressure is applied, as the lens is practically permitted to rotate from the upward pull of the wheel alone. Speed of rotation is much quicker.

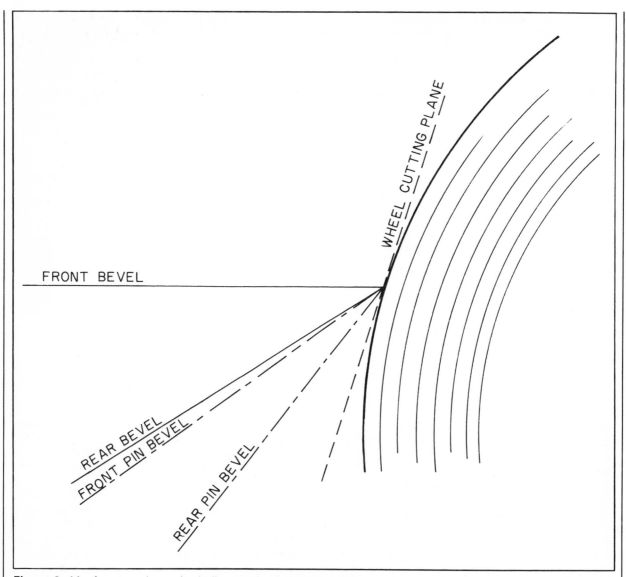

FRONT BEVEL

WHEEL CUTTING PLANE

REAR BEVEL

FRONT PIN BEVEL

REAR PIN BEVEL

Figure 9–11. *A comparison of grinding angles in hand edging.*

When completed, the pin bevel should only be noticed by the absence of edge sharpness and microchips, rather than by measurable visibility.

The rear pin bevel may prove difficult if the lens has a high meniscus curve combined with a narrow *B* dimension. The rear center spans the surface of the wheel and cannot be reached without using the edge of the wheel. Figure 9–12 demonstrates that some wheels have purposely rounded edges to permit pin bevelling in just such instances.

Because face type hand edgers do not have an exposed edge, a spherically shaped central wheel area is provided. This spherical central portion is used exclusively for the rear pin bevel, as in Figure 9–13.

To pin bevel the apex, hold the lens vertically with

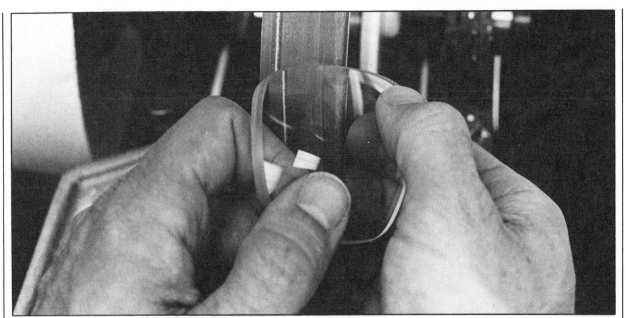

Figure 9–12. *When pin-bevelling the back edge of the lens on the rounded corner of the wheel, care must be taken to reduce pressure. The small lens/wheel contact area quickly raises the pressure per unit area.*

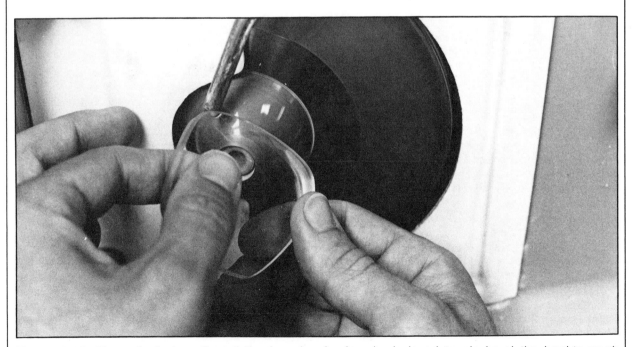

Figure 9–13. *The spherical section of the face hand edger is designed to pin bevel the hard-to-reach back edge of high-minus lenses.*

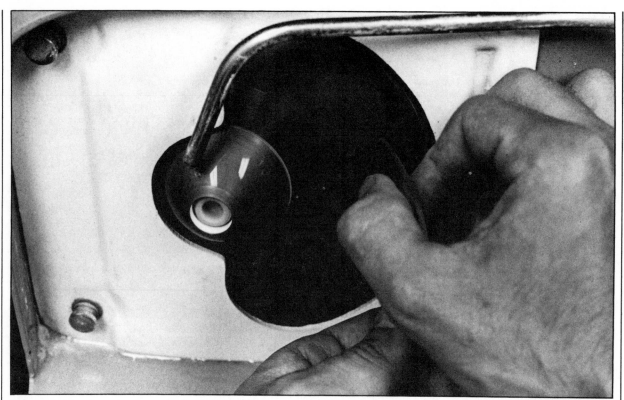

Figure 9–14. *Pin bevelling the bevel apex is done with very little pressure.*

the right hand. The lens may be guided with the left but should be held loosely enough to allow free rotation. See Figure 9–14 for an example of this procedure. Some operators are able to safety bevel the apex with one hand only.

Pin Bevelling for Rimless Lenses
A pin bevel has an angle that is halfway between the two surfaces it separates. Therefore, when safety bevelling a flat-edged rimless lens, it should be evident that the steep angles necessary for conventionally bevelled lenses are not used. Instead the lens is angled as conventional lenses are during the edge smoothing process. Rimless pin bevels are permitted to be slightly more visible than conventional pin bevels.

Hand Edging the Franklin Style Lens
The Franklin style lens lends itself to easy spoilage in the hands of inexperienced operators. Because of lens design, a large portion of the front bevel ends abruptly with the seg ledge on nasal and temporal sides of the lens. During the process of smoothing the front bevel surface, apply only light pressure to this section. Because ledge corners form small points, lens material is removed extremely rapidly. This same precaution must be observed during the pin bevelling process. Unless care is taken, the lens will prove to be more suitable when mounted directly in the frame *without* hand edging.

Automatic Pin Bevellers
Because of the relative skill required in hand edging, machines that pin bevel lenses automatically are available. If such equipment is used, the edge smoothing process is skipped (as it sometimes is when pin bevelling is done by hand). Whether or not the hand smoothing process is used depends upon the grit of the automatic edger's finishing wheel and the demand for craftsmanship.

An automatic pin beveller may serve a useful function in some situations, but cannot be expected to work well for each varying type of lens. Its chief advantage is that it does not necessitate operator training.

Hand Edging for Metal Frames

One of the most difficult tasks in hand edging is to reduce the size of an edged lens to fit a metal frame. Much skill is required to maintain the integrity of the lens shape during the process. The ideal situation is to have a sensitive automatic edger that allows small changes in lens size. However, despite the best of precautions, the necessity of making lenses fit through hand edging methods invariably arises.

Size reduction is accomplished by applying pressure to the rear bevel surface (as during a smoothing operation) and moving the bevel slightly farther forward than desired. The front bevel is then smoothed until the bevel returns to its proper position. If only a slight size reduction is required, repeating the edge smoothing process without attempting to move the bevel position could prove sufficient.

Even a small lens size reduction can make a large difference in how well it fits. If the frame is available, the lens should be checked often by placing it in the frame and closing the eyewire. If the eyewire screw is used, it may be backed out just far enough to allow the lens to be removed and reinserted. Size may also be checked by squeezing the eyewire barrels together with a pair of thin-nosed pliers, as seen in Figure 7–36.

The ability to screw the eyewire barrels flush together, or nearly so, does not indicate a good fit. There may be undue pressure on the lens by the eyewire. In plastic lenses this will cause warpage, and in glass a stress pattern will be set up within the lens. If nothing is done to relieve the stress, edge flaking (surface chipping at the lens edge) will occur if the rims receive even a slight blow.

Stress may also result when the meniscus curve of the lens does not match the curve of the eyewire. In this case, either the eyewire must be shaped to match the lens bevel curve, or the bevel must be repositioned by hand to match the curve of the frame. The distance from the front edge of the lens to the bevel apex will then vary around the circumference of the lens.

Check for stress within the lens by placing the lens between two crossed polaroids (as would be done to check for a heat hardened lens). Viewing the lens in this state will show a zig-zag color fringed pattern around the lens edge wherever there is a stress buildup. If this encompasses the lens completely, as Figure 7–38 illustrated, the lens is still large. It should

be taken down evenly on all sides. If, however, the pattern occurs only in one area, that area should be noted and edge stock removed.

When "lenses only" are ordered for a metal rimmed frame, some practitioners have found it helpful to have a variety of "metal sizers" on hand. These are simply frame fronts or metal chassis of some of the most commonly used frames. If the lenses fit the sizer, they should also fit the wearer's frame. Whether this proves to be the case or not depends upon tolerances in frame manufacturing.

An alternative to metal sizers that enjoyed some use in the past and has been reintroduced is the circumference gauge. Using this small gadget, the lens rotates one complete turn while a measuring wheel rolls. Thus, exact circumference of the edged lens is measured and can be compared to the previously recorded standard value for a correctly sized lens.

Hand Edging Hidden Bevels

Up to this point, processes described have applied only to those lenses having a V-bevel. Lenses having a hidden bevel do not lend themselves to conventional rear surface edge smoothing techniques—if edge smoothing is attempted, it can be carried out on the front surface alone. Only a minimum amount of pressure may be exerted in order to keep from moving the bevel back. Pin bevelling is done normally.

Because of the need to reduce the size of the lens having a hidden bevel, hand edger wheels with V-grooves are now available. To reduce the size of a lens having a hidden bevel, hold the lens perpendicular to the wheel with its bevel in the V-groove; Figure 9–15 shows how this is done. Use of the groove to smooth lens edges is possible if the groove angle matches that of the automatic edger. Edge smoothing for hidden bevels requires a steady hand. There must also have been an allowance made during automatic edging for the slight size reduction that occurs during edge smoothing.

Hand Edging of Polycarbonate

After automatic edging, polycarbonate lenses will have a residue of plastic material clinging to the lens surface/bevel surface interface. This buildup is known as *flash* or *swarf* and has been described as looking like white shredded wheat. (The amount of swarf remaining on the lens can be reduced by increasing edger head pressure.) Remove the swarf by scraping the lens edge with a razor or knife blade held perpendicular to the lens surface.

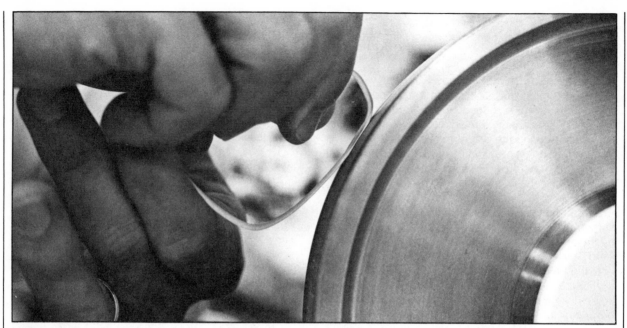

Figure 9–15. *It is helpful to brace one hand on the tray while reducing size or reshaping a lens with a hidden bevel edge configuration on a grooved wheel.*

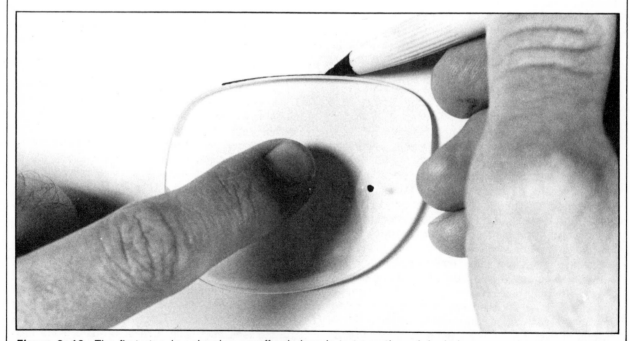

Figure 9–16. *The first step in salvaging an off-axis lens is to trace the original shape.*

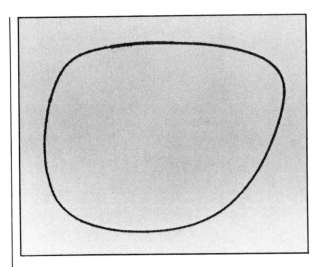

There are hand edger wheels especially made for polycarbonate, but since these may not be available in every lab, an alternative is necessary. Some suggested procedures to use in pin bevelling polycarbonate include:

1. using a dry, blue ceramic wheel. The disadvantage is that edging on regular wheels will quickly load them.
2. using the side of a conventional ceramic wheel.
3. mounting fine sandpaper on a hard, flat surface, and turning the edge on the sandpaper.

CORRECTIONAL MODIFICATIONS

Once an operator masters smoothing and pin bevelling, much versatility is gained. These skills make otherwise unachievable corrections and modifications in lens shapes possible.

Removing Chips
When a larger than average chip appears at the lens surface/lens bevel border, it should not be ground out by pin bevelling. This creates a double bevel appearance clearly visible to both wearer and observer. If the lens is to be salvaged, the procedure is to gradually steepen the rear bevel angle as the chip is approached. In other words, without moving the bevel apex forward, the rear bevel surface is smoothed in the chip area until it just disappears. Light pin bevelling is then done.

Salvaging an Off-Axis Lens
After mounting a lens in a plastic frame it may be discovered that the lens is off axis. If the lens shape is rounded, it may be possible to twist it slightly with lens rotating pliers without disturbing the appearance of the frame.

Shapes having distinct corners do not allow a lens that has actually been edged off axis to be twisted much, as rotated corners cause an unusual humping. If humping is evident, attempt to correct it as follows:

1. Trace the lens on a piece of paper as it would appear were the axis correct (Figures 9–16 and 9–17).
2. Turn the lens on the tracing to the correct axis (Figure 9–18).
3. Note which areas of the lens are outside the tracing and mark them, taking overall shape into consideration (Figure 9–19).
4. Hand edge these areas away.

If the integrity of the lens shape is restored and the lens still fits snugly in the frame, it may be used. With only a little experience it will no longer be necessary to construct a tracing.

This same procedure may be used for straight top spherical bifocals when the upper bifocal edges do not align horizontally. Unfortunately, this practice is limited to plastic frames, as metal frames do not have the elasticity required.

Correcting for Vertical Prism
When a high-powered pair of lenses is edged, a very small amount of error in vertical positioning during layout or blocking can induce vertical prism. Assuming that the prescription is for a plastic frame, it may be possible to hand edge the lenses to reduce vertical prism to zero. To determine if this is possible, remove the lenses from the frame and respot them on their major reference points.

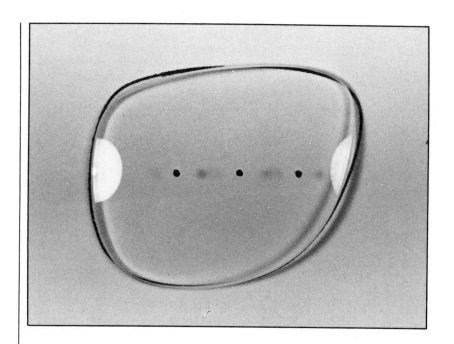

Figure 9–18. The lens is placed on the tracing and the 180-degree cutting line oriented until perfectly horizontal. The lens will be "trimmed" wherever the traced line shows through the lens. The areas to be removed should be outlined with a non-water-soluble pen.

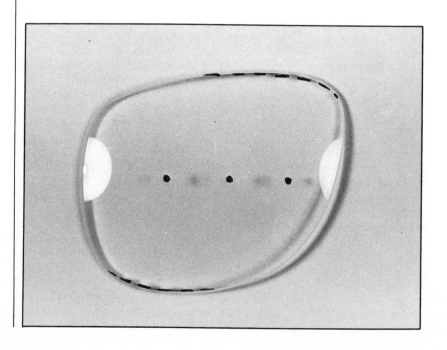

Figure 9–19. Once marked, the indicated areas of the lens can be removed by hand edging. The lens then fits into the frame without causing the frame to hump up or be distorted.

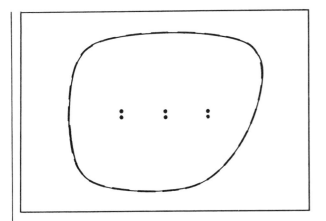

Figure 9–20. *This lens pair has been edged, then respotted. When the lenses are held "back-to-back," the dots should exactly overlap one another. If they do not, vertical prism will be manifested in the mounted prescription.*

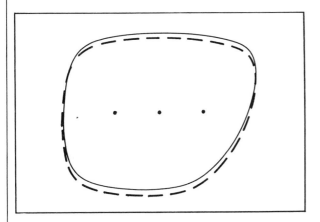

Figure 9–21. *To salvage a lens pair with manifested vertical prism, the result must be an overlapping set of Lensometer dots. By sliding one lens up until an overlap is achieved, it is now possible to visualize which lens area must be "trimmed" away. The left lens is represented by dotted lines, the right by a solid line.*

Next hold the lenses back to back so that their shapes exactly overlap one another. With lenses so aligned, as in Figure 9–20, the spotted MRP's will be seen one above the other. (If they overlap exactly, then the measured imbalance was due to a frame irregularity, rather than to the lenses.) Now slide one lens up or down until the MRP's overlap, as in Figure 9–21. Extra lens material that extends above and below the areas of overlap must be removed, as marked in Figure 9–22. If this reduces the overall *B* dimension too much, then a new lens must be prepared. The total *B* dimension reduction will equal the amount which the two MRP's were separated initially.

Hand Shaping a Minus Lenticular

A *negative lenticular* form lens (often known by the name *myodisc*) is a high-minus lens that has had the peripheral portion flattened for the purpose of reducing weight and edge thickness. The central optical portion is referred to as the *aperture* and the flattened portion as the *carrier*. When a round or oval aperture is desired, the lens is produced in the surfacing laboratory. It is also possible to produce an aperture with a shape that duplicates the frame shape. (See Figure 9–23.) This must be done by hand.

To produce a so-called *hand-flattened lenticular*, the peripheral portion of the rear surface of an edged lens is smoothed down on the hand stone until a conventional edge thickness and the desired aperture size is reached. The carrier portion will have a plus lens configuration. (See Figure 9–24.)

After the correct lens shape has been achieved, the carrier will have the frosted look common to hand-smoothed bevel surfaces. It should then be polished to a clarity that matches that of the aperture portion using a rag buffing wheel and a white polishing compound. (Red compounds may discolor plastic lenses.)

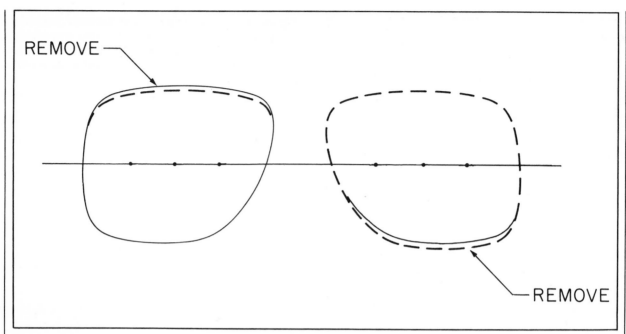

Figure 9–22. *By removing the upper portion of the wearer's right lens and the lower portion of the left, the B dimension of each lens is reduced equally. The amount of material to be removed from each lens equals the amount of separation between the two sets of dots, as first noted in Figure 9–20.*

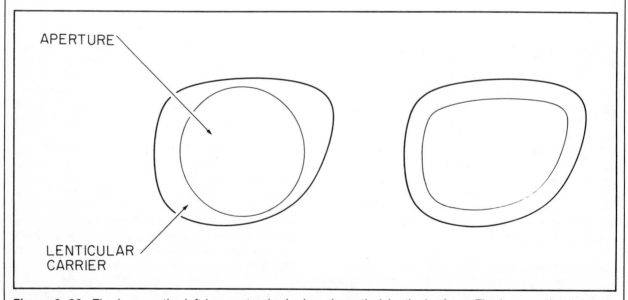

Figure 9–23. *The lens on the left has a standard minus (negative) lenticular form. The lens on the right is a hand-flattened lenticular, requiring considerable skill to produce.*

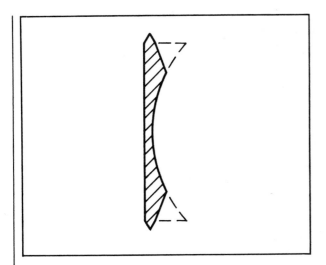

EDGE POLISHING

The term *edge polishing* can have different definitions, depending upon the material being described.

Glass Lenses

When speaking of glass lenses, edge polishing refers to the edge smoothing process carried out on a fine or extra-fine grit wheel. This was described previously. In the true sense of the term, this process is not edge polishing, but is generally the highest degree of polish that glass lens edgers are allowed. It would be possible for a practitioner to increase edge gloss on glass lenses by buffing the edges with a rotating drum tool while using the same type of polishing compound as for lens surfacing. This would be extremely time consuming and is currently neither cost effective nor in demand.

Plastic Lenses

When speaking of plastic CR-39 lenses, it is difficult to know whether edge polishing is used to refer to edge smoothing or if the edges have truly been brought to a high degree of luster. There are several different methods being used that yield satisfactory results.

One method is to simply use an extra-fine hand edger wheel. If the lens has a hidden bevel, a grooved wheel must be used. The lens is left approximately .25 mm large when edged, in anticipation of size reduction on the hand wheel. Edges are attractive, but translucent.

A second method that may be used does not require a grooved wheel. Initially the edge is buffed on a rag wheel using a white buffing compound; Figure 9–25 shows how this is done. (If the edges are especially rough or heavily frosted, hold the lens edge against the side surface of the rag wheel for a preliminary first buff.) A hand buffing may tend to round the bevel apex. Restore a distinct edge shape by smoothing the front bevel surface on a ceramic or extra-fine diamond wheel.

A third method makes use of a flat rotating drum tool. The felt surface of the tool is charged with a bar of white polishing compound. The edge surface is then pressed against the rotating tool and a polished edge achieved in approximately 2 minutes.

A most effective edge polishing method uses surface polishing compound. (This is the same polishing slurry as used to polish out the optical surface of plastic lenses.) Units are available that polish plastic lens edges automatically in three minutes. The lens is not deblocked after edging and is mounted in the unit on its finishing block. (See Figure 9–26.)

Polycarbonate Lenses

The edges of polycarbonate lenses can be hand polished. However, edge glazes[3] are available that give a finished appearance. Not every type of edge coating is appropriate, as solvents used in many such products will adversely affect the polycarbonate material.

---

[3]One such glaze is PC Lens Glaze, manufactured by Inland Diamond Products Co.

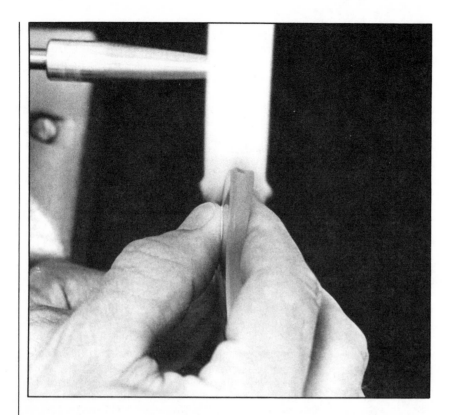

Figure 9–25. *Using buffing compound on a rag wheel, a smooth luster can be achieved on plastic lens edges.*

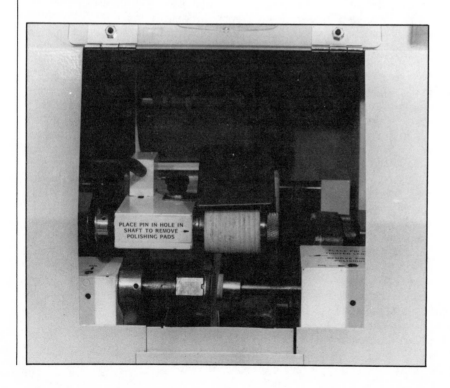

Figure 9–26. *A lens edge may also be polished with the same type of polish as is used for lens surfaces. Here the process is done automatically. (Photo courtesy Coburn Optical.)*

CHANGING SHAPES

Re-edging a Lens for a Different Frame

Most wearers erroneously assume that putting old lenses into a new frame is a simple matter; however, several factors must be considered ahead of time. Even if old lenses *do* fit into the new frame without re-edging, if the distance between lenses (DBL) of the new frame differs from that of the old, the PD will no longer be correct.

Customarily lenses are not re-edged if the frame can be stretched to accept the old lenses. In this manner unwanted air spaces between lens and frame are eliminated.

If the new frame is metal, or if the integrity of the plastic frame shape is to be preserved, then the old lens must be of sufficient size so that the entire lens opening is covered, with the following conditions met:

1. Spherocylinder lenses may not be turned from their prescribed axis.
2. The lens MRP must be located at the wearer's PD.

The best policy is to spot the lenses in the Lensometer according to the prescription. Measure from the center of the frame bridge to half the prescribed PD and hold the lens with its MRP in this position. The lens opening must still be completely covered by the lens.

If the lens previously has been heat treated (as evidenced by a maltese cross pattern observable through crossed polaroids), then it must be dehardened before edging.[4] Chemically hardened lenses may be re-edged as they are. Both types need to be rehardened before dispensing.

If possible, block and re-edge the lenses with an automatic edger and the new pattern. If this is not possible, then hold one lens up to the frame and note those areas of overhang that must be edged away. Reshape the lens on a hand edger. Once the first lens has been satisfactorily shaped, use it as a model for the second in order to assure left-right symmetry.

Changing Frame Shapes

It is reasonable to expect that modifications of lens shapes for a specific frame will be requested. The simplest type of change specifies that a certain well-known lens shape be mounted in another company's frame. The purpose for substituting shape is to obtain a better bridge fit or a slightly larger *B* dimension.

On the other hand, the practitioner may know the desired effect, but be unable to suggest a specific alternate pattern. Commonly requested alterations are for nasal cuts, nasal adds, and increases in the *B* dimension.

The Nasal Cut

A nasal cut is requested when the wearer's nose broadens more toward the nostril area than the frame does. Were the frame left unaltered, it would rest on the nose on the lower nasal corners of the rims instead of on the pads. The amount of nasal cut desired is specified in millimeters, as Figure 9–27 shows.

If the frame specified is rimless, the matter is simple. Assuming an extra pattern is available, the pattern is marked for a nasal cut and the marked area filed away; Figure 9–28 is an example of this method. The lens is run normally. If the lens is for a plastic frame, this procedure will not work. Filing the pattern with no other compensation will only cause an inferior nasal gap between lens and frame groove. Following is a list of some alternatives to filing.

1. Heat the frame and reshape for a nasal cut effect. Make a new pattern for this shape. The main disadvantage is that often the frame takes on a different look than the practitioner anticipated.
2. Modify the pattern as described for rimless lenses above. This time, however, edge the lenses somewhat larger to take up slack in the rim. CAUTION: Any time a change in eyesize is made, decentration must be recalculated. For example, if the frame to be used had an *A* dimension of 50 and a DBL of 18, for a wearer having a 65-mm PD, decentration per eye will be

$$\frac{50 + 18 - 65}{2} = 1.5\,\text{mm}.$$

But if the lenses were edged at 51 mm to allow for a nasal cut, decentration per lens would be

$$\frac{51 + 18 - 65}{2}$$

or 2 mm per lens.
3. Edge the lenses slightly large using the normal pattern and do the nasal cut on the hand edger. Determine if enough lens stock has been removed by comparing the lens to the frame and the paired lens. When results are satisfactory, hand edge the paired lens to conform to the new shape.

---

[4]Dehardening is done by placing the lens in the heat treating unit for the same length as is required for hardening. As the lens is removed from the furnace area, instead of fast cooling with forced air to create the customary stress pattern, the air is turned off and the lens allowed to cool slowly.

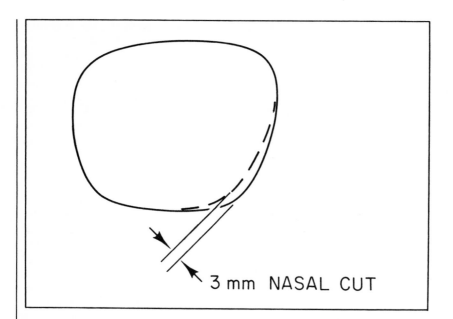

Figure 9–27. *If the frame shape does not have a sufficient amount of flare, the lens may be reshaped.*

3 mm NASAL CUT

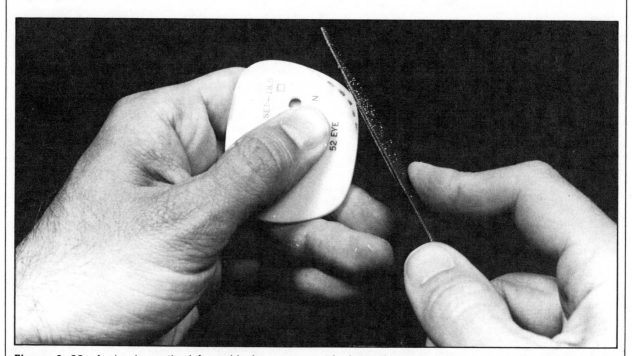

Figure 9–28. *A simple method for achieving a symmetrical nasal cut on both lenses is by reshaping the pattern.*

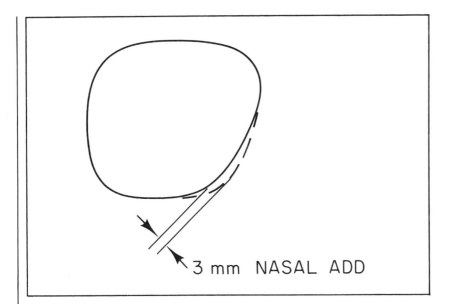

3 mm NASAL ADD

Figure 9–29. A nasal add is more difficult to achieve by hand, since the lens must be edged large, then reduced everywhere but in the nasal add area.

Compensation for decentration should be considered here as well.

The Nasal Add

The nasal cut has been used to reshape for a wide nose. The reverse modification is to add to the inferior nasal portion of the lens shape in an effort to achieve a better fit for wearers who have less than the normal amount of nasal flare; Figure 9–29 illustrates how a lens is edged for the add. Results are somewhat less predictable than with the nasal cut from both a cosmetic and fitting viewpoint. The amount of *nasal add* is also specified in millimeters.

Best results are obtained by finding a pattern that comes close to duplicating the desired shape. If an exact pattern cannot be found, a closely related shape can be used and the lenses modified on the hand edger to conform to the shape desired.

When only a small amount of add is required, the lenses can be first edged large without compensating the decentrations. The lens is then reduced back to size on the hand edger on all sides, sparing only the area of the requested nasal add.

Yet another method is to find a spare pattern which duplicates the needed nasal add shape. The lower nasal quarter is cut off and glued securely to the front of the original pattern, creating the new shape.[5]

---

[5]Contributed by Gerald Gaustad, Madison, WI.

Increasing the B

When frame styles are large, there is seldom a need for requesting an increase in the *B* dimension. Narrow frame styles, though, are known to prevent effective use of trifocals and progressive addition lenses. Increasing the *B* dimension can be carried out by finding an appropriate pattern. If none is to be found, the lenses may be edged large using the normal pattern. Then, hand edge them to reduce their size back to the correct *A* dimension. However, only the nasal, temporal, and upper edges should be worked, leaving the lower edges untouched.

When inserting the lens with an increased *B* dimension, the upper frame rim is not heated as extensively as the rest of the frame. All of the increase in *B* should be at the bottom.

CLEANING LENSES

After the lenses have been deblocked and hand edged, they are almost ready for tinting, coating, drilling, or hardening. Before further processing, they must be cleaned well and inspected for visible flaws.

Glass Lens Cleaning

If a non-water-soluble lens spray has been used to aid in lens blocking, then a solvent such as acetone or alcohol must be used on the lens surface. The lens is generally dipped in an open container of the solution and wiped with a tissue or lint-free soft cloth. When no sprays have been used, a solution of detergent will be effective.

Occasionally after cleaning a small spot remains on the lens. It can, at times, be difficult to tell whether this spot is a surface imperfection or superficial foreign material. In such cases the best test device may prove to be an ordinary pencil. The pencil point is hard enough to give a good feel for whether the spot is external, yet soft enough not to scratch the glass. If foreign material is stuck to the surface, it may be removed simply by the action of the pencil lead. If the spot is not a surface flaw, but will not break free with the pencil point, turn the pencil around and attempt to erase it.

If none of the solutions or methods removes the spot, wet pumice rubbing compound (as is used on wood furniture) may be effective. It should only be used gently to avoid abrading the surface.

Plastic Lens Cleaning

Acetone is used extensively for cleaning CR-39 lenses, but should not be allowed to come in contact with plastic frame parts. Detergents also clean plastic lenses well.

By far the most effective cleaning method for glass or plastic is an ultrasonic bath. Major manufacturers of uncut lenses use a series of hot ultrasonic baths with different cleaning agents to achieve an extremely clean surface. For small operations ultrasonic facilities are usually not cost effective.

Inspecting a plastic lens that has been alloy blocked may reveal the presence of an indentation at the location of the block. To eliminate the indentation, place the lens in an oven[6] at 200°F for a minimum of 20 minutes. This same method is also used when plastic lens warpage is detected. When an oven is unavailable, the lens may be placed in water near the boiling point for an equal amount of time.

Polycarbonate Lens Cleaning

Polycarbonate lenses are coated to make them more scratch resistant. With conventional lenses, lens coatings are more subject to solvent damage than the actual lenses; however, with polycarbonates the exposed bevel shows damage before the coated surface. Because of this, use only a liquid detergent such as dishwashing liquid. Most alcohols will work, but should only be considered secondarily.

Under no circumstances should methylene chloride, methyl ethyl ketone, any of the ketone family, or acetone be used. Highly volatile chlorinated or aromatic hydrocarbons must also be avoided.[7]

---

[6]Small ovens are made especially for lens laboratories, but regular ovens work perfectly well.

[7]Optical Laboratory Marketing Plan, Gentex, Section 4, Finishing and Glazing, 1980.

PROFICIENCY TEST QUESTIONS

1. For a thick edge lens with a hand edged bevel, the bevel apex should be approximately how far back from the front lens surface?
   a. ½
   b. ⅓
   c. ⅔
   d. ¾

2. An extra-fine grit hand edger would be least suited for which of the following?
   a. Removing edge stock
   b. Edge smoothing
   c. Pin bevelling

3. What is the correct sequence of steps in hand edging?
   a. 2, 3, 4, 1, 5   1. front pin bevel
   b. 4, 1, 5, 2, 3   2. smooth front face of bevel
   c. 4, 1, 2, 3, 5   3. smooth rear face of bevel
   d. 5, 4, 1, 2, 3   4. rear pin bevel
   e. 3, 2, 1, 4, 5   5. apex pin bevel

4. T or F   It is advantageous to travel as far as possible around the periphery of the lens during hand edging before lifting the lens from the wheel.

5. What is the accepted apical angle that should be produced during the hand edging process?
   a. 85 degrees
   b. 90 degrees
   c. 100 degrees
   d. 110 degrees
   e. 115 degrees

6. During the hand edging process, the lens is held at varying angles to the cutting plane of the wheel. Which two hand edging operations require holding the lens at nearly the same angle?
   a. 1 + 2   1. Front bevel edge smoothing
   b. 2 + 3   2. Rear bevel edge smoothing
   c. 3 + 4   3. Front pin bevel
   d. 1 + 4   4. Rear pin bevel
   e. 2 + 4

7. Which factor causes hand edging cutting speed to increase?
   a. Decreasing speed of rotation of lens
   b. Using a finer grit wheel
   c. Approaching a thicker section of the lens
   d. Decreasing pressure against the wheel
   e. All of the above cause cutting speed to decrease.

8. When inserting a lens with an increased *B* dimension in a plastic frame,
   a. the whole eyewire should be heated evenly.
   b. the upper eyewire should be heated more than the lower, as it is generally thicker.
   c. the lower portion of the eyewire is heated more than the upper rim.

9. A lens pair manifests vertical prism. It is determined that the right lens OC is 1 mm higher than the left lens OC. How should a practitioner correct the problem?
   a. Take .5 mm off the top of the right lens and .5 mm off the bottom of the left lens.
   b. Take .5 mm off the top of the left lens and .5 mm off the bottom of the right lens.
   c. Take 1 mm off the top of the right lens and 1 mm off the bottom of the left lens.
   d. Take 1 mm off the top of the left lens and 1 mm off the bottom of the right lens.

10. What is a metal sizer?
    a. A diameter marker
    b. A pattern made from metal
    c. An edge thickness measuring device
    d. A frame front or chassis from a metal or combination frame
    e. An *A* dimension measuring device

11. T or F   Acetone cleans polycarbonate lenses well.

12. If a plastic lens is warped,
    a. drop ball test it to see if it will be acceptable.
    b. put it in an oven at 200°F for awhile.
    c. send the lens on anyway, as warpage in plastic lenses is unimportant.
    d. throw it out, as such lenses are both unacceptable and unsalvageable.

13. Assume that a lens has been found off axis and an attempt to salvage it is made. If the lens reads as axis 5 and should be axis 180, where would lens stock commonly be removed to correct the problem?
    a. Top edge (left half) and bottom edge (right half)
    b. Top edge (right half) and bottom edge (left half)

    c. Top edge (right half) and bottom edge (right half)

    d. Top edge (left half) and right edge (top half)

14. T or F   If a small spot remains on a glass lens after cleaning, an attempt may be made to erase it with a pencil eraser.

Chapter 10

Maintenance and Calibration

Having the very best in up-to-date equipment will not ensure prescription accuracy and quality craftsmanship if that equipment is not properly maintained and correctly calibrated. Many fine apprenticeship programs in optical craftsmanship begin, not with an explanation of optics, but with instruction on cleaning and care of the equipment vital to the functioning of the laboratory. Do not consider the material presented in the next two chapters as reference material to consult only in an emergency situation—the maintenance of equipment is just as important to the successful operation of an optical laboratory as an understanding of optical principles.

MAINTENANCE SCHEDULES

It is helpful to keep a master maintenance schedule that outlines how often each piece of equipment should be lubricated, greased, cleaned, or calibrated. This master list should not only contain how often each of these tasks must be done, but should leave enough space to regularly enter the date when the service was performed and the signature or initials of the individual who performed it. In this way deficiencies may be noted at a glance.

A second backup reminder system is to put a sticker on each piece of equipment that lists the service performed and the date. (What works for automotive oil changes should work for edger coolant changes as well!)

As much as is possible, maintenance services should be done on a regularly scheduled basis, so that each work day concludes with cleaning and wiping of equipment. The end of the week could, for example, be devoted to more thorough maintenance, coolant changes, and calibration checks.

CARE OF THE LENSOMETER

Prescription accuracy begins and ends with the Lensometer. A laboratory Lensometer must have fine timepiece accuracy. Those operators who work directly with the Lensometer must know how to adjust it for exact measurements so that they are confident that the refractive power they are reading is exactly the power the lens actually has. Many a disagreement between laboratory and account would never have occurred if both instruments had been correctly used and rightly calibrated.

Calibration of Power

Before any instrument is calibrated, the individual must be certain that it is properly adjusted for his or her eye. The eye's accommodative (focusing) mechanism and refractive error can directly influence lens power readings. Turn the eyepiece out (counterclockwise) and slowly turn it inward until the black reticle lines *first* come into focus. It is helpful to look at the 1.0Δ ring for best reference.

With no lens in the instrument, turn the power wheel from a minus direction until the target clears. Do not rock the wheel back and forth to obtain a focus, but simply stop it when the target first clears. (This rule applies equally during neutralization of lenses.) The power should read zero. If the instrument does not read zero, repeat the process several times to be certain of obtaining a clear target. If the target still does not focus at zero, the instrument must be recalibrated.

When assured that the target is accurately sharp and zeroed, recalibrate the power reading by loosening the power wheel with the appropriate tool, such as a screwdriver or Allen wrench. The zero setting is turned to the index mark and the wheel retightened. (Some instruments allow for correction of small errors by an adjustment of the index mark.)

Prism

With both reticle and target in focus, check the instrument for prism accuracy. With no lens in the instrument, the target should cross exactly at the center of the reticle. (If an auxillary rotary prism

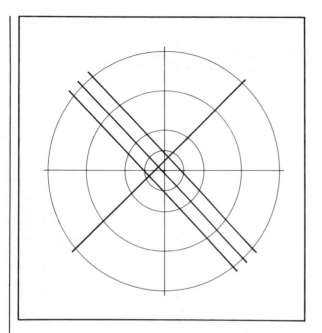

Figure 10–1. *An off-center target is difficult to compensate for and should be fixed as soon as possible. (Instruments with prism compensation devices should be checked to ascertain that the device registers zero.)*

system is present, also check this system to be certain that it is not inducing prism via the rotary prism.)

If the prism is evident without lenses present, as is seen in Figure 10–1, consult the instrument manual for corrective measures. It may require factory realignment.

Optics
The optics of a Lensometer or other optical instrument may be blown free of dust using a syringe or canned compressed air (such as is employed for photography lenses). Alternatively, a camel's hair brush may be used to wipe dust from the lenses. Alcohol, or any solution that would not damage a fine, vacuum-coated camera lens, may be used to clean away oily film or smudges.

Exterior
Smooth-finish exteriors may be cleaned with a damp cloth. To restore polish to enamel exteriors on Lensometers, edgers, or other instruments having a shiny enamelled look, use a high-quality automotive paste wax.

Wipe black crackle-finish exteriors clean with a damp cloth, then polish with mineral oil to return their original luster.

Inking
If the spotting mechanism is giving splotchy and incomplete dots, or is depositing too much ink on the lens, clean the pad and reservoir; then reink the pad. Ordinary stamp pad ink works well.

CENTRATION DEVICES (MARKERS)

Accuracy of Axis
Centration devices must be checked for accuracy in marking. The stamp must correctly mark the 180-degree line. If the stamp mechanism is turned slightly, as Figure 10–2 illustrates, every cylinder lens will be off axis and every bifocal top tilted. The axis may be checked by simply looking through the instrument *after* the lens has been stamped. The stamp must overlap the 180-degree reference line in the instrument. If it does not, the stamp itself must be adjusted.

Accuracy of Decentration
The instrument must also mark accurately for decentration. Within most centering devices there is a movable vertical line (and in many devices, there is a movable horizontal line as well). The background grid or hash-marked line system used to measure off decentration is stationary. To check for horizontal and vertical stamping accuracy, stamp a lens and,

194

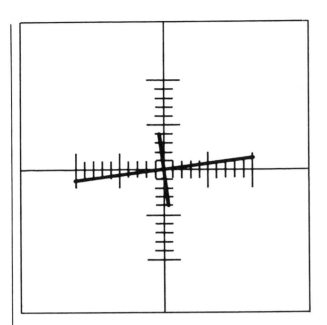

being careful not to move it, look into the instrument. The stamp must exactly correspond to the center of the stationary grid. If the stamp is horizontally or vertically displaced, as in Figure 10–3, decentration will not be accurate.

It is theoretically possible to compensate for the error during layout, but generally it is considerably easier to readjust the instrument for accurate stamping. Readjustment is usually done with setscrews that control the position of the stationary grid, as Figure 10–4 shows. Take care not to rotate the grid during alignment. The movable vertical line may be used for reference to ensure that no rotation occurs.

Cleaning the Stamp

The pad within the instrument must be cleaned and reinked periodically. If the instrument is not making a thin, clear mark, it is possible that the pad has amassed thick, gooey ink as a result of evaporation. If the ink is water soluble, apply water to the pad instead of more ink. If the ink is of the non-water-soluble variety, an appropriate thinner could be applied. (In marking for edging, some practitioners use ordinary office stamp pad ink. If this is done, caution must be taken in handling the marked lenses, as the ink smears easily.)

To produce a clear, distinct mark, the rubber stamp must be cleaned regularly. This can be done with water or alcohol on a damp cloth. (Do *not* use acetone, as this and other similar solvents will attack the rubber.)

Marker/Blocker Accuracy

To check the accuracy of a marker/blocker, begin by hand-marking a lens. A flexible ruler should be used to ensure that the line is straight. Align the hand-drawn mark on the grid as if there were no decentration, taking care to place the mark exactly on the origin. Block the lens in the customary manner.

After blocking, the mark on the lens should be exactly in the center of the block. Figure 10–5 illustrates how the 180-degree line marked on the lens should be coincident with and parallel to the 180-degree reference line on the block.

Adhesive pad blocks have a small central hole used in some blocking alignment systems. This hole should be at the center of the hand-drawn mark. If the marker/blocker is blocking inaccurately, correct the problem in the same manner as for other centration devices.

Blockers

Blockers for adhesive pad blocking are either combined with a marking system or are so simple in design that no special adjustment considerations are necessary. Metal alloy blockers, whether combined with a centration device or not, require attention in some areas.

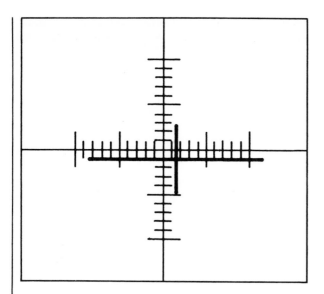

Figure 10–3. *Centration devices must periodically be checked. Occasionally the lens should be left in place after being stamped and examined to determine if the instrument is stamping at the grid origin. If not, repositioning of the grid is required.*

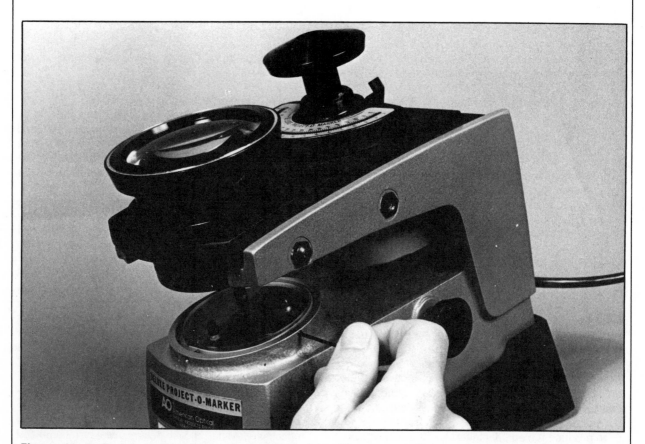

Figure 10–4. *Translucent grids may be readjusted by Allen screws (setscrews), or other similar means. Here the adjustment is for horizontal alignment.*

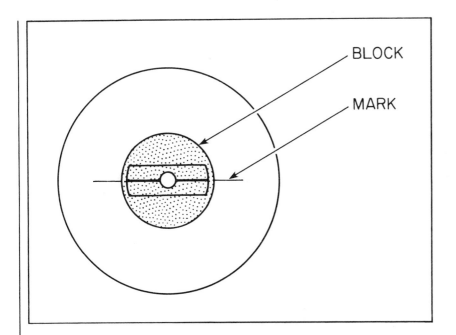

BLOCK

MARK

Figure 10–5. *Centration devices with direct blocking capability may be checked by first hand-marking the lens, then placing the mark on the grid origin and blocking. If the block conforms to the marked 180-degree line both horizontally and vertically, the centration device is in adjustment.*

The Alloy

Alloy is subject to contamination. To reduce inevitable contamination to a minimum, blocks should be rinsed clean and dried before being returned to the alloy pot. Fortunately, because of the weight (density) of the alloy, most contaminates are lighter than alloy and "float" to the top. The contaminates, along with oxidized foam, may be scraped off with a spoon as shown in Figure 10–6, until a mirror-like surface is restored.

The alloy pot should not be allowed to be drawn off to the point where it is almost empty, as contaminates that normally float on top are then drawn through the feeder tube, increasing the risk of clogging the system.

Overfilling

If the mold overfills during blocking, mushrooming into a small ball above the fill hole, excess alloy should be quickly wiped away with the finger. Even though it is "molten metal," the temperature is well below the point where there is any danger of causing burns.

If the alloy is not wiped away, it will solidify, in which case the hardened alloy must be broken away before the blocked lens can be removed from the holding fork.

In the event that alignment viewing holes or other blocker parts should become clogged with alloy, the clogged part can be removed and placed in the hot salt bath used in frame warming. Alloy will quickly liquify and flow out of the clogged section.

Axis Misalignment in Blocking

In alloy blocking, the block is molded directly to the lens. The molds used are a rubber material and must be replaced when they become worn. Molds fit into a metal or plastic part of the blocker that may be aligned to ensure that the block will be molded with its long axis along the 180-degree line. Ordinarily, setscrews are loosened to allow for realignment.

Accuracy of axis alignment may be checked after blocking by using the previously marked cross on the lens for reference. If the mark does not parallel the 180-degree line on the block, as in Figure 10–7, the mold must be realigned.

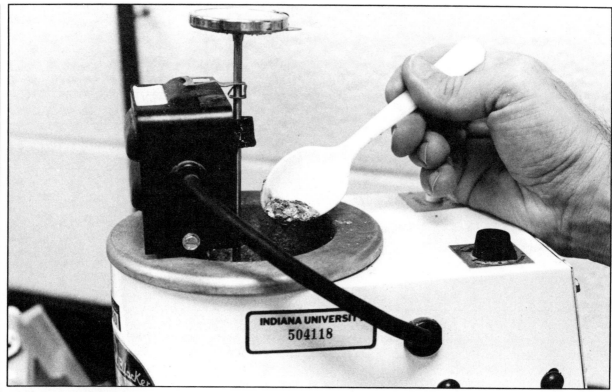

Figure 10–6. Oxidized froth should be removed from the surface of the liquid alloy.

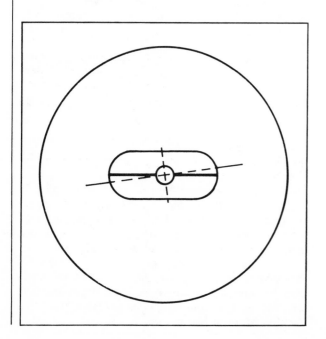

Figure 10–7. When block and mark do not correspond, either the lens was held in a rotated position for blocking or the blocker mold is off axis.

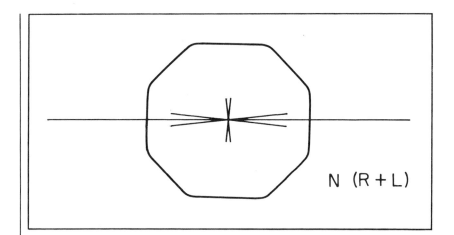

CALIBRATION OF EDGERS

When considering calibration and maintenance of edgers, keep in mind that textual material discussed here cannot be considered an adequate substitute for familiarity with the individual characteristics of each edger. This discussion should rather be regarded as a generic basis to which more specific knowledge should be added.

Checking Axis Accuracy

In edging lenses, it is essential that the 180-degree datum line on the pattern always parallel the 180-degree datum line on the lens. However, because the pattern and lens are some distance apart and each is held in place by a separate mechanism, the possibility of misalignment is understandable. For this reason edgers are made so that axis alignment may be fine-tuned for repeatable accuracy.

To check for accuracy of the axis, choose a pattern whose shape comes close to being a square or octagon. It is helpful if pattern corners are squared-off and distinct, with sides, tops, and bottoms as straight as possible.

Carefully mark a pair of lenses along the 180-degree cutting line in the customary manner. The mark must be either non-water-soluble or protected with tape or spray so as to withstand the washing effect of the coolant. (Test lenses do not need to be cylindrical, since the point of reference is the marked cutting line and not the cylinder axis.)

Next, edge the lenses. As the two lenses must be held back-to-back exactly over one another when cut, it is helpful to have a flat edge. Therefore, the lenses should be either cut on the rimless program or stopped after they have been roughed. (Reminder: Lenses are being edged as if they were a pair; therefore the pattern must be turned after edging the first lens.)

When edging is completed, hold the lenses concave side against concave side. Their shapes must match exactly. If the marked cutting lines exactly match each other, the edger axis is properly set. (The sequence for checking the edger axis is reviewed below in Table 10–1.) If, however, these marked lines are *not* coincident (as in Figure 10–8), then the axis of either the edger or the blocker must be readjusted. This is further clarified in Figure 10–9A and should not be confused with axis problems caused by other pieces of equipment. Thus, before making any adjustments, make absolutely certain that the problem is indeed caused by the edger. Review Figure 10–9 and Table 10–2 carefully to understand the possible sources of error.

Readjusting the Edger Axis

Although methods of readjustment vary, most edger

Table 10–1. Edger Axis Checking Sequence

1. Clearly mark one lens pair with non-water-soluble ink.
2. Accurately block both lenses.
3. Choose a squared pattern.
4. Flat edge or rough only.
5. Hold edged lenses back to back.
6. Marks on lenses must overlap.

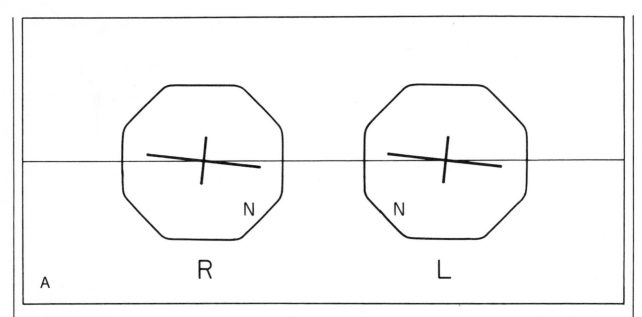

Figure 10–9. A. *The lenses are placed face up and correctly turned; the marks are off axis. (These lenses are the same as those shown in Figure 10–8.) When the error manifests itself in this manner, the problem could stem from an axis error in either the edger or the blocker.*

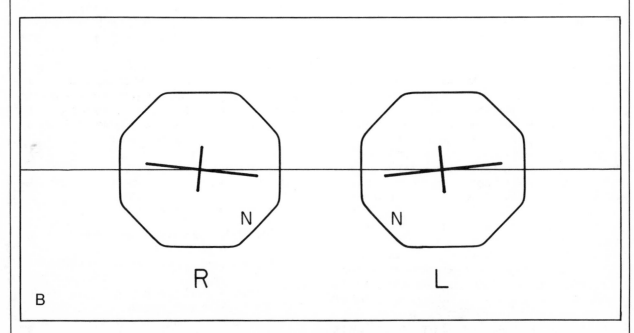

B. *Were these lenses placed back-to-back, the two marks would overlap exactly, masking the problem. The possible source of this error is a pattern that has been cut off axis. (It could be that the lenses are actually correct, but the frame shape has been misinterpreted and the lenses are twisted wrong.)*

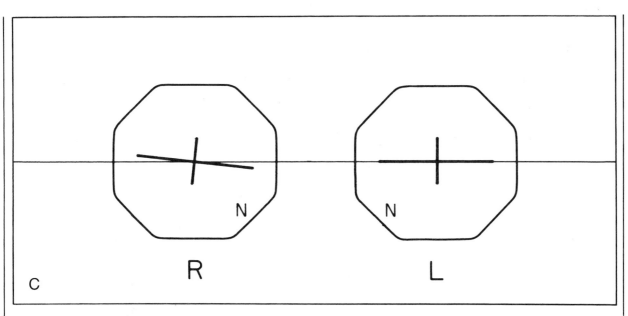

C. *Three sources of error are possible here: human error; the block slipped during edging; or one side of a paired alloy blocking unit is off axis.*

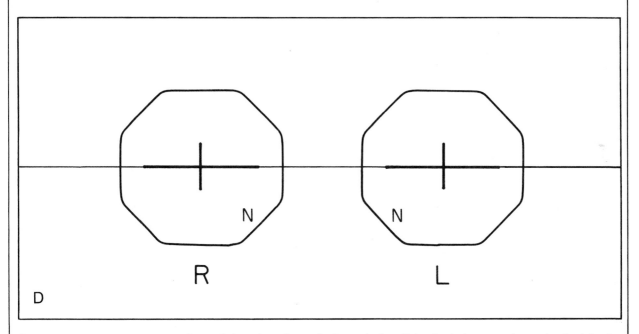

D. *If the marks are correct after edging, but the cylinder axis is off for both lenses when checked in the Lensometer, then the problem lies with the centration device. (It does not matter if the centration device is being used purely as a marker, or as a marker/blocker.)*

Table 10–2. Possible Sources of Axis Errors

Checkpoints	Source of Error
Axis error discovered on another Lensometer	Compare Lensometer axes
Axis error shows on same Lensometer as was used for spotting	Lensometer error ruled out; could be edger, marker, or blocker
To check *edger,* hold edged, marked lenses back to back	If marks not coincident, edger at fault
To check *marker,* mark lens and look into marker before removing lens	If mark not on the 180-degree line, marker is at fault
To check *blocker;* block marked lens	If 180-degree line on block is not parallel to mark on lens, blocker is at fault

axis adjustments are made by turning two or more Allen screws on the pattern holder assembly. Their location is shown in Figure 10–10. Most generally the procedure involves loosening setscrews, turning adjustment screws in the requisite direction, and retightening setscrews.

Checking Wheel Differential (Grinding Allowance)
Wheel differential is the difference in size of a lens after it has been rough edged compared to its final size. Because the finishing wheel uses fine-grit diamond particles, it cuts slowly and has the potential of wearing down quickly if used excessively. For maximum speed and best wheel life, the lens should be cut as small as possible on the coarse-grit roughing wheel first.

Roughing wheels cut rapidly but coarsely, leaving chips along the lens periphery. These edge chips should be removed on the finishing wheel. Generally the roughed lens must be reduced in size by about 2 mm in order to ensure the complete removal of all chips. (Recommendations for wheel differentials vary for different edgers and various bevel styles. Flat bevels require the largest differentials and V-bevels the smallest. The operator may wish to start with the manufacturer's recommendations and experimentally see if these can be reduced.)

Wheel differential will increase as the roughing wheel wears down, and this must of necessity be periodically monitored. Failure to monitor wheel dif-

ferential will cause an unnecessary increase in edging time with a corresponding decrease in edge quality and finishing wheel life.

How to Measure Wheel Differential
There are two ways in which to measure wheel differential. The first method begins when the operator places a blocked lens blank in the edger and starts the edging cycle. After the roughing cycle is completed, but before the finishing cycle starts, the edger is turned off. The roughed lens is removed and its A dimension measured. Afterwards the lens is returned to the edger and the cycle is allowed to continue until the lens is fully bevelled. Upon completion of the cycle, the lens is measured a second time. The difference in size between the first and second measurements is the wheel differential. (Figure 10–11 shows a lens being measured using a Box-o-Graph. However, still higher accuracy can be obtained using a vernier caliper in combination with a round lens.)

The second method for checking wheel differential allows the machine itself to aid in the measuring process. In this method, a lens blank is blocked and edged completely. It is not removed from the edger. Instead, without ever changing the edger setting, the whole cycle is begun again. This time as the edger begins the roughing cycle, the power is cut. When the wheel stops, the edger setting is reduced until the lens bevel comes in contact with the roughing

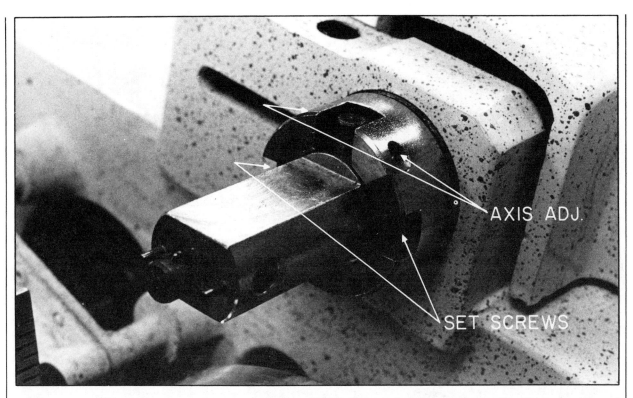

Figure 10–10. *The exact method for realignment of the edger axis will vary depending upon model and manufacturer. However it is not unusual to have setscrews to hold the setting correctly. These are first loosened, then the axis adjustment screws turned. In general only slight turning of the axis adjustment screws is required to effect a change. Setscrews are then retightened to hold the new position.*

wheel. The difference between this new edger setting and the original setting is the wheel differential.

The sequence is shown in Figure 10–12. (Table 10–3 summarizes both methods.)

Table 10–3. Wheel Differential Checking Sequence

Method 1

1. Start to edge a lens.
2. Stop the cycle after roughing.
3. Measure the eyesize of the roughed lens.
4. Replace the lens and complete the cycle.
5. Measure the finished lens eyesize.
6. (Wheel differential) = (roughed eyesize) − (finished eyesize)

Method 2

1. Edge a lens.
2. Do not remove the lens or change the edger setting.
3. Begin the cycle again.
4. Stop the edger in mid-roughing cycle.
5. Turn the eyesize dial until the lens bevel touches the roughing wheel.
6. (Wheel differential) = (original eyesize) − (step 5 eyesize)

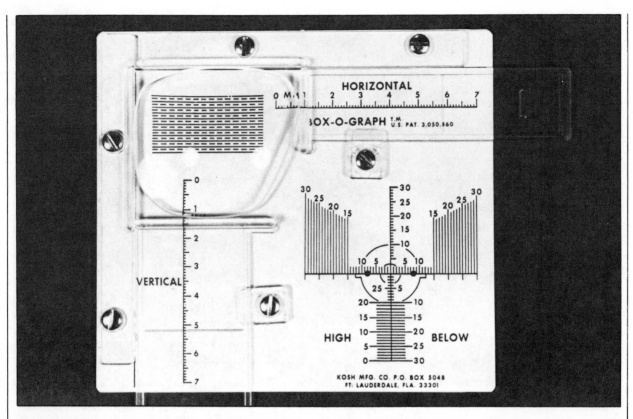

Figure 10–11. *For a lens or pattern to be measured correctly using a Box-o-Graph, it must not be turned. (If spotted, the three dots should all fall parallel to the horizontal lines on the device.) Both horizontal and vertical bars are pushed securely against the lens and the A and B dimensions read from the scale. In the example lens, A = 58 mm and B = 52 mm.*

Example:

A lens is edged to a 50-mm eyesize. Since the pattern is a "set-10" pattern, the edger is set for 40.0. Without changing the setting, the cycle is begun again and stopped during roughing. Now, the edger setting is reduced until the lens touches the roughing wheel. When this happens, the dial reads 37.2. Therefore,

$$\text{wheel differential} = 40 \text{ mm} - 37.2 \text{ mm}$$
$$= 2.8 \text{ mm}.$$

Since this is larger than recommended, the wheel differential must be reduced.

Adjusting for Wheel Differential

Methods for wheel differential adjustment vary considerably from edger to edger. Often the position of the wear plate upon which the pattern turns during roughing must be readjusted. These plates must also be reset after installing new or retrued wheels. (Exact procedures will be found in the manual that accompanies each edger.) Make no attempt to recalibrate eyesize until the correct wheel differential has been properly set.

Eyesize Adjustments

In simplest terms, eyesize is checked by edging a lens, then measuring it to see if its size corresponds

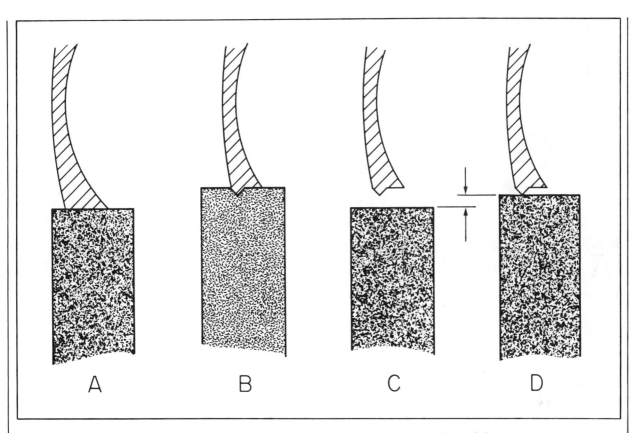

Figure 10–12. *The wheel differential (grinding allowance) measuring system is as follows:*
A. *Rough the lens.*
B. *Finish the lens.*
C. *Start cycle again.*
D. *Stop the edger during roughing and turn the eyesize setting dial until the lens just touches the roughing wheel. The difference between the two settings equals the wheel differential.*

to what was intended.

When checking eyesize accuracy it is best to use a round pattern, or at least one that is easily measured. Make certain that the pattern chosen is widest at the midline, so less error in measurement is likely. The pattern should be measured with vernier calipers and its set number figured.

Recall that figuring the set number is done by subtracting the pattern *A* dimension from the standard size. In the USA this is 36.5 mm. If a pattern measures 41.5 mm, the set number would be 36.5 −41.5 = −5. Therefore, the set number is −5.

The pattern is placed on the edger and a commonly used setting (such as 45) is chosen. With a test lens in place, the edger is run through its complete cycle. The edged lens is removed and measured with the vernier caliper in the same manner as was done for the pattern. Edged lens size should correspond to the anticipated value.

In summary, to check eyesize setting accuracy:
1. Choose a round or easily measured pattern.
2. Measure the pattern.
3. Set the edger to an "average" value eyesize setting for that pattern.
4. Edge a test lens.
5. Measure the test lens.

For example, if the edger is set at 45 using a pattern having a −5 set number, the eyesize anticipated will be

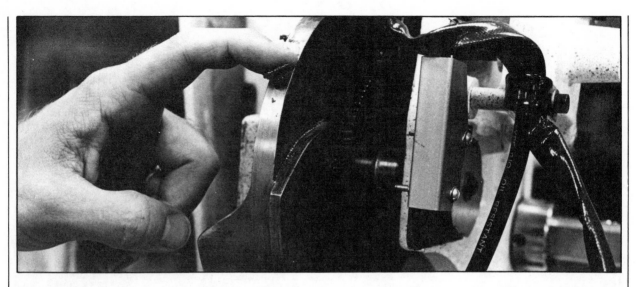

Figure 10–13. *Unless moving parts are cleaned and regreased regularly, machine life and efficiency is rapidly reduced.*

edger setting = eyesize + set number

or

45 = eyesize −5.

Therefore,

eyesize = 45 + 5 = 50.

If the eyesize is incorrect, the setscrew on the eyesize dial is loosened, allowing the dial to turn freely. The dial is turned to the *setting that corresponds to the eyesize actually produced* by the edger and the setscrew is tightened up again.

To illustrate: Suppose that the lens was edged to a 50.5-mm eyesize instead of a 50-mm eyesize. The setting that *should* produce a 50.5-mm lens using a set −5 pattern is

edger setting = eyesize + set number

or

edger setting = 50.5 −5

= 45.5.

Therefore the dial is loosened, turned to 45.5, and retightened.

Edger Leveling

Free-float edger bevelling systems require that the machine be level in order to allow the lens to slip into the groove correctly. If the edger is tilted, the bevel may be too far to the front or rear of the lens.

Beyond the use of a carpenter's level to assure both front-to-back and side-to-side leveling, the manufacturer's instructions should be consulted.

CLEANING AND LUBRICATING EDGERS

Glass and plastic sludge should not be allowed to build up hard deposits anywhere within or upon the edger, as they can only be removed through mechanical action that is damaging to machine surfaces (see Figure 10–13).

To clean the edger, flush the grinding chamber with water so that excess glass or plastic sludge is flushed down into the coolant tank for removal. A small hose run from a faucet or other source is most effective. Take care not to overfill the coolant tank while flushing the chamber.

It is best to lightly clean the edger at the end of each day by rinsing off excess sludge and wiping the exterior with a damp cloth. The machine should be cleaned thoroughly at least once a week, or as often as the coolant is changed, whichever occurs more frequently. To clean the edger thoroughly:

1. Remove all glass or plastic sludge from the chamber by rinsing and wiping.
2. Clean the exterior thoroughly.

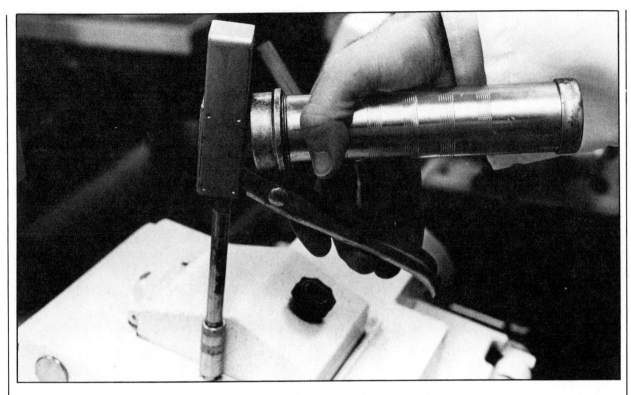

Figure 10–14. *Zirk fittings allow ease in greasing internal moving parts using a grease gun.*

3. Wipe grease from exposed gears or moving parts and regrease where required.
4. Apply grease from a grease gun to all grease fittings. (Figure 10–14)
5. Grease the clapper plate surface with Vaseline for smoother pattern turning. (Figure 10–15)
6. Oil those areas indicated in the manual such as hinges and springs using a light machine oil like those suitable for sewing machines. (Some areas require oiling only once every few months. Record these maintenance requirements on a master maintenance sheet.)

If thorough greasing is not carried out when indicated, glass can creep into moving parts, causing excessive wear and possible freeze-up.

Regluing Pads

Maintenance procedures also include replacement of felt chucking pads. Replacement becomes necessary when pads have become too thin, hardened through glass sludge saturation, or simply unglued and fallen off. It is advisable to have an extra chuck adapter already padded and on hand, since regluing

is not an instantaneous process. There is no reason to experience downtime for such a small matter.

Regluing is done as follows:
1. Clean the chuck adapter to remove any old glue or pieces of pad.
2. To decrease drying time, heat the adapter in a flame or in the salt pan frame warmer.
3. Apply glue to both the pad and the chuck adapter and allow to set for just under a minute before placing the pad on the adapter.
4. Center the new pad on the adapter and press it into place.
5. Place the pad and adapter into the edger and chuck a lens as if it were to be edged. This presses the pad and adapter firmly together.
6. Finally, allow the pad to dry. Drying time may vary from 15 minutes to overnight, depending upon the type of glue being used.[1]

---

[1] Any of a variety of glues may prove equally suitable. One type of glue often used is Scotch-Grip Rubber Adhesive 1300. It is certain that more effective adhesives will continue to be developed.

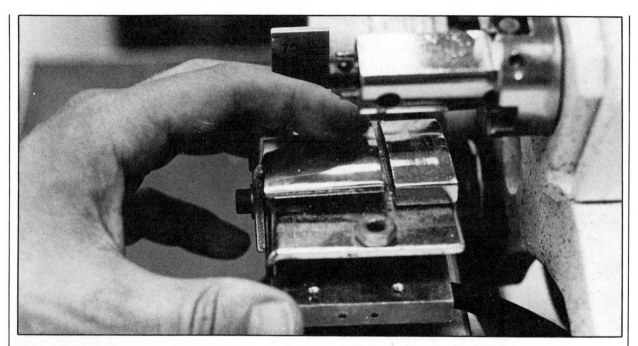

Figure 10–15. *Apply petroleum jelly to the clapper plate to allow for ease in pattern rotation.*

EDGER COOLANTS

Coolant is absolutely essential in the conventional edging operation, as it serves several different purposes. The most obvious purpose is to reduce heat generated in the edging process. This prevents lens cracking or excessive chipping. In addition, though, the coolant serves to flush abraded glass or plastic material off the wheel. Ground lens material eventually settles in the coolant tank below.

Coolants have a certain lubricating effect as well and are important in maintaining good wheel life. The more coolant used, the better the wheel grinds.

Trying to shortcut on coolants can have hidden costs that more than offset any "savings" brought about by using substitutes or dilute solutions. One such substitution has been the use of automotive antifreeze. Besides being poisonous because of the chromates that it contains, antifreeze was never designed to promote lens cutting or increase diamond wheel life. Considering the value of edgers and their diamond wheels (not to mention their operators!) such substitutions can hardly be considered thrifty.

Changing the Coolant

The coolant tank is usually a five-gallon bucket that can be pulled out from under the edger. The liquid is drained off, leaving sludge in the plastic bag liner. The sludge-filled liner is removed and tied at the top for disposal.

Before adding new coolant, cleanse the coolant pump and rinse any residue from drains and electrical cords. If this is done regularly, it is done with ease. If not, residues become increasingly difficult to remove.

Coolants come in varying concentrations that are added to fresh water. Remember that coolant replacement is the *last* in a series of maintenance procedures. Some procedures that may precede coolant changes are:
1. stoning (dressing) the diamond wheel
2. cleaning the coolant chamber
3. lubrication of the edger.

Since the coolant pump is located inside and toward the top of the coolant tank, coolant level should be checked to ensure that the pump remains covered. Water may be added to raise the coolant back up to the required level to compensate for evaporation.

PROFICIENCY TEST QUESTIONS

1. T or F Focusing the Lensometer eyepiece allows the instrument to compensate for either the lack of accommodation or for a refractive error on the part of the operator. This means two individuals may well require two different eyepiece settings. Failure to refocus the eyepiece before using the instrument may cause discomfort to the operator, but it in no way affects the accuracy of the reading.

2. Which of the following is not normally recommended for cleaning lenses in an optical instrument?
   a. Alcohol
   b. Camel's hair brush
   c. Ammonia
   d. Canned compressed air

3. T or F It is possible to use ordinary stamp pad ink in the Lensometer marking device when plastic lenses are being marked.

4. Which of the following method(s) properly clean(s) the rubber stamp in a lens marking device?
   a. Wiping pad clean with alcohol on a cloth
   b. Wiping pad clean with acetone on a cloth
   c. Wiping pad clean with water on a cloth

5. T or F The metallic foam that periodically collects on the surface of alloy used in lens blocking can be reduced by stirring a small amount of salt into the liquid alloy.

6. T or F When the axis becomes misaligned in an alloy blocking unit, it always indicates the need for replacing the rubber mold.

7. Which shape lens is best for checking edger axis accuracy?
   a. Round
   b. Square
   c. Oval

8. When is it most helpful to have a flat edge on test lenses?
   a. When checking edger eyesize.
   b. When checking Lensometer accuracy
   c. When checking edger axis

9. When verifying completed work in the finishing lab and using the same Lensometer as was used in marking up the lenses, it is discovered that there are errors in axis as follows:

should be	actually is
R $+2.00 -1.00 \times 180$	$+2.00 -1.00 \times 008$
L $+2.25 -1.25 \times 5$	$+2.25 -1.25 \times 13$
R $-3.75 -2.00 \times 48$	$-3.75 -2.00 \times 56$
L $-4.00 -1.75 \times 136$	$-4.00 -1.75 \times 144$

   All lenses are edged for metal frames. The lenses are straight in the frame. Which pieces or piece of equipment may be responsible for the errors?
   a. 1, 2, 3, or 4   1. Lensometer
   b. 1, 2, or 3   2. Marker
   c. 2, 3, or 4   3. Blocker
   d. 2 or 3   4. Edger
   e. 4

10. Both left and right lenses are correctly inserted into a metal frame with their marking crosses still intact. Assuming the frame is properly manufactured, if the right and left lenses both show the marking cross at 10 degrees instead of 180 degrees, where might the error lie?
    a. The edger axis may be out of adjustment.
    b. The lens marker stamp may be rotated.
    c. The pattern may have been cut off axis.
    d. Any of the above could have caused the problem.

11. Both left and right lenses are correctly inserted into a metal frame with their marking crosses still intact. Assuming the frame is properly manufactured, if the right lens marking cross is turned to axis 10 and the left marking cross turned to axis 170, where might the error lie?
    a. The edger axis may be out of adjustment.
    b. The lens marker stamp may be rotated.
    c. The pattern may have been cut off axis.
    d. Any of the above could have caused the problem.

12. While checking the edger for eyesize accuracy, it is discovered that the wheel differential is also in need of adjustment. Which should normally be corrected first?
    a. Eyesize
    b. Wheel differential

13. What is the wheel differential in reference to automatic edgers?
    a. Difference in the width of the wheel edge

between roughing and finishing wheels

b. The ratio between the speed of rotation of the lens drive motor and the speed of rotation of the edger wheel itself

c. The wheel speed of the edger in question as compared to a standard wheel speed

d. The size difference a lens has after being rough edged on the roughing wheel in comparison to the size it has after being edged on the finishing wheel

e. The difference between the wheel speed as measured at the edge of the roughing wheel in comparison to the speed as measured at the edge of the finishing wheel

14. A lens is edged to 47 mm using a "set-15" pattern. To check wheel differential the lens is once more started through the cycle. During roughing, power is cut and the edger setting dial turned until the lens touches the roughing wheel. At this point the dial reading is 29.5. What is the wheel differential?
a. Cannot be determined with the information given
b. 2.5 mm
c. 3.5 mm
d. 7.0 mm
e. None of the above is correct.

15. A lens is edged to a 52-mm eyesize using a "set-10" pattern. To check wheel differential, the same lens is rerun and stopped in the middle of the roughing cycle. Turning the eyesize dial until the lens touches the roughing wheel produces a dial reading of 38.8 mm. What is the wheel differential?
a. Cannot be determined with the information given
b. 2.8 mm
c. 3.2 mm
d. 3.8 mm
e. None of the above is correct.

16. An edger is checked for accuracy of eyesize. An accurate pattern with a "set-12" size is used. The edger dial is set for 45. What should the lens *A* dimension measure when cut?
a. 45
b. 33

c. 57
d. 36.5
e. None of the above is correct.

17. A sizing pattern which has an *A* dimension of 46.5 is used to check the edger for correctness in cutting eyesize. The edger is set on 45 and a trial lens edged. When removed and measured, the lens is found to be 54.5 mm. To reset the edger, the thumb screw is loosened and the sizing dial knob turned. The thumb screw is then retightened and the edger now cuts a test lens correctly. What does the edger read now that it cuts properly?
a. 45
b. 54
c. 54.5
d. 44.5
e. 55.5

18. To check for edger eyesize accuracy, a "set-15" pattern is used. When edged, the lens measures 49.2 instead of the 49.0 mm that was called for by the dial setting. To correctly calibrate the edger, its eyesize dial is loosened. To what should it be turned in order to be correctly recalibrated?
a. 49.2
b. 48.8
c. 33.8
d. 34.2
e. None of the above is correct.

19. T or F   One suitable substitute for edger coolant is four parts water to one part automotive antifreeze.

20. Place the following edger maintenance jobs in their optimum order, from first job to be carried out, to last.
1. Cleaning the grinding chamber
2. Changing the coolant
3. Stoning the wheel
4. Lubricating the edger
a. 1, 3, 4, 2
b. 4, 3, 2, 1
c. 2, 1, 3, 4
d. 3, 1, 4, 2
e. 1, 4, 2, 3

Chapter 11

Diamond Wheels

There are quite a number of diamond wheels marketed through a variety of sources. Without a knowledge of wheel construction and factors that may vary, a practitioner may find it difficult to compare wheels. In addition, the care that diamond wheels must be given varies according to type. Even if a wheel is chosen with great care, if it is not properly maintained, it will not give the service that otherwise would have been obtained.

FOUR CONSTRUCTION FACTORS

There are four main variable factors in the construction of diamond wheel surfaces, including grit size, diamond concentration, depth of the diamond layer, and type of bond used to hold the diamond to the wheel.

Grit Size

A diamond abrasive works in much the same manner as does ordinary sandpaper. Coarse grade sandpaper contains large chunks of abrasive and will remove surface material rapidly. A surface coarsely sanded will show visible grooves and feel rough to the touch. On the other hand, fine grade sandpaper gives a smooth, clean finish. Yet because it can only abrade away small amounts of material, it is inappropriate for anything but a fine finish.

The same is true for diamond wheels. If the main task of the wheel is to grind away large quantities of material, large, chunky diamond particles are appropriate.

Wheels having a coarse grit grind rapidly but leave ragged edges with a certain amount of flaking. Large grit diamond particles are used for making roughing wheels. Finer particle sizes are used for finishing wheels and, though slower grinding, produce edges with very few chips.

Before they are used as industrial abrasives, diamond particles are sorted by size. This may be done by a screening process, using progressively finer mesh to trap larger particles. If a diamond particle is small enough to fall through one screen, but is stopped by the next, then its size is known to be between the two sieve sizes. Because sieves are measured by the number of wires or fibers per unit area, diamond grit numbers are based on this system as well. Therefore, the *higher* the diamond code number, the *smaller* the diamond particle size.

When grit size is extremely small, the diamond material takes on a flour-like consistency and is referred to as *diamond powder.*

It is feasible to use two or more different grit sizes in combination on the same wheel. In this manner a better cutting speed can be achieved while producing a more acceptable edge finish.

Segregating two different single grits on separate sectors of the same wheel may also be used to advantage. A finer grit is used on the face of the V-groove, which cuts the front of the bevel, while a slightly rougher, faster cutting grit is used on the surface of the groove cutting the minus side of the bevel. Since the minus side of the lens is cut faster than the plus, the bevel is moved forward. (This was described earlier in the chapter on edging and is shown in Figure 7–23).

Grit size also becomes a factor in how well a wheel holds its form. The finer the grit used in a wheel, the faster it will be worn away during the edging process. As would be expected, V-bevels and hidden bevels lose their configuration as the wheel wears. There is thus a compromise between how smooth and flake-free the bevel will be, in contrast to how long the wheel will cut distinct edges before retruing is necessitated.

Concentration

The second factor in diamond wheel evaluation is the amount of diamond per cubic unit. A wheel having only a small amount of diamond in comparison to bonding material is of low concentration.

The highest concentration wheel normally used in the optical industry contains 25% diamond and 75% bonding material. This concentration is designated by volume and is given a code number of 100, as in Table 11–1.

Table 11–1. Diamond Concentration

Concentration number	Carats*/ Cubic inch	Carats/Cubic centimeter	% diamond by volume
100	72	4.4	25
75	54	3.3	18.75
50	36	2.2	12.5
25	18	1.1	6.25

*One carat of diamond is considered to be 0.2 g.

Which Concentration Is Best?

When considering which wheel to use for a given edging situation, it should not be automatically assumed that a high concentration wheel is the best wheel for all situations.

For example, roughing wheels having a high concentration of diamond are excellent for edgers with a heavy head pressure (i.e., over 10 lbs.). If the same high concentration wheel is used on edgers having light pressure, the exposed diamonds tend to dull quickly. Thus, a high concentration wheel on a low pressure edger will cut poorly. Therefore, the standard concentration is much more efficient for edgers having the lower (5 to 10 lbs) head pressure.

Effect of Concentration on Wheel Wear

As would be expected, high concentration wheels wear slower. Therefore, they are the correct choice for finishing wheels made to cut distinct edge shapes. If a medium or low concentration of diamond were to be used, sharp bevel angles would soon begin to round. This necessitates all-too-frequent retruings of the wheel, which could be avoided by using a higher diamond concentration. See Table 11–2, which compares wheels by grit types.

Standard concentration[1] finishing wheels are acceptable in low volume situations where 10 pair of lenses or less[2] per day are being edged. In this situation, wheel life and groove shape are extended to acceptable lengths by virtue of their low usage.

Concentration can be varied over the face of the wheel. This is done on some roughing wheels with the highest diamond concentration being located in the area of most frequent wear.

Depth of Layer

Were a wheel to have a good concentration of the proper grit diamond material, it would still have no lasting value if the depth of layer were too thin. (See Figure 11–1.) A wheel is only useful while abrasive material remains on the core. Once this layer has worn thin, the wheel must be replaced. For edger wheels, normal depth of layer usually ranges from $\frac{1}{16}$ to $\frac{1}{4}$ inch.[3]

Type of Bonding

Diamond material must be solidly bound to the core of the wheel and simultaneously allow exposure of sharp diamond edges. Bonding is usually accomplished in one of two ways.

1. *Impregnated or metal bonded* wheels are made by mixing diamond material with powdered metal. This mixture is placed in a mold containing the core of the wheel. The filled mold is heated in a furnace until the metal begins to melt. When cooling takes place, the diamond grit is bound to the core of the wheel with solidified metal.
2. *Electroplated or electrometallic* wheels are made by electrolytically depositing metal onto the wheel.

---

[1] "Standard" concentration wheels will vary from manufacturer to manufacturer, but often have a concentration number of around 75.

[2] "A.I.T. Optical Diamond Wheels," A.I.T. Industries, Inc., Skokie, Illinois, p. 13.

[3] Hans Hirschhorn, "Diamond Edging Wheels," *Optical Index*, Vol. 53, No. 9, September 1978, p. 132.

During this process diamond particles are encompassed by a thickening layer of metal that is electrolytically transferred from the ion-laden plating solution.

Generally, impregnated wheels are used to grind glass lenses, although they may be used for conventional plastic lenses as well. Electroplated wheels, though, are used almost exclusively for plastic lenses. The wheel types are shown in Figure 11–2. Edging a hard glass lens on an electroplated wheel causes an extreme reduction in wheel life, as diamond particles are easily torn from the electroplated metal.

Although the edging of plastic lenses on impregnated wheels intended primarily for glass is acceptable, results are satisfactory only up to a point. If the ratio of plastic to glass is too high, the wheel clogs with plastic between the diamonds (i.e., the wheel glazes). When this occurs, cutting speed drops for plastic and flaking occurs on glass lenses.

Electroplated wheels are available for both roughing and finishing.

During the finishing cycle, excellent results may be obtained for plastic lenses using either an electroplated or an impregnated wheel. (Some impregnated wheels are designed exclusively for plastic.) Table 11–3 summarizes the process.

Table 11–2. Grit and Concentration Factors in Selecting Finishing Wheels

Advantages	Disadvantages
Fine Grit	
Smooth bevels Flake-free edges	Quicker loss of distinct bevel shape, necessitating more frequent retrues
Medium Fine	
Size and shape definition are retained longer	Slight flake line at edge requires pin bevelling
High Concentration	
Better edge shape Retruing required less often	Higher price "Overkill" in low production setting.

DRESSING OF DIAMOND WHEELS

From time to time a diamond wheel begins to lose some of the sharp cutting ability that it had when new. This is generally a result of a "glazed" wheel or diamonds that have become dull.

The Glazed Wheel

When the empty spaces between exposed diamond particles begin to fill up with ground lens material, the diamonds are unable to dig or bite into the lens as deeply. This condition is known as *glazing* and is most common when plastic lenses are being run on a metal bonded roughing wheel intended primarily for glass. A glazed wheel looks smooth and feels relatively smooth to the touch.

This condition may be prevented, or at least slowed, by running glass lenses often enough and in sufficient volume to produce a self-cleaning effect. There is not total agreement as to the best procedure to prevent glazing. Some practitioners maintain that glass and plastic should be alternated as often as possible to obtain the best cleaning effect with minimal extra effort. Others take the opposite extreme in their concern for not scratching plastic lenses. They advise that the edger be flushed with water, the wheel dressed, and the coolant changed before plastic lenses are run.

It would seem that if no adverse scratching were detected, alternating of lens types would have advantages. However, if scratching is manifested, steps toward the second extreme may be implemented until problems disappear.

When a wheel becomes fully glazed, preventive techniques are no longer useful and it must be cleaned by dressing.

Dressing the Wheel

Wheels may lose their cutting ability because their exposed diamonds have dulled through use.

If the outermost diamonds can be removed to allow exposure of ones slightly deeper in the bond, cutting integrity can be restored. This is done by attacking the outer surface of the metal bond that holds the diamond in place and is referred to as *dressing*. The most common method used to dress a wheel is called *stoning* and is done by holding an abrasive stick against the spinning wheel. Figure 11–3 shows the abrasive stick, most often made up of aluminum oxide or silicon carbide grit formed into a squared stick and held together by means of a soft bonding material. When the abrasive stick is held against the wheel, exposed diamonds easily furrow

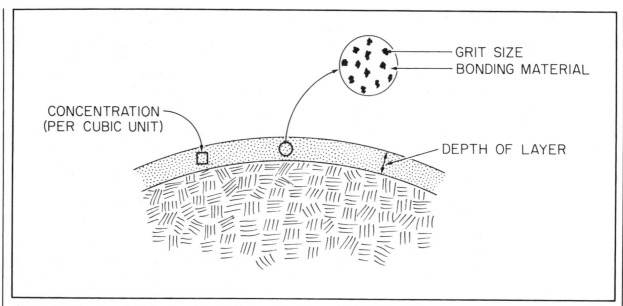

Figure 11–1. Important factors in specifying wheel type include concentration (particles per cubic unit of area), grit size (how big the abrasive particles are), bonding material (what is used to hold the abrasive particles in place), and depth of layer (how thick the abrasive particle layer is).

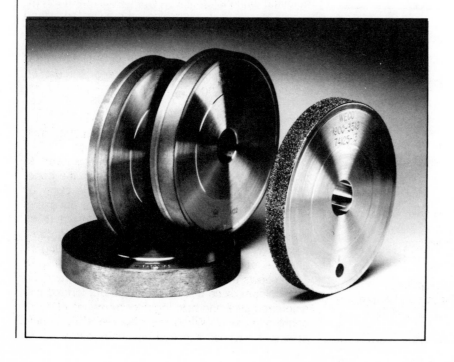

Figure 11–2. The three wheels on the left are impregnated diamond wheels. The wheel on the right is an electroplated roughing wheel intended only for plastic (but not polycarbonate) lenses. (Photo courtesy of WECO.)

Table 11–3. Types of Wheels and Sequence Used in the Edging of Glass and Plastic Lenses*

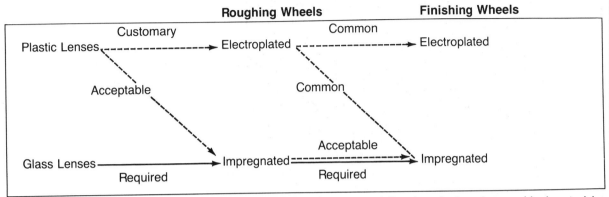

*This table represents possible paths plastic (designated by dashed lines) and glass lenses (designated by solid lines) may take in the edging process. It may be readily seen that there is much more latitude in the processing of plastic lenses.

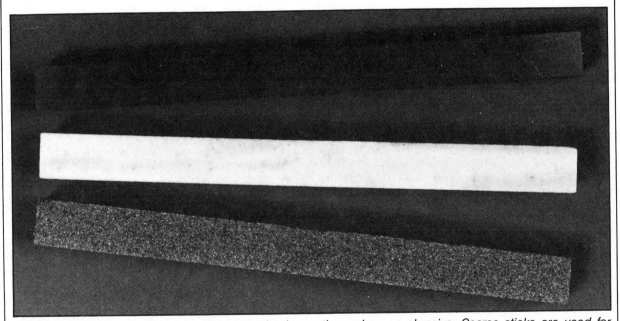

Figure 11–3. Dressing sticks for diamond wheels are themselves an abrasive. Coarse sticks are used for roughing wheels, fine sticks for finishing wheels.

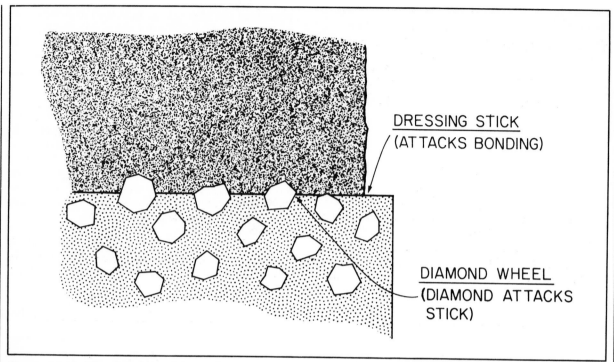

Figure 11–4. *The dressing stick attacks the softer bonding material, allowing worn diamonds to drop out and exposing fresh, new diamond particles.*

through the loosely bonded stick surface. This allows the stick to rub against the bonding material surrounding the diamond particles. The bonding is ground down far enough that old, dull diamonds no longer are embedded in enough bonding material to hold them and so they drop off. As Figure 11–4 shows, other diamonds embedded more deeply in the bonding are exposed, giving a fresh, sharp cutting surface.

Dressing of an edger wheel should be done *before* changing coolant. In this manner, the spent abrasive material from stick and wheel is not left to recirculate in the coolant, increasing the risk of scratching. The proper sequence is:

1. Dress the wheel.
2. Cycle the machine empty to flush abrasive material from the wheel.
3. Rinse or clean the grinding chamber.
4. Change the coolant.

Dressing of Roughing Wheels

Only impregnated wheels are to be stoned, as attempts to stone an electroplated wheel cause the soft bonding material to glaze over the diamonds, *decreasing* wheel effectiveness.

The procedure for stoning an impregnated roughing wheel begins by soaking a correctly chosen abrasive stick in coolant. A coarse grit is the appropriate choice and most sticks are recognizable by color. If the stick is not soaked, there is no lubricating effect. Then the edger coolant pump is disconnected and the wheel turned on. Since roughing wheels should *not* be stoned at full speed, the power is turned off and the abrasive stick pressed firmly against the wheel until rotation is halted, as in Figure 11–5. This is repeated until the stick is rapidly and easily consumed by the wheel, indicating exposure of fresh cutting surfaces. *Do not* attempt to drag the stick laterally across the wheel! Do one section at a

Table 11–4. Controlling Bevel Apex Location

Outcome desired	Action
To move the bevel apex forward	Dull the front (plus) side of the groove or Sharpen (stone) the rear (minus) side of the groove
To move the bevel apex back on the lens	Sharpen the front (plus) side of the groove or Dull the rear (minus) side of the groove

time. Table 11–4 illustrates this process.

In summary, to stone impregnated roughing wheels:
1. Soak coarse grit abrasive stick in coolant.
2. Disconnect edger pump.
3. Turn wheel on till full speed is achieved.
4. Turn wheel off.
5. Stop wheel quickly with stick.
6. Repeat till stick is consumed quickly.

Roughing wheels may also be dressed using a sandblasting unit that may be found in laboratories processing safety lenses. (The small sandblasting unit is used to etch the laboratory trademark and other required code letters on safety lens surfaces.) Sandblasting an edger wheel also attacks the bonding material, achieving the same end as an abrasive stick.

Dressing of Impregnated Finishing Wheels

Finishing wheels require dressing when their cutting speed slows or when the bevel produced in a free-float situation no longer properly situates itself even when the machine is level. Finishing wheels should not be dressed unless there is clear evidence of need. Just because one wheel needs stoning does not mean that all wheels in the lab should be done as a preventive measure. Do not stone a wheel until it needs it.

To stone a finishing wheel, begin with a pumice or fine grit stick that has been soaked in coolant. (Exercise extreme caution in stoning finishing wheels, as bevel configuration can be ruined if improper procedures are followed.) A round pattern is placed on the edger and the size setting increased to a maximum so that the edger head is out of the way. For finishing wheels the coolant is left *on* and the wheel runs at *full power.* Power is not turned off during stoning. In this way the rapidly spinning exposed diamonds tend to protect the bonding from excessive erosion and loss of bevel form.

With both coolant and power on, the stick is *lightly* pressed against the wheel for a few seconds. All portions of both flat and V portions should be touched, one after the other. Only ½ to 1 inch of stick should be required to stone the wheel. When stoning is complete there should be no shiny portions left on the wheel. The entire surface should have an even, matte appearance.

In summary, to stone impregnated finishing wheels:
1. Soak fine grit abrasive stick in coolant.
2. Put round pattern on edger.
3. Set to large eyesize.
4. Turn wheel and coolant on. (*Do not turn off!*)
5. Lightly press stick against wheel for a few seconds.

Changing the Lens Bevel Location

Since stoning an edger wheel causes it to cut faster, it stands to reason that if only one side of a finishing wheel groove were stoned, the stoned side would cut faster. Were this the side corresponding to the front bevel, more lens material would be ground from the front than the rear, placing the bevel apex toward the back of the lens. This, of course, would be undesirable. However, by selectively dressing only portions of the edger wheel, the bevel apex can be moved either forward or backward to advantage.

For example, suppose that an edger is consistently edging lenses with the bevel either exactly in the middle or somewhat farther back. It is desirable to place the bevel apex more at the ⅓–⅔ location. This may be done by selectively stoning the rear (minus) surface of the groove. Thus, the minus side of the lens is cut away faster; the lens shifts *back* toward the dressed half of the groove; and the bevel apex moves forward. See Figure 11–6 for a summary of the procedure.

Bevel apex location can also be shifted by selectively *dulling* one section of the finishing wheel. *D*ulling serves to *d*raw the bevel apex toward the dulled side, just as *s*harpening *s*hoves the apex to the sharp side. Control the location of the bevel apex as listed in Table 11–4.

Selectively dulling one portion of the edger wheel may be accomplished using a tungsten carbide tool,

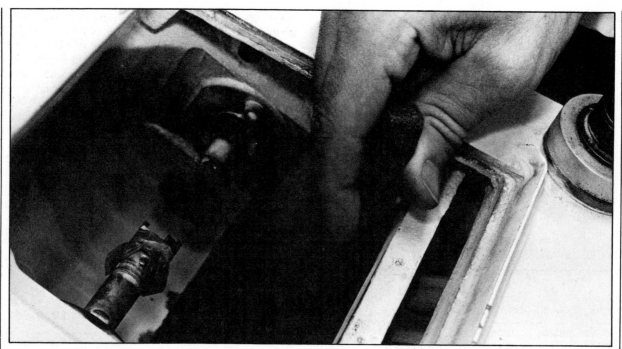

Figure 11–5. *In stoning the roughing wheel, the power is turned off and the stick pressed against the stone until rotation stops.*

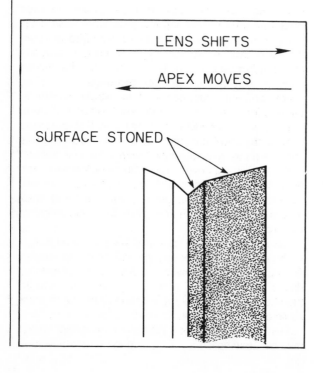

LENS SHIFTS →

← APEX MOVES

SURFACE STONED

Figure 11–6. *Stoning the righthand side of the wheel causes it to cut more aggressively. Therefore the rear surface of the lens bevel is ground away more rapidly, moving the bevel apex forward.*

a carbide chip, or even an Allen wrench. Without coolant and with the wheel at full power, the tool is touched to the side of the groove. To make certain that the desired result has been obtained, a test lens may be run. If the bevel apex has moved too far, the surface may be resharpened a bit by holding the proper abrasive stick against both sides of the groove simultaneously.

In summary, to position the bevel apex:
1. Stone the impregnated finishing wheel.
2. Run the test lens.
3. If the bevel is still improperly positioned, dull the side toward which the bevel apex is to be drawn. This is done by
   a. turning off the coolant
   b. turning on power to the wheel
   c. holding dulling tool against the predetermined side of the groove.
4. Run the test lens, again turning the coolant back on.
5. If the bevel apex has moved too far, stone both groove sides simultaneously.

Cleaning of Electroplated Wheels
In the event that electroplated wheels show a tendency to become glazed, they must be cleaned, rather than dressed. Cleaning may be accomplished by using a stiff bristle brush in combination with a scrubbing kitchen cleanser. Any attempt to stone an electroplated wheel will result in further glazing, because the soft bonding material will be forced over the diamond cutting surfaces.

TRUING OF DIAMOND WHEELS

When edger wheels no longer cut to the proper configuration despite careful attention to proper machine maintenance and correct dressing of wheels, then consideration must be given to having the wheel trued. For diamond wheels this must be done at the factory rather than in the lab.

The truing process itself consists of recutting a new surface on the wheel that duplicates the shape of the original surface. After truing, the wheel surface is shaped like new, but the wheel radius is slightly smaller than it was originally.

Retruing of Roughing Wheels
Retruing of roughing wheels is of questionable value and should be done only after all other options have been tried. (Some of the options were discussed in

Chapter 7, "Edging.") Possibilities for getting better wear from a roughing wheel include:
1. turning the wheel around periodically. (A turned wheel must be dressed before being used in the new direction.)
2. using a split wheel so that right and left halves can be interchanged as the wheel wears centrally.

Because the roughing wheel does not give the lens edge its final configuration, the fact that the wheel has become grooved is not a major consideration. Truing would only be considered if it were felt that the uneven edge shape produced on the lens after roughing was creating too much wear in one location on the finishing wheel. Usually, however, excessive finishing wheel wear is a result of failure to compensate for a worn down roughing wheel by resetting the wheel differential.

Keep in mind that when a roughing wheel is factory retrued, all diamond surface that extends above the lowest level of the worn trough will be removed.

If no program of wheel rotation or differential adjustment is carried out, excessive wheel grooving and lens edge chipping will result. In such circumstances, retruing of the roughing wheel is in order.

Finishing Wheel Retruing
Finishing wheels should be retrued when it is noted that bevels are poorly formed. This could manifest itself as rounded bevel apices or loss of a sharp demarcation between bevel and hidden-bevel ledge, as shown in Figure 11–7. Failure of lenses to fit well in metal frame eyewires can also be an indication for a needed retrue.

Do not allow finishing wheels to deteriorate excessively between retrues. Excessive deterioration necessitates removing a great deal of diamond material in order to bring the wheel back to its correct shape, thus reducing the number of times a wheel may be trued. The alternative will result in consistent high quality workmanship and more retrues from each wheel.

When feasible, it is best to have an extra finishing wheel. If two finishing wheels can be interchanged, a freshly trued wheel will always be available when wear begins to manifest itself as a reduction in quality. With a spare wheel on hand, the temptation to forestall the process "just a while longer" is reduced.

A retruing kit is available that allows the finishing wheel groove to be sharpened in-house. This small truing wheel mounts in the edger chucking system so that truing may be carried out without having to

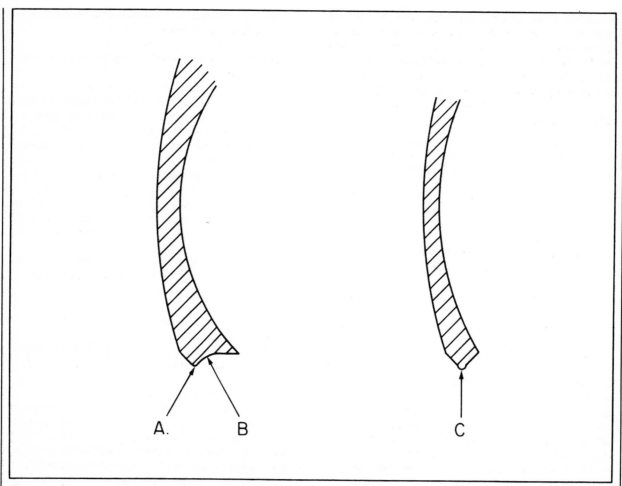

Figure 11–7. *Failure to retrue finishing wheels often enough will result in loss of sharp, distinct edges (A and B), or a rutting out of the groove apex of the V-bevel (C).*

remove the edger wheel from the machine. With such an option it is possible to maintain good bevel shapes for a longer time before sending the wheel to the factory for complete retruing.

PROFICIENCY TEST QUESTIONS

1. How does a diamond wheel having a coarse grit cut in comparison to one having a fine grit?
   a. At a faster speed
   b. At a slower speed
   c. At the same speed

2. Assuming equal diamond concentrations, a fine grit diamond wheel that will produce edges practically free from flakes:
   a. can be expected to produce well-defined, distinct lens bevels for longer periods of time before retruing is necessary than a wheel that causes slightly more edge flaking.
   b. cannot be expected to produce well-defined, distinct lens bevels for longer periods of time before retruing is necessary than a wheel that causes slightly more edge flaking.

3. Numbers used in decribing diamond grit size for use in optical grinding wheels become:
   a. larger as the particle size becomes smaller.
   b. larger as the particle size becomes larger.

4. A diamond wheel described as having a concentration of 50 contains what percent of diamond by volume?
   a. 75%
   b. 50%
   c. 25%
   d. 12.5%
   e. None of the above, as percent is always specified by weight

5. What diamond concentration code number would be given to an edger wheel having a percentage of 18.75% diamond and 81.25% bonding material by volume?
   a. 100
   b. 75
   c. 23
   d. 18.75
   e. 12.25

6. When are "standard" concentration finishing wheels a good option?
   a. When a high percentage of polycarbonate lenses are being edged
   b. When more than 10 lens pairs are edged on a daily basis
   c. When 10 or less lens pairs are edged on a daily basis

   d. When the edger has a high (over 10 pounds) head pressure

7. Bounded metal diamond wheels are made by:
   a. bonding diamonds to the wheel through an electrolytic process.
   b. fusing a powdered metal and diamond particle mixture together at a high temperature.

8. Glass is best edged using which of the following?
   a. A bonded wheel
   b. An electroplated wheel
   c. A milling cutter
   d. A router blade
   e. Any of the above are acceptable, although some methods are better than others.

9. What diamond concentration is best for the roughing wheel of a light pressure edger (5–10 lbs)?
   a. Medium concentration
   b. High concentration

10. In ophthalmic use, for what are electroplated wheels used more often?
    a. Photochromic lenses
    b. Crown glass lenses
    c. High-index lenses
    d. CR-39® plastic lenses

11. When referring to ophthalmic lens grinding wheels, what best defines the term *glazing*?
    a. Dressing of the wheel with an abrasive stick.
    b. Accumulation of lens material between abrasive particles on the edger wheel surface.
    c. Turning of the wheel so that it spins in the opposite direction.
    d. Dulling of a portion of the groove with a hard, blunt instrument, for purposes of controlling bevel placement.

12. T or F   A small number of plastic lenses may be edged periodically on metal bonded diamond roughing wheels designed to be used primarily for edging a large number of photochromic glass lenses.

13. T or F   A small number of crown glass lenses may be regularly edged on electroplated wheels designed primarily for CR-39 plastic lenses, so long as the wheel is properly dressed afterwards.

14. Which is the proper sequence for doing each of the jobs listed?
    1. Rinse or clean the grinding chamber.
    2. Change the coolant.
    3. Dress the wheel.
    4. Cycle the machine empty.
    a. 3, 1, 2, 4
    b. 2, 4, 1, 3,
    c. 2, 3, 1, 4
    d. 3, 4, 1, 2

15. T or F   When stoning an edger wheel, drag the stick across the wheel laterally until the stick is rapidly and easily consumed by the wheel.

16. What type of dressing stick should be used to dress an electroplated finishing wheel?
    a. White (fine grit) used wet
    b. White (fine grit) used dry
    c. Brown (80 grit) used wet
    d. Brown (80 grit) used dry
    e. Electroplated finishing wheels should not be dressed.

17. Sandblasting may be used in the optical laboratory for how many of the following functions?
    a. To clean off excess low-temperature metal alloy that may have become adhered to hand tools
    b. To mark safety lenses
    c. To dress a bonded diamond wheel
    d. All of the above functions are valid.
    e. None of the options listed in a–c are valid.

18. T or F   Wheels should only be stoned when they show signs of needing it, and not as part of a regular maintenance schedule.

Matching (an answer may be used more than one time)

19. What type of wheel is stoned when it is running under full power? _____
20. What type of wheel is stoned after turning power off? _____
21. What type of wheel is stoned with coolant running? _____
22. What type of wheel is stoned with coolant off? _____

23. What type of wheel is not stoned? _____
    a. Bonded (impregnated) roughing wheel
    b. Bonded (impregnated) finishing wheel
    c. Electroplated roughing wheel
    d. None of the other responses is appropriate

24. What will stoning only the front side of a finishing wheel groove cause the bevel apex to do?
    a. Move forward toward F_1.
    b. Move backward toward F_2.
    c. Become somewhat more pointed.
    d. Move forward for plus lenses and backward for minus lenses.

25. If the effect of dulling one side of the finishing wheel groove has caused the bevel position to move *too* far in the desired direction, the best correction procedure is to:
    a. resharpen just the dulled side with an abrasive stick.
    b. dull the opposite side of the groove slightly.
    c. resharpen *both* sides of the groove with an abrasive stick simultaneously.

26. In the event that an electroplated diamond wheel shows a tendency to become glazed, it may be corrected by:
    a. using a pumice abrasive stick.
    b. using a coarse grit abrasive stick.
    c. using a stiff bristle brush and scrubbing cleanser.

27. Which type of wheel requires the most frequent retruing?
    a. Impregnated (metal bonded) roughing wheel
    b. Impregnated (metal bonded) finishing wheel
    c. Electroplated roughing wheel
    d. Electroplated finishing wheel

28. Which of the following is the best statement about the truing of impregnated diamond roughing wheels?
    a. Impregnated roughing wheels should be regularly trued to prevent grooving of the surface.
    b. Roughing wheels should be trued when grooving first appears.
    c. Retruing of impregnated roughing wheels is of questionable value.
    d. Impregnated roughing wheels cannot be retrued.

29. T or F   Dress the roughing wheel on a diamond edger with the wheel running at full RPM.

Appendix 1

Standards of Lens and Frame Measurement

How much lenses are decentered for edging depends entirely upon the method by which lenses and frames are measured. Two main systems are used throughout the English-speaking world, one based upon a "boxed" lens size and another upon a mid-lens width measurement. The *boxing system* is pictured in Figure A1–1 and is used in the United States and Canada. The *datum system,* as further defined in the *British Standards,* is used in England and many of the British Commonwealth nations. It is

imperative that one standard or the other be used consistently, since the pattern is made for either one standard or the other and cannot be used interchangeably.

In the boxing system the *eye* or *lens* size is determined by the horizontal distance between two vertical tangents enclosing the lens on the left and right. The point halfway between these vertical tangents and also halfway between horizontal tangents enclosing the lens in a box is the primary reference

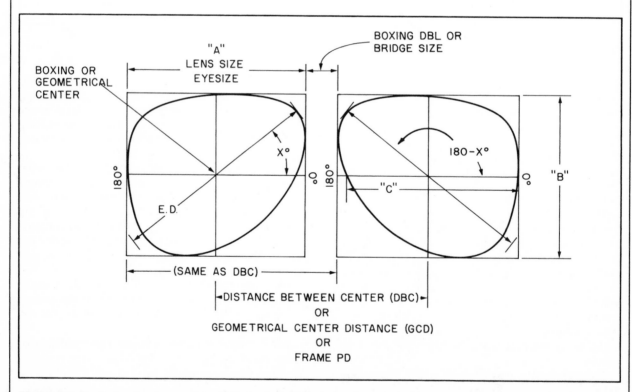

Figure A1–1. *In the boxing system, E.D. is the abbreviation for effective diameter, which is twice the longest radius of the shape as measured from the boxing (geometrical) center. The angle from the zero-degree side of the 180-degree line to the effective diameter axis is X for the right lens. The measure is used in accurate calculation of the minimum lens blank size and blank thickness required to fabricate the prescription.*

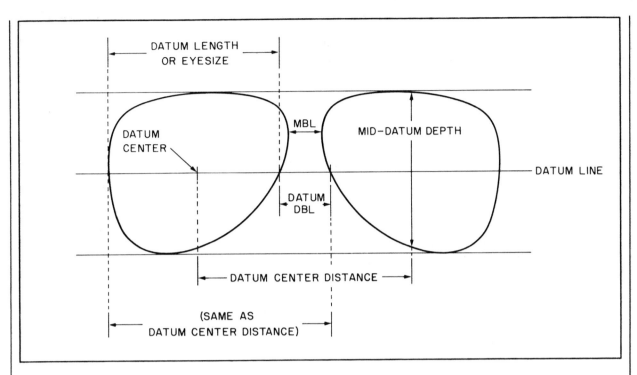

Figure A1–2. The datum system.

point. This is known as the *boxing center,* since it is the center of the box enclosing the lens. It is alternately referred to as the *geometrical center,* because *after* the lens is edged, it is the geometrical center point. (The term geometrical center must usually be qualified, since the geometrical center of an uncut lens blank will not be at the geometrical center of the lens once it has been edged.)

The *British Standards* (see Figure A1–2) define the lens or eyesize as being the width of the lens along the datum line. The *datum line* is a horizontal line halfway between the two horizontal tangents that border the top and bottom of the lens. This measure corresponds to the so-called *C* dimension of the boxing system and is known as the *datum length,* or simply the *eyesize.* The central reference point in the datum system is halfway across the lens as measured along the datum line and is called the *datum center.*

The distance between lenses (DBL) is measured differently between the two standards as well. The British Standard measures this along the datum line. As can be seen from Figure A1–2, this distance between lenses may not necessarily be the *smallest* distance between lenses. Therefore, the British Stan-

dards define the smallest measurable distance between the two lenses (regardless of the level where this minimum occurs) as the *minimum between lenses* (MBL). The datum MBL is the same as the boxing system's DBL.

When patterns are being manufactured, the center of rotation is drilled to correspond to the central reference point of the standard being used. And because the boxing center is not located at the same point for a given shape as the datum center, a pattern drilled for the boxing system won't work if the British Standard is being used to calculate lens decentration and vice versa.

Fortunately, decentration calculations are made in exactly the same manner, regardless of the system being used. However, the results must not be interchanged.

For example, suppose a frame has the following dimensions:

boxing eyesize (A) = 52
boxing DBL = 15
datum length = 48
datum DBL = 19
wearer's PD = 63.

Decentration for the boxing system is

225

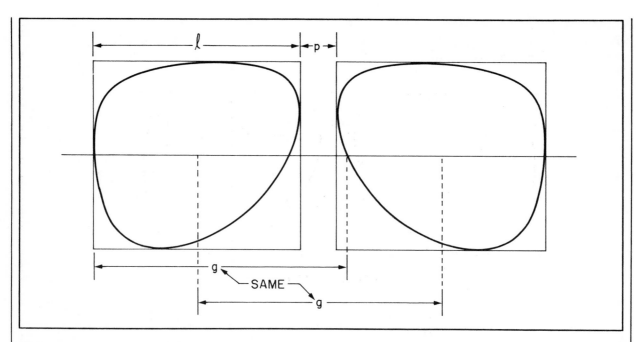

Figure A1–3. The GOMAC system.

ℓ = boxed length of lens ("largeur totale du verre")

p = boxing DBL ("distance minima entre verres," or "pont")

g = datum center distance ("grandeur, ou taille de la monture")

Not pictured:

n = base of the frame bridge on the datum line, a type of anatomical inside bridge measure ("largeur nasale anatomique").

t = width of a rimless mounting front measured from barrel center to barrel center ["largeur temporale de la face, mesurée entre les axes d'articulation (seulement pour les monture glaces)"].[1]

---

[1]Sasieni, L. S., "Optical Standards," *Manufacturing Optics International*, Vol. 25, No. 10, May 1972, pp. 395–398.

$$\frac{(\text{eyesize} + \text{DBL}) - \text{PD}}{2} = \frac{(52 + 15) - 63}{2},$$
$$\text{decentration} = 2 \text{ mm per lens.}$$

Decentration for British Standards is

$$\frac{(\text{eyesize} + \text{DBL}) - \text{PD}}{2} = \frac{(49 + 19) - 63}{2},$$
$$\text{decentration} = 2.5 \text{ mm per lens.}$$

Now if a pattern intended for the boxing standard is used when British Standard calculations have been made, the distance between the two lens optical centers will be 1 mm smaller than ordered.

A third system was established by a group representing the European Economic Community and referred to as the Groupement des Opticiens du Marché Commun (GOMAC). As Figure A1–3 shows, the attempt was to reach a compromise between boxing and datum systems. The results have not been universally accepted, even among Common Market countries.

Differences and similarities in systems are summarized in Figure A1–4, while corresponding terms are listed in table A1–1. Similarities and differences between U.S. and British multifocal placement terminology are summarized in Figures A1–5 and A1–6.

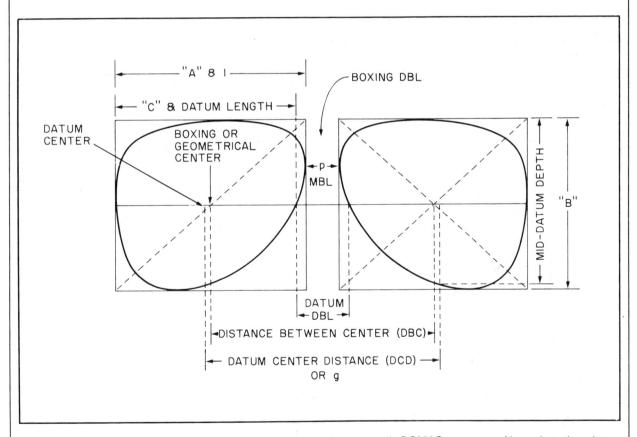

Figure A1–4. Diagrammatical comparison of boxing, datum, and GOMAC systems. *Note that the datum center will not always be outset with respect to the boxing center. For an upswept harlequin shape, the datum center will be inset as compared to the boxing center.*

Table A1–1. Comparison of Standard Terms.

Boxing	Datum or British Standards	GOMAC
Mechanical Center		P.
A	—	ℓ
B	—	—
C	Datum length	—
Boxing DBL	MBL	p
—	Datum DBL	—
—	Datum center distance (DCD)	g
Distance between centers (DBC) (Geometrical center distance) (GCD) ("Frame PD") (Boxing center distance)	—	—
—	Mid-datum depth	—
Major reference point (MRP)	Distance centration point (DCP) (or simply centration point)	

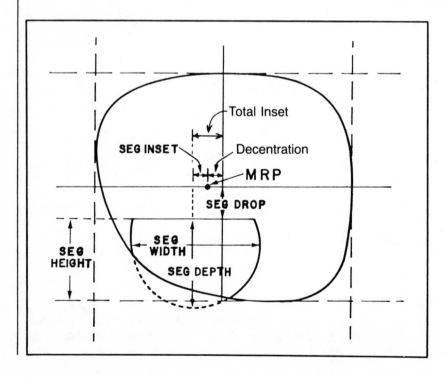

Figure A1–5. *Accepted U.S. multifocal placement terminology. Decentration is sometimes referred to as* inset. *This must not be confused with* seg inset *or* total inset.

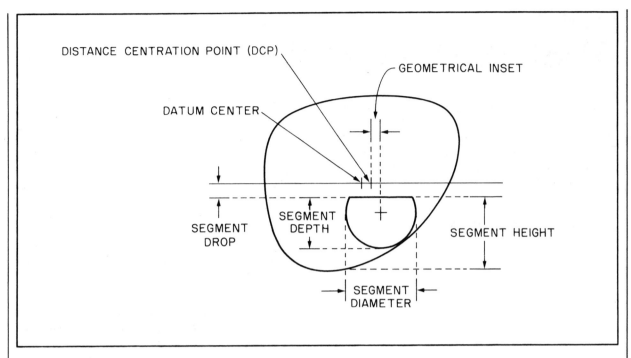

Figure A1–6. *Accepted British multifocal placement terminology. (It will be noted that a right lens is shown in this diagram, whereas a left lens was shown in Figure A1–5.) Because the datum center and boxing center do not necessarily correspond, the decentration required for the MRP (DCP) will not likely be the same.*

ANSI Z80 Standards

Standards established by the American National Standards Institute are summarized here in tabular form. The tables are not meant to be all-inclusive. For complete information consult *American National Standard Recommendations for Prescription Ophthalmic Lenses,* Z80.1 It may be obtained from:

American National Standards
1430 Broadway
New York, New York 10018

Table A2–1. ANSI Refractive Power Tolerances*

Refractive Power	Tolerance
For the sphere component	
From 0.00 to ±6.50D	±0.13D
Above ± 6.50D	2% of the sphere power
For the cylinder component	
From 0.00 to 2.00D cyl	±0.13D
From 2.12 to 4.50D cyl	±0.15D
Above 4.50D cyl	4% of the cylinder power
For the near addition	
For multifocals whose *distance* powers are 8.00D and below, the add power tolerance is	±0.13D
For multifocals whose *distance* powers are above 8.00D, the add power tolerance is	±0.18D

*Based on *American Standard Recommendations for Prescription Ophthalmic Lenses,* Z80.1-1979, American National Standards Institute, Inc., New York, 1979, p. 10.

Table A2–2. Tolerance for Cylinder Axis*

Cylinder power	Tolerance
0.125D to 0.375D	±7 degrees
0.500D to 0.750D	±5 degrees
0.875D to 1.50D	±3 degrees
1.625D and above	±2 degrees

*Tolerances are based on *American National Standard Recommendations for Prescription Ophthalmic Lenses,* Z80.1 – 1979, p. 10.

Table A2–3. ANSI Prism Power and Major Reference Point Location (Provisional Standards)*

	Tolerance
For lenses in the frame	
Vertical prism or MRP placement	⅓ prism diopter *or* 1.0 mm difference between left and right MRP height's in high power Rx with no prism ordered
Horizontal prism or MRP placement	⅔ prism diopter (Total from both lenses combined) *or* ±2.5 mm variation from the specified distance PD for high powered Rx's
For "lenses only" (not yet mounted) *and* Uncut multifocals	
Prism power	± ⅓ prism diopter in any direction on the lens.
MRP position placement	±1.0 mm in any direction for high powered lenses.

*Based on *American National Standard Recommendations for Prescription Ophthalmic Lenses,* Z80.1-1979, p. 11.

Table A2–4. ANSI Segment Location Tolerances* (Provisional Standards)

Vertical (segment height)	Tolerance
Unmounted single lens	±1.0 mm
Lens pair: mounted or unmounted	±1.0 mm (but both lenses in pair should be at matching heights)

Horizontal (segment inset)	
Unmounted single lenses	±1.0 mm
Mounted lens pair	±2.5 mm Inset should appear symmetrical and balanced

*Based on *American National Standard Recommendations for Prescription Ophthalmic Lenses,* Z80.1-1979, p. 11.

Table A2–5. ANSI Miscellaneous Tolerances* Tolerance

Thickness	±0.3 mm (when specified on order)
Warpage	1.00D (does not apply within 6 mm of eyewire)
Base curve	±0.75D (when specified or order)

*Based on *American National Standard Recommendations for Prescription Ophthalmic Lenses,* Z80.1-1979, pp. 11-12.

British Standards

Appendix 3
British Standards

Standards established by the British Standards Institution are summarized here in tabular form. The tables are not meant to be all-inclusive. For complete information consult *British Standard 2738:1962, Specification for Spectacle Lenses.* It may be obtained from:

> British Standards Institution
> British Standards House
> 2 Park Street
> London, W.1, England

or from national standards bodies.

Table A3–1. British Standards Refractive Power Tolerances*

Component	Tolerance
Sphere	
From 0.00 to ±4.00D[1]	±0.06D
From ±4.12 to ±8.00D[1]	±0.12D
From ±8.12 to ±13.00D[2]	±0.12D
From ±13.12 to ±20.00D[2]	±0.25D
Over ±20.00D[2]	±0.50D
Cylinder	
From 0.00 to ±4.00D	±0.06D
From ±4.12 to ±13.00D	±0.12D
From ±13.12 to ±20.00D	±0.25D
Over ±20.00D	±0.50D
Near addition	
The bifocal addition power is expressed as the difference between the back vertex power in the distance prescription and the back vertex power of the near power when the bifocal or multifocal segment is incorporated on the back of the lens. When the segment is incorporated on the front of the lens, the addition is expressed as the difference between distance and near front vertex powers.	±0.09D

---

*Adapted with permission from *British Standard 2738:1962, Specification for Spectacle Lenses,* British Standards Institution, London, p. 6.

[1]The power of the sphere component depends upon the form in which the prescription is written, i.e., either plus or minus cylinder form. For tolerance purposes, lenses up to 8.00D produced with a concave toric surface are considered as if written in minus cylinder form, whereas lenses produced with a convex toric surface are considered as if written in plus cylinder form.

[2]Lenses above 8.00D are evaluated for tolerance according to the way the prescription was originally written, regardless of whether produced with a concave or convex toric surface.

Table A3–2. British Standards Tolerance for Cylinder Axis*

Cylinder power	Tolerance
0.00 to 0.25D	±5 degrees
0.37 to 1.25D	±2½ degrees
Over 1.25D	±1¼ degrees

*Adapted with permission from *British Standard 2738:1962, Specification for Spectacle Lenses,* p. 6.

Table A3–3. British Standards for Optical Centration of Finished Lenses: For Lenses in the Frame, "Lenses Only" (Not Yet Mounted), and Uncut Multifocals*

Refractive power in meridian of displacement	Horizontal[1] displacement	Vertical displacement
0.00 to ±0.75D (multifocals only[2])	3.0 mm	1.5 mm
0.00 to ±1.25D	2.0 mm	1.0 mm
±1.37 to ±2.50D	1.0 mm	0.5 mm
Over ±2.50D	0.5 mm	0.5 mm

Paired lenses	Horizontal prismatic effect	Vertical prismatic effect
In addition to the above, when lenses are paired, their maximum combined unwanted prismatic effect must not exceed	1.0Δ	0.25Δ

*Adapted with permission from *British Standard 2738:1962, Specification for Spectacle Lenses,* p. 7.
[1]To obtain the equivalent maximum acceptable unwanted prism, use Prentice's rule. For example, a 1.25D lens would allow a maximum of 0.25Δ of horizontal prism per lens for a per-pair total of 0.50Δ. [$\Delta = (0.2 \text{ cm})(1.25)$.]
[2]Above 0.75D, multifocal lenses have the same centration standards as single vision lenses.

Table A3–4. British Standards Segment Location Tolerances*

Vertical (segment height) and Horizontal (geometrical inset) location	*Tolerance*
Unmounted or mounted single lens	±0.5 mm
Mounted lens pair	Reasonable match on visual inspection

*Adapted with permission from *British Standard 2738:1962, Specification for Spectacle Lenses,* p. 8.

Table A3–5. British Standards for Plano Prisms*

Prism power	Tolerance of base setting	Tolerance of prism power
0.00Δ		
1.00Δ	5 degrees	±0.12Δ
2.00Δ		
3.00Δ		
4.00Δ	2½ degrees	±0.25Δ
5.00Δ		
6.00Δ		
10.00Δ	1¼ degrees	±0.50Δ
Up		

*Adapted with permission from *British Standard 2738:1962, Specification for Spectacle Lenses.* p. 8.

Appendix 4

F.D.A. Policy

Appendix 4
Federal Regulation on Impact-Resistant Lenses*

Code of Federal Regulations
**Title 21—Food and Drugs
Chapter I—
Food and Drug Administration
PART 801—LABELING
Subpart H–Special Requirements for
Specific Devices**

§801.410 Use of impact-resistant lenses in eyeglasses and sunglasses.

(a) Examination of data available on the frequency of eye injuries resulting from the shattering of ordinary crown glass lenses indicates that the use of such lenses constitutes an avoidable hazard to the eye of the wearer.

(b) The consensus of the ophthalmic community is that the number of eye injuries would be substantially reduced by the use in eyeglasses and sunglasses of impact-resistant lenses.

(c)(1) To protect the public more adequately from potential eye injury, eyeglasses and sunglasses must be fitted with impact-resistant lenses, except in those cases where the physician or optometrist finds that such lenses will not fulfill the visual requirements of the particular patient, directs in writing the use of other lenses, and gives written notification thereof to the patient.

(2) The physician or optometrist shall have the option of ordering glass lenses, plastic lenses, or laminated glass lenses made impact resistant by any method; however, all such lenses shall be capable of withstanding the impact test described in paragraph (d)(2) of this section.

(3) Each finished impact-resistant glass lens for prescription use shall be individually tested for impact resistance and shall be capable of withstanding the impact test described in paragraph (d)(2) of this section. Raised multifocal lenses shall be impact resistant but need not be tested beyond initial design testing. Prism· segment multifocal, slab-off prism,

lenticular cataract, iseikonic, depressed segment one-piece multifocal, bi-concave, myodisc and minus lenticular, custom laminate and cemented assembly lenses shall be impact resistant but need not be subjected to impact testing. To demonstrate that all other types of impact-resistant lenses, including impact-resistant laminated glass lenses (i.e., lenses other than those described in the three preceding sentences of this paragraph (c)(3)), are capable of withstanding the impact test described in this regulation, the manufacturer of these lenses shall subject to an impact test a statistically significant sampling of lenses from each production batch, and the lenses so tested shall be representative of the finished forms as worn by the wearer, including finished forms that are of minimal lens thickness and have been subjected to any treatment used to impart impact resistance. All nonprescription lenses and plastic prescription lenses tested on the basis of statistical significance shall be tested in uncut-finished or finished form.

(d)(1) For the purpose of this regulation, the impact test described in paragraph (d)(2) of this section shall be the "referee test," defined as "one which will be utilized to determine compliance with a regulation." The referee test provides the Food and Drug Administration with the means of examining a medical device for performance and does not inhibit the manufacturer from using equal or superior test methods. A lens manufacturer shall conduct tests of lenses using the impact test described in paragraph (d)(2) of this section or any equal or superior test. Whatever test is used, the lenses shall be capable of withstanding the impact test described in paragraph (d)(2) of this section if the Food and Drug Administration examines them for performance.

(2) In the impact test, a ⅝-inch steel ball weighing approximately 0.56 ounce is dropped from a height of 50 inches upon the horizontal upper surface of the lens. The ball shall strike within a ⅝-inch diameter circle located at the geometric center of the lens. The ball may be guided but not restricted in its fall by being dropped through a tube extending to within approximately 4 inches of the lens. To pass the test,

the lens must not fracture; for the purpose of this section, a lens will be considered to have fractured if it cracks through its entire thickness, including a laminar layer, if any, and across a complete diameter into two or more separate pieces, or if any lens material visible to the naked eye becomes detached from the ocular surface. The test shall be conducted with the lens supported by a tube (1-inch inside diameter, 1¼-inch outside diameter, and approximately 1-inch high) affixed to a rigid iron or steel base plate. The total weight of the base plate and its rigidly attached fixtures shall be not less than 27 pounds. For lenses of small minimum diameter, a support tube having an outside diameter of less than 1¼-inches may be used. The support tube shall be made of rigid acrylic plastic, steel, or other suitable substance and shall have securely bonded on the top edge a ⅛ by ⅛-inch neoprene gasket having a hardness of 40 ± 5, as determined by ASTM Method D 1415;[1] a minimum tensile strength of 1,200 pounds, as determined by ASTM Method D 412;[1] and a minimum ultimate elongation of 400 percent, as determined by ASTM Method D 412 (ASTM Methods D 412 and D 1415 are incorporated by reference). The diameter or contour of the lens support may be modified as necessary so that the ⅛ - by ⅛-inch neoprene gasket supports the lens at its periphery.

(e) Copies of invoice(s), shipping document(s), and records of sale or distribution of all impact-resistant lenses, including finished eyeglasses and sunglasses, shall be kept and maintained for a period of 3 years; however, the names and addresses of individuals purchasing nonprescription eyeglasses and sunglasses at the retail level need not be kept and maintained by the retailer. The records kept in compliance with this paragraph shall be made available upon request at all reasonable hours by any officer or employee of the Food and Drug Administration or by any other officer or employee acting on behalf of the Secretary of Health and Human Services and such officer or employee shall be permitted to inspect and copy such records, to make such inventories of stock as he deems necessary, and otherwise to check the correctness of such inventories.

(f) In addition, those persons conducting tests in accordance with paragraph (d) of this section shall maintain the results thereof and a description of the test method and of the test apparatus for a period of 3 years. These records shall be made available upon request at any reasonable hour by any officer or employee acting on behalf of the Secretary of Health and Human Services. The persons conducting tests shall permit the officer or employee to inspect and copy the records, to make such inventories of stock as the officer or employee deems necessary, and otherwise to check the correctness of the inventories.

(g) For the purpose of this section, the term "manufacturer" includes an importer for resale. Such importer may have the tests required by paragraph (d) of this section conducted in the country of origin but must make the results thereof available, upon request, to the Food and Drug Administration, as soon as practicable.

(h) All lenses must be impact-resistant except when the physician or optometrist finds that impact-resistant lenses will not fulfill the visual requirements for a particular patient.

(i) This statement of policy does not apply to contact lenses.

(Secs. 201, 501, 502, 519, 701(a), 52 Stat. 1040-1042 as amended, 1049-1051 as amended, 1055, 90 Stat. 564-565 (21 U.S.C. 321, 351, 352, 360i, 371 (a))

[41 FR 6896, Feb. 13, 1976, as amended at 44 FR 20678, Apr. 6, 1979]

---

*Reprinted with permission from *Questions and Answers: Impact Resistant Lenses,* Appendix D, U.S. Department of Health and Human Services, Public Health Service/Food and Drug Administration, Bureau of Medical Devices, December 1981.

[1]Copies may be obtained from: American Society for Testing Materials (ASTM), 1916 Race St., Philadelphia, PA 19103.

Bibliography

"A.I.T. Optical Diamond Wheels," A.I.T. Industries Catalog No. 576, Skokie, Illinois.

American National Standard Recommendations for Prescription Ophthalmic Lenses, ANSI Z80.1-1979, American National Standards Institute, Inc., New York, 1979.

Bonsett-Veal, John D., "Enhancing the Cosmetic Appearance of High-Minus Spectacle Lenses," unpublished paper, Feb. 1980.

Brooks, C. W., and Borish, I. M., *System for Ophthalmic Dispensing,* The Professional Press, Inc., Chicago, 1979.

"Centrator VS/80," Fomap, Rimini, Italy.

"Coburn Plastic Edge Polisher Parts Catalog and Operation Manual," Coburn Optical Industries, Inc., Muskogee, Oklahoma.

Denison, Jack, "Finishing Optical Plastic Lenses Made from CR-39® Monomer—Part 2," *Optical Index,* Vol. 55, No. 9, September 1980, pp. 72–76.

"Description Weco 170" (hand edger) Stand 1980, Wernicke & Co. GMBH, Düsseldorf, West Germany.

"Description Weco 1061," Edition 1980, Wernicke & Co. GMBH, Düsseldorf, West Germany.

"Description Weco FHG4 Automatic Pattern Maker," Wernicke & Co. GMBH, Düsseldorf, West Germany.

"Description Weco ZG2 Centering Device," Stand 1980, Wernicke & Co. GMBH, Düsseldorf, West Germany.

"Diamond Wheels for the Optical Industry," Inland Diamond Products Co., Troy, Michigan.

"Everything You Always Wanted to Know About Diamond Wheels . . . But Didn't Know Who to Ask . . .," Inland Diamond Products Co., Troy, Michigan.

FM 8-37 Optical Laboratory Technician, Headquarters, Department of the Army, Washington, DC, Aug. 1976.

Geeren, Hans, *Werkstattbuch,* Verlag Neues Optikerjournal, Pforzheim, West Germany, 1981.

Hernandez, William, *Practical Systems Inc., Catalog and Technical Bulletin Manual,* Tarpon Springs, Florida.

"High-Lite, S-1005 High Index, Low Density," Schott Optical Glass, Inc., Duryea, Pennsylvania, 1979.

Hirschhorn, Hans, "Diamond Edging Wheels," *Optical Index,* Vol. 53, No. 9, Sept. 1978, pp. 131–34.

Hirschhorn, Hans, "Modern Edging Methods—Part 1," *Optical Index,* Vol. 55, No. 4, April 1980, pp. 93–95.

Hirschhorn, Hans, "Modern Edging Methods—Part 2," *Optical Index,* Vol. 55, No. 5, May 1980, pp. 81–86.

Horne, D. F., *Spectacle Lens Technology,* Adam Hilger Ltd, Bristol, England, 1978.

"Information Manual Optronics R–7 Bevel Edger," National Optronics, Inc., Charlottesville, Virginia.

"Instructions and Maintenance Manual A.I.T. Super Swifty Metal Blocker 317A," A.I.T. Industries, Skokie, Illinois, April 1977 revision.

"Instructions and Parts List for Model 18440 Deluxe Project-O-Marker," 18840–45B, American Optical Corporation, Southbridge, Massachusetts.

"Instructions for the '325' Face Type Hand Edger," A.I.T. Industries, Schaumburg, Illinois, Sept. 1979.

"Job Coach for Prescription Laboratory Operations, Bausch & Lomb, Rochester, New York, 1946 (reprinted 1970).

"Lens Learning System, Nova Communications, Inc. for Titmus Optical, Petersburg, Virginia.

Marco Lensometer Instruction Handbook, 1276-5M, Marco, Jacksonville, Florida. 1976.

"MBX," Essilor International, R.C. B712 049 618 1.22.4, Paris, France.

"MD1" (hand edger), Essilor International R.C. B712 049 618 EDI655, Paris, France.

"MD2" (hand edger), Essilor International R.C. B712 049 618-4/75 EDI 542, Paris, France.

Murphy, H. Lee, "A New Look at Some Advancements in Lens Grinding," *Optical Index,* Vol. 56, No. 2, Feb. 1981, pp. 36-37.

"Notice Technique Centreur C2000," Asselin Machines Briot, Elbeuf, France.

"Operating Instructions for the 2000 Bevelling Machines," Asselin, Machines Briot, Elbeuf, France.

"Operation and Maintenance Instructions for the 355 Metal Blocker," A.I.T. Industries, Schaumburg, Illinois, Dec. 1979.

"Operation and Maintenance Instructions for the 501 Marker-Blocker," A.I.T. Industries, Schaumburg, Illinois, Sept. 1980.

"Operation and Maintenance Instructions for the

Grande Mark Bevel Edgers Model No. 660 and 660A (Air)," A.I.T. Industries, Schaumburg, Illinois, Oct. 1980.

Operation and Maintenance Instructions for the Mark IV-A Mark V Air Chucking Super Dyna-Myte Bevel Edgers," A.I.T. Industries, Skokie, Illinois, Sept. 1971.

Operation and Maintenance Instructions for the Mark VI B, C, and E Bevel Edgers Featuring Continuous Force Principle," A.I.T. Industries, Schaumburg, Illinois, Nov. 1979.

"Optical Diamond Products," Dixie Diamond Manufacturing, Inc., Atlanta, Georgia.

Optical Laboratory Marketing Plan, Gentex, [R] *The Toughest Prescription Lens Made,* Gentex Corporation, Dudley, Massachusetts, 1980.

"Patternmaker XL 120," Fomap, Rimini, Italy.

"Polimatic Series LV," Fomap, Rimini, Italy.

Requirements for Dress Ophthalmic Frames, ANSI Z80.5. New York, American National Standards Institute, 1979.

Sasieni, L. S., "Optical Standards," *Manufacturing Optics International,* Vol. 25, No. 8, Feb. 1972, pp. 304-5.

Sasieni, L. S., "Optical Standards," *Manufacturing Optics International,* Vol. 25, May 1972, pp. 395–98.

"3M Leap System Adhesive Blocking System for Finishing," Armorlite, San Marcos, California.

Tomasetti, T. A., Bauer, F. A., "Testing of Molded Parts for Residual Molding Stresses—Solvent Stress Analysis," MR69PTM–29, General Electric Plastics Department, Polycarbonate Technical Marketing, Memo Report, Pittsfield, Massachusetts, October 23, 1969.

Westgate, Jud, "Edging Tough Polycarbonate is a Matter of Technique," *Optical Index,* Vol. 56, No. 1, Jan. 1981, pp. 37–42.

Wiand, Ronald C., "New Methods for Edging Polycarbonate Lenses," a paper given at the Optical Laboratories Association annual meeting, Atlanta, Georgia, November 20–22, 1980.

Woodcock, F. R., "Prescription Shop Machinery, Part 9: Automatic Diamond Edging Machines," *Manufacturing Optics International,* Vol. 27, No. 10, Oct. 1974, pp. 487–506.

"X63" (centration device), Essilor International R. C. B712 049 618; 45-0380, Paris, France.

Proficiency Test Questions Key

CHAPTER 1

1. F
2. F
3. T
4. b
5. b
6. d

CHAPTER 2

1. e
2. a and c
3. F
4. d
5. a
6. c
7. F
8. c
9. F
10. c
11. d
12. c and d
13. d
14. F
15. T
16. T
17. d
18. a
19. c
20. a and b
21. a
22. c

CHAPTER 3

1. a) 4 total in, b) 8 total in, c) 1 total in
2. b
3. R: 3 mm in
   L: 1.5 mm in
4. e
5. b

6. d
7. 2 mm in and 2 mm up
8. d
9. 1 mm out
10. d
11. 4 mm to the right of and 2 mm above the cross
12. a) .6△ base out
    b) 1.5△ base in
    c) 1.725△ base out

CHAPTER 4

1. c
2. c
3. a
4. 2.5 mm above, 1.5 mm out
5. c
6. c
7. d
8. d
9. e
10. a
11. b
12. b, d, and e
13. c
14. d
15. a
16. T
17. R: 3 mm inset, 2.5 mm raise
    L: 1 mm inset, 1.5 mm raise
18. 3 mm in and 3 mm down
19. b and c
20. b and d
21. e

CHAPTER 5

1. consult textual material
2. a
3. b, c, and d
4. F
5. c

6. d
7. b
8. c
9. c
10. c
11. e
12. T
13. d
14. b
15. b
16. d
17. T
18. 1 mm in
19. OC is 2 mm from the MRP

CHAPTER 6

1. a
2. 2.5 mm
3. 45 mm
4. 5.5 mm
5. a
6. c
7. b, c, and e
8. F
9. b
10. 2 in, 1.5 down
11. d
12. a
13. d
14. c
15. a
16. b
17. d
18. c

CHAPTER 7

1. a. 0
   b. 50
   c. 46.5
   d. 38
   e. 44.5
   f. -8
   g. 52
   h. -8
   i. 0
   j. 50
   k. 62
   l. 41.5
   m. -15

n. 35
o. -13.5
p. 38.5
2. d
3. b
4. a
5. c
6. d
7. b
8. 2.5 mm
9. c
10. d
11. c
12. a
13. b
14. F
15. c
16. b
17. e
18. b
19. b
20. b
21. a and c
22. a
23. c, e, b, g
24. b
25. F
26. d
27. a
28. T
29. b

CHAPTER 8

1. b
2. F
3. d
4. b
5. F
6. T

CHAPTER 9

1. b
2. a
3. e
4. T
5. e
6. b
7. a
8. c

9. d
10. d
11. F
12. b
13. a
14. T

CHAPTER 10

1. F
2. c
3. T
4. a and c
5. F
6. F
7. b
8. c
9. c
10. a
11. c
12. b
13. d
14. b
15. c
16. c
17. d
18. d
19. F
20. d

CHAPTER 11

1. a
2. b
3. a
4. d
5. b
6. c
7. b
8. a
9. a
10. d
11. b
12. T
13. F
14. e
15. F
16. e
17. b and c
18. T
19. b

20. a
21. b
22. a
23. c
24. b
25. c
26. c
27. b
28. c
29. F

Glossary

Δ
The symbol for prism. When following a number it denotes the units known as prism diopters.

– A –

A
the horizontal dimension of the boxing system rectangle that encloses a lens or lens opening

add
see addition, near

add, nasal
the modification of an existing lens shape by allowing more lens material to remain in the inferior, nasal position than would be indicated otherwise for the purpose of creating a better frame fit

addition, near
the power that a lens segment has in addition to that power already present in the main portion of the lens

allowance, grinding
synonym for wheel differential

anisometropia
a condition in which one eye differs significantly in refractive power from the other

aperture
an opening or hole that admits only a portion of light from a given source or sources

aperture, lens
the portion of the spectacle frame that accepts the lens (synonym: *lens opening*)

apex
the junction point at which the two nonparallel surfaces of a prism meet

astigmatism
the presence of two different curves on a single refracting surface on or within the eye causing light to focus as two line images instead of a single point

axis, of a cylinder
an imaginary reference line used to specify cylinder or spherocylinder lens orientation and corresponding to the meridian perpendicular to that of maximum cylinder power

– B –

B
the vertical dimension of the boxing system rectangle that encloses a lens or lens opening

barrel
the housing for a screw on a pair of glasses

base
in a prism, the edge of maximum surface separation opposite the apex

base curve
see curve, base

base down
vertical placement of prism such that the base is at 270° on a degree scale

base in
horizontal placement of prism such that the base is toward the nose

base out
horizontal placement of prism such that the base is toward the side of the head

base up
vertical placement of prism such that the base is at 90° on a degree scale

BCD
boxing center distance, *see* distance, boxing center

bevel
the angled edge of the spectacle lens

bevel, hidden
an edged lens configuration that attempts to reduce the appearance of thickness by creating a small bevel with the rest of the lens edge remaining flat

bevel, pin
synonym for safety bevel

bevel, safety
(1) to remove the sharp interface between lens surface and bevel surface and the sharp point at the bevel apex; (2) the smoothed interface between lens surface and bevel surface and the smoothed lens bevel apex

bevel, V
a lens edge configuration having the form of a V across the whole breadth of the lens edge

bifocals
lenses having two areas for viewing, each with its own focal power. Usually the upper portion of the lens is for distance vision, the lower for near vision

bifocals, blended
a bifocal lens constructed from one piece of lens material and having the demarcation line smoothed out so as not to be visible to an observer

blank, finished lens
a lens having both front and back surfaces ground to the desired powers, but not yet edged to the shape of the frame

blank, pattern
a predrilled, flat piece of plastic from which a pattern may be cut

blank, rough
a lens-shaped piece of glass with neither side having the finished curvature. Both sides must yet be surfaced in order to bring the lens to its desired power and thickness

blank, semi-finished lens
a lens with only one side having the desired curvature. The second side must yet be surfaced in order to bring the lens to its desired power and thickness

block
that which is attached to the surface of a lens in order to hold it in place during the surfacing or edging process

blocker
the device used to place a block on the lens in order to hold the lens in place during the edging process

blocker, layout
a centering device with the capability of also blocking the lens. The layout blocker does not mark the lens first, nor does it have a conversion capacity to allow marking of the lens

blocking, finish
the application of a holding block to an ophthalmic lens so that it may be edged to fit a frame

blocking, surface
the application of a holding block to an ophthalmic lens so that one side may be ground to the correct curvature and polished

Boley gauge
see gauge, Boley

Box-o-Graph
a flat device containing grids and slides, used in the measurement of pattern and edged lens size

boxing center distance
see distance, boxing center

boxing system
see system, boxing

bridge
that area of the frame front between the lenses

–C–

C
the horizontal width of a lens at a level half-way between the two horizontal tangents to the top and bottom of the lens shape (synonym: datum length)

caliper, vernier
a hand-held width measuring device with a short graduated scale that slides along a longer graduated

scale allowing a measure of fractional parts or decimals

carrier
the optically unusable outer portion of a lenticular lens that "carries" the optically usable central portion

center, boxing
the midpoint of the rectangle that encloses a lens in the boxing system

center, cutting
synonym for mechanical center

center, datum
the midpoint of the datum length (C dimension) of a lens along the datum line

center, edging
synonym for mechanical center

center, geometrical
(1) the boxing center, (2) the middle point on an uncut lens blank

center, mechanical
the rotational center of a pattern found at the midpoint of the central hole

center, optical
that point on an ophthalmic prescription lens through which no prismatic effect is manifested

center, rotational
the point on a pattern around which it rotates during edging

centration
the act of positioning a lens for edging such that it will optically conform to prescription specifications

colmascope
an instrument that utilizes polarized light to show strain patterns in glass or plastic

concave
an inward-curved surface

convergence
(1) an inward turning of the eyes as when looking at a near object; (2) the action of light rays travelling toward a specific real image point

convex
an outward-curved surface

coolant
a recirculating liquid used to cool and lubricate the lens/grinding wheel interface during the grinding process

CR-39
a registered trademark of Pittsburgh Plate Glass Co. for an optical plastic known as Columbia Resin 39

cribbing
the process of reducing a semi-finished lens blank to a smaller size in order to speed the surfacing process or reduce the probability of difficulty

cross curve
see curve, cross

cross, fitting
a reference point 2 to 4 mm above the major reference point on some progressive addition lenses. The fitting cross is to be positioned in front of the pupil

cross, power
a schematic representation upon which the two major meridians of a lens or lens surface are depicted

curve, base
the surface curve of a lens that becomes the basis from which the other remaining curves are calculated

curve, cross
the stronger curve of a toric lens surface

cut, nasal
the removal of an inferior, nasal portion of the lens shape for purposes of creating a better frame fit

cutting line
see line, cutting

cylinder
a lens having refractive power in one meridian only and used in the correction of astigmatism

–D–

datum center distance
see distance, datum center

datum line
see line, datum

datum system
see system, datum

DBC
distance between centers

DBL
distance between lenses

DCD
datum center distance

decentration
(1) the displacement of the lens optical center or MRP away from the boxing or datum center of the frame's lens aperture; (2) the displacement of a lens optical center away from the wearer's line of sight for the purpose of creating a prismatic effect

depth, mid-datum
the depth of the lens measured through the datum center

depth, seg
the longest vertical dimension of the lens segment

diameter, effective
twice the longest radius of a frame's lens aperture as measured from the boxing center

difference, frame
in the boxing system, the difference between frame *A* and *B* dimensions, expressed in millimeters

difference, pattern
in the boxing system, the difference between pattern *A* and *B* dimensions, expressed in millimeters

differential, wheel
the difference in millimeters between the size of lens produced in roughing and finishing operations during edging

diopter, lens (D)
unit of lens refractive power equal to the reciprocal of the lens focal length in meters

diopter, prism
the unit of measurement that quantifies prism deviating power; one prism diopter (1Δ) is the power required to deviate a ray of light one centimeter from the position it would otherwise strike at a point one meter away from the prism

distance between centers
in a frame or finished pair of glasses, the distance between the boxing (geometrical) centers

distance between lenses
(1) in the boxing system, the distance between the two boxed lenses as positioned in the frame (synonym; datum minimum between lenses [MBL]); (2) in the datum system, the distance between lenses in the frame as measured at the level of the datum line

distance, boxing center
synonym for distance between centers

distance, datum center
the distance between the datum centers in a frame or pair of glasses

distance, frame center
synonym for distance between centers

distance, geometrical center
the distance between the boxing (geometrical) centers of a frame

distance, interpupillary
the distance from the center of one pupil to the center of the other

distance, near centration
the distance between the geometrical centers of the near segments

distortion, pattern
the loss of correct lens shape resulting from use of a pattern which is too large or small in comparison to the lens size being edged

dress
to resharpen the cutting surface of a grinding wheel

drop, seg
(1) the vertical distance from the major reference point to the top of the seg when the seg top is lower than the MRP; (2) (laboratory usage) the vertical distance from the datum line to the top of the seg when the seg top is lower than the datum line (opposite: seg raise)

–E–

ED
effective diameter

edger
that piece of machinery used to physically grind the uncut lens blank to fit the shape of the frame

edger, hand
a grinding wheel made especially for grinding lenses by hand

effective diameter
see diameter, effective

electrometallic wheel
see wheel, electrometallic

electroplated wheel
see wheel, electroplated

eyesize
(1) in the boxing system, the *A* dimension; (2) in the datum system, the datum length

eyewire
the rim of the frame that goes around the lenses

–F–

F
denotes lens refractive power in diopters

facet
an edge configuration used with high-minus lenses to reduce edge thickness and weight

fining
a process by which a roughly cut lens surface is smoothed to the point where polishing is possible

finishing
that process in the production of spectacles that begins with a pair of lenses of the correct refractive power, and ends with a completed pair of spectacles

fitting cross
see cross, fitting

flash
synonym for swarf

fork, centering
a fork-like device used to hold a lens in position for blocking or for placing a lens in an edger at a specific orientation

form, minus cylinder
the form a prescription takes when written such that the value of the cylinder is expressed as a negative number

form, plus cylinder
the form a prescription takes when written such that the value of the cylinder is expressed as a positive number

former
British equivalent of *pattern*

frame center distance
see distance, frame center

frame difference
see difference, frame

frame PD
see PD, frame

–G–

g
symbol for the GOMAC system equivalent of the datum center distance

gauge, Boley
a gauge used to measure width of lenses or frame lens apertures

GCD
geometrical center distance

generating
the process of rapidly cutting the desired surface curvature onto a semi-finished lens blank

geometrical center distance
see distance, geometrical center

geometrically centered pattern
see pattern, geometrically centered

glazing
(1) the insertion of lenses into a spectacle frame; (2) the clogging of empty spaces between the exposed abrasive particles of an abrasive wheel resulting in reduced grinding ability

GOMAC
Groupement des Opticiens du Marché Commun. (A committee of Common Market opticians formed for the purpose of establishing European optical standards)

GOMAC system
see system. GOMAC

grinding allowance
synonym for wheel differential

–H–

hand edger
see edger, hand

hand stone
see stone, hand

height, seg
the vertically measured distance from the lowest point on the lens or lens opening to the level of the top of the seg

Hide-a-Bevel
tradename for an edge grinding system producing a shelf-effect behind the bevel on thick edge lenses

–I–

impregnated wheel
see wheel, impregnated

index, refractive
the ratio of the speed of light in a medium (such as air) to the speed of light in another medium (such as glass)

inset
the amount of lens decentration nasally from the boxing (or datum) center of the frame's lens aperture (opposite: outset)

inset, geometrical
the lateral distance from the distance centration point to the geometrical center of the segment (synonym: seg inset)

inset, seg
the lateral distance from the major reference point to the geometrical center of the segment

inset, total
the amount the near segment must move from the boxing (or datum) center to place it at the near PD (near centration distance)

interpupillary distance
see distance, interpupillary

–L–

l
symbol for the GOMAC system eyesize measure. It is equal to the boxed length of the lens (*A* dimension)

lap
a tool having a curvature matching that of the curvature desired for a lens surface. The lens surface is rubbed across the face of the tool and, with the aid of pads, abrasives and polishes, the lens surface is brought to optical quality

layout
the process of preparing a lens for blocking and edging

layout blocker
see blocker, layout; *also* marker/blocker

LEAP™
a 3M Company adhesive pad blocking system

length, datum
the horizontal width of a lens or lens opening as measured along the datum line

lens, laminate
a lens composed of 2 or more materials layered together

lens, mineral
synonym for glass lens

lens, minus cylinder form
a lens ground such that it obtains its cylinder power from a difference in surface curvature between two back surface meridians

lens, photochromic
a lens that changes in its transmission when exposed to light

lens, plus cylinder form
a lens ground such that it obtains its cylinder power from a difference in surface curvature between two front surface meridians

lens, progressive addition
a lens having optics which vary in power gradually from the distance to the near zones

lens, single vision
a lens with the same sphere and/or cylinder power throughout the whole lens, as distinguished from multifocal lenses

lens size
see size, lens

Lensometer
the tradename for an instrument used for finding power and prism in spectacle lenses

lenticular
a high powered lens with the desired prescription power found only in the central portion. The outer carrier portion is ground so as to reduce edge thickness and weight in minus prescriptions and center thickness and weight in plus prescriptions

lenticular, hand-flattened
a negative lenticular produced on a hand stone and hand polished

lenticular, negative
a high-minus lens that has had the peripheral portion flattened for the purpose of reducing weight and edge thickness (synonym: myodisc)

line, cutting
the 180-degree line marked on a lens after it has been properly positioned for cylinder axis orientation and decentration. It is used for reference in blocking and edging a lens.

line, datum
a line drawn parallel to and halfway between horizontal lines tangent to the lowest and highest edges of the lens

line, mounting
(1) the horizontal reference line that intersects the mechanical center of a lens pattern; (2) on metal or rimless spectacles the line that passes through the points at which the guard arms are attached, and which serves as a line of reference for horizontal alignment

– M –

major reference point
see point, major reference

marker
a centering device used to accurately position a lens and stamp it with horizontal and vertical reference lines for use in accurate lens blocking

marker/blocker
a device used to accurately position a lens and either stamp it with horizontal and vertical reference lines for use in accurate lens blocking, or block it directly while still in the device; i.e., a centering device with stamping and blocking capability.

MBL
minimum between lenses

MBS
minimum blank size; *see* size, minimum blank

meridian, axis
the meridian of least power of a cylinder or spherocylinder lens; for a minus cylinder the least minus meridian, for a plus cylinder the least plus meridian

meridian, major
one of two meridians in a cylinder or spherocylinder lens. These meridians are 90 degrees apart and

correspond to the maximum and minimum powers in the lens

meridian, power
the meridian of maximum power of a cylinder or spherocylinder lens; for a minus cylinder the most minus meridian, for a plus cylinder the most plus meridian

metal bonded wheel
see wheel, metal bonded

mid-datum depth
see depth, mid-datum

minimum between lenses
the datum equivalent of the boxing distance between lenses

minus cylinder form
see form, minus cylinder

minus cylinder form lens
see lens, minus cylinder form

mounting
(1) a rimless or semi-rimless spectacle frame; (2) the attaching of lenses to a rimless or semi-rimless spectacle frame

mounting line
see line, mounting

MRP
major reference point

multifocal
a lens having a sector or sectors where the refractive power is different from the rest of the lens, such as bifocals or trifocals

myodisc
synonym for negative lenticular

–N–

nasal
that side of lens or frame that is toward the nose (inner edge)

nasal add
see add, nasal

nasal cut
see cut, nasal

neutralize
to determine the refractive power of a lens

number, set
the compensating number used with a pattern to arrive at a compensated eyesize setting for the edger

–O–

OC
optical center

OD
Latin, oculus dexter (right eye)

opening, lens
the portion of the spectacle frame that accepts the spectacle lens (synonym: lens aperture)

optical center
see center, optical

optically centered pattern
see pattern, optically centered

Optyl
the tradename for an epoxy resin material used to make spectacle frames

OS
Latin, oculus sinister (left eye)

outset
the amount of lens decentration temporally from the boxing (or datum) center of the frame's lens aperture (opposite: inset)

–P–

p
symbol for the GOMAC system distance between lenses. It is equal to the boxing DBL

parallax
the apparent change in position of an object as the result of a change in viewing angle

pattern
a plastic or metal piece having the same shape as the lens aperture for a given frame. Used in lens edging as a guide for shaping the lens to fit the frame

pattern difference
see difference, pattern

pattern, optically centered
a pattern with its mechanical center above boxing center

pattern, geometrically centered
a pattern with mechanical and geometrical centers on the same horizontal plane

PD
interpupillary distance. The distance from the center of one pupil to the center of the other

PD, binocular
the interpupillary distance specified as a single number, without reference to the center of the frame

PD, distance
the wearer's interpupillary distance specified for a situation equivalent to when the wearer is viewing a distant object

PD, frame
synonym for distance between centers

PD, monocular
half the interpupillary distance as specified for each eye individually with the center of the frame's bridge as a reference point

PD, near
the interpupillary distance as specified for a near viewing situation

photochromic lens
see lens, photochromic

plano
a term referring to a lens or lens surface having a zero refracting power

pliers, chipping
pliers used to chip or break away the outer portions of an uncut or semi-finished lens in order to either reduce its size or bring it into the rough shape needed to approximate the finished shape

plus cylinder form
see form, plus cylinder

plus cylinder form lens
see lens, plus cylinder form

point, distance centration
the British equivalent of the major reference point

point, major reference
the point on a lens where the prism equals that called for by the prescription

polycarbonate
a strong, plastic lens material often used for safety eyewear

power cross
see cross, power

precoat
a spray or brush-on liquid that when applied to a lens, protects the surface during processing, and/or makes the adhesion of a block to the lens possible

Prentice's rule
see rule, Prentice's

prism
that part of an optical lens or system that deviates the path of light

protractor, lens
a millimeter grid on a 360 degree protractor used in the lens centration process for both surfacing and finishing

–R–

raise, seg
(1) the vertical distance from the major reference point to the top of the seg when the seg top is higher than the MRP; (2) (laboratory usage) the vertical distance from the datum line to the top of the seg

when the seg top is higher than the datum line (opposite: seg drop)

refraction
(1) the bending of light by a lens or optical system; (2) the process of determining the needed power of a prescription lens for an individual

refractive index
see index, refractive

rimless
having to do with frames (mountings) that hold lenses in place by some method other than eyewires. Most rimless mountings have 2 points of attachment per lens

rule, Prentice's
a rule that states that the decentration of a lens in centimeters times the power of the lens is equal to the prismatic effect ($\Delta = cF$)

–S–

safety bevel
see bevel, safety

seg
see segment

seg depth
see depth, seg

seg drop
see drop, seg

seg height
see height, seg

seg inset
see inset, seg

seg width
see width, seg

segment (seg)
an area of a spectacle lens with power differing from that of the main portion

semi-finished blank
see blank, semi-finished

set number
see number, set

shop, back
synonym for surfacing laboratory

shop, front
synonym for finishing laboratory

single vision lens
see lens, single vision

size, lens
(1) according to the boxing system, the *A* dimension of a lens or lens opening; (2) according to the datum system, the datum length of a lens

size, minimum blank
the smallest lens blank that can be used for a given prescription lens and frame combination

sizer
a frame chassis or frame front used exclusively for checking edged lens size accuracy

smoothing, edge
the process of bringing the bevel surfaces of an edged lens to a finer, smoother finish

sphere
a lens having a single refractive power in all meridians

spherocylinder
the combination of a sphere lens and a cylinder, combined into a single lens

spotting
the placing of spots on a lens correctly oriented for axis in order to indicate the location of major reference point and horizontal meridian

stars
microchips at the lens surface/lens bevel interface

stone
(1) an abrasive grinding wheel; (2) to sharpen the cutting ability of a grinding wheel by honing it with an abrasive stick

stone, hand
synonym for hand edger

surfacing
the process of creating the prescribed refractive power, prism, and major reference point location on a lens by generating the required curves and bringing the surface to a polished state

swarf
accumulated waste material present as a result of the grinding process

system, boxing
a system of lens measurement based upon the enclosure of a lens by horizontal and vertical tangents that form a box or rectangle

system, datum
a system of lens measurement that defines the lens or eyesize as being the width of the lens along the datum line

system, GOMAC
a European Economic Community standard incorporating portions of both boxing and datum systems

–T–

temporal
that area of lens or frame that is toward the temples (outer edge)

toric transposition
see transposition, toric

total inset
see inset, total

transposition, toric
the process of transposing a prescription from the form in which it is written to another, such as from plus to minus cylinder form

trifocals
lenses having three areas of viewing, each with its own focal power. Usually the upper portion is for distance viewing, the lower for near, and the middle or intermediate portion for distances inbetween

true
(1) to reshape the cutting surface of a worn edger wheel so that it cuts at the angles and in the manner

originally intended; (2) to bring a pair of glasses into a position of correct alignment

–U–

uncut
a lens that has been surfaced on both sides, but not yet edged for a frame

–V–

V-bevel
see bevel, V

–W–

wheel differential
see differential, wheel

wheel, electrometallic
synonym for electroplated wheel

wheel, electroplated
an abrasive wheel made by electrolytically depositing metal on the wheel in such a manner as to encompass diamond particles. This type of wheel is often used to grind plastic lenses

wheel, finishing
the wheel used in edging to bring the lens edge to its final configuration

wheel, hogging
synonym for roughing wheel

wheel, impregnated
abrasive wheels made by mixing diamond material with powdered metal which is heated in a mold until fusion of the metal occurs

wheel, metal bonded
synonym for an impregnated wheel

wheel, roughing
an edger wheel that rapidly cuts a lens to near its finished size

width, seg
the size of a seg measured horizontally across its widest section

–Z–

zone, blended
the blurred area of an "invisible" bifocal between distance and near portions. (Not to be confused with the progressive zone of a progressive add lens)

zone, progressive
that portion of a progressive addition lens between distance and near portions where lens power is gradually increasing

Index